FUNDAMENTAL NEUROANATOMY

FUNDAMENTAL
NEUROANATOMY

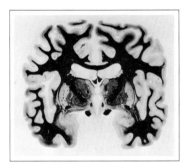

Walle J. H. Nauta

Department of Psychology and Brain Science
Massachusetts Institute of Technology

Michael Feirtag

Board of Editors
Scientific American

• • •

Anatomical drawings by Carol Donner

W. H. FREEMAN AND COMPANY / NEW YORK

Library of Congress Cataloging in Publication Data

Nauta, Walle J. H.   Fundamental neuroanatomy. Includes bibliography and index.
1. Neuroanatomy.   I. Feirtag, Michael.   II. Title. [DNLM: 1. Neuroanatomy.   WL 101 N314f]
QM451.N38   1986   611′.8   84-28675   ISBN 0-7167-1722-0   ISBN 0-7167-1723-9 (pbk.)

Printed in the United States of America
1 2 3 4 5 6 7 8 9 0   KP   3 2 1 0 8 9 8 7 6

For Ellie

For Deborah

Contents

FUNDAMENTAL NEUROANATOMY

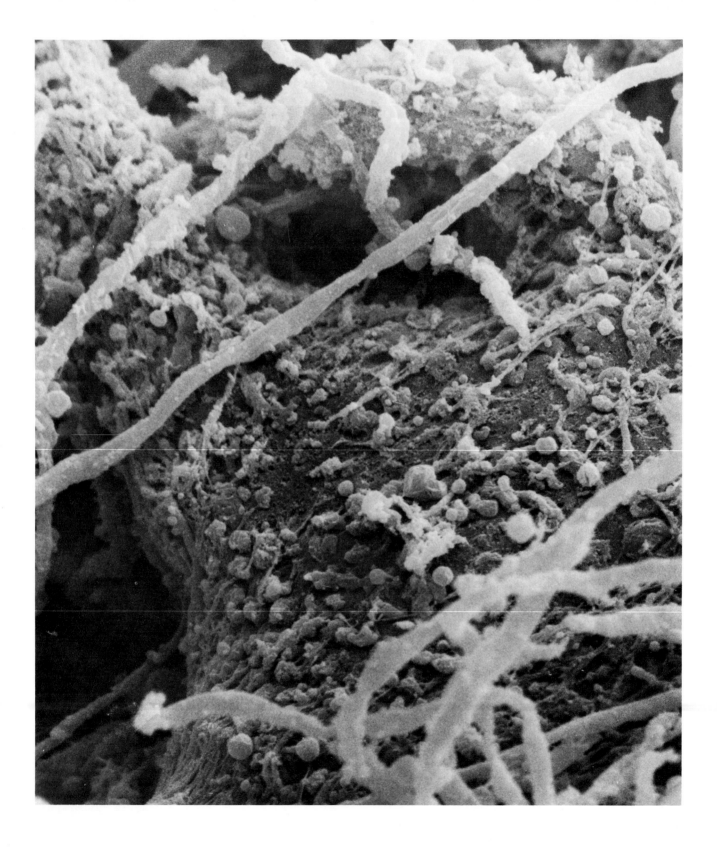

Part I

PRELIMINARIES

Facing page: **Surface of a nerve cell** occupies much of this scanning electron micrograph, which shows a nerve cell, or neuron, from the brain of a cat. (In particular, the neuron is from the part of the brainstem designated the nucleus reticularis magnocellularis.) Toward the bottom is the neuron's cell body; it is some 60 micrometers across, which makes it large as neurons go. Toward the top are the neuronal protrusions called dendrites; one dendritic trunk curves behind the other. Arrayed on both the cell body and its dendritic protrusions are a multitude of rounded swellings. They range from .5 to two micrometers in diameter. They are synaptic terminals: the sites at which the cell gets chemical signals from the axons, or nerve fibers, emitted by other neurons. A given neuron may have thousands of such connections. Indeed, neurons are embedded in neuropil, a feltwork of axons and dendrites. Here much of the felt has been stripped away. Still, a number of axons course across the field of view. The micrograph was made by Linda Paul, Itzhak Fried, Peter Duong, and Arnold B. Scheibel of the School of Medicine of the University of California at Los Angeles.

Chapter One

Early Phylogeny; The Great Intermediate Net

This book is an introduction to the structure of the brain and the spinal cord, with special reference to the brain and the spinal cord of mammals, notably man. It is, first and foremost, a medical text: it describes anatomy that medical students are called on to master. But we hope it does more than that. We hope a student of physiology, or chemistry, or psychology, or computer science and artificial intelligence — in fact we hope that anyone seeking familiarity with the tissues inside the skull and at the center of the vertebral column will find guidance in these pages. Thus we assume no special knowledge on the part of the reader; we start from scratch. At times we venture into neurophysiology, into neurochemistry, into neuroembryology, and into neurology, and there again we start from scratch. To that extent the book is an introduction not to neuroanatomy alone but to the neurosciences. The book, it must be said, is far from encyclopedic. Most notably, it slights the molecular basis of neural activity and the intricate local patterns in which nerve cells are organized. Instead it makes broad sweeps through the brain and the spinal cord, and even on that scale it offers examples, not catalogs. But then, we want to treat the nervous system conceptually, not as a mass of detail. Accordingly, the book is unorthodox: it presents the brain and the spinal cord first as a network of communications established by the fibers that nerve cells emit, and only then as a three-dimensional structure of complex architecture. The first part of the book — this part — is a set of preliminaries. It discusses the evolutionary advent of the nervous system, the nature of the nerve cell and of the cells that support its activity, the chief anatomical divisions of the brain, and the techniques that enable investigators to trace the connections a nerve

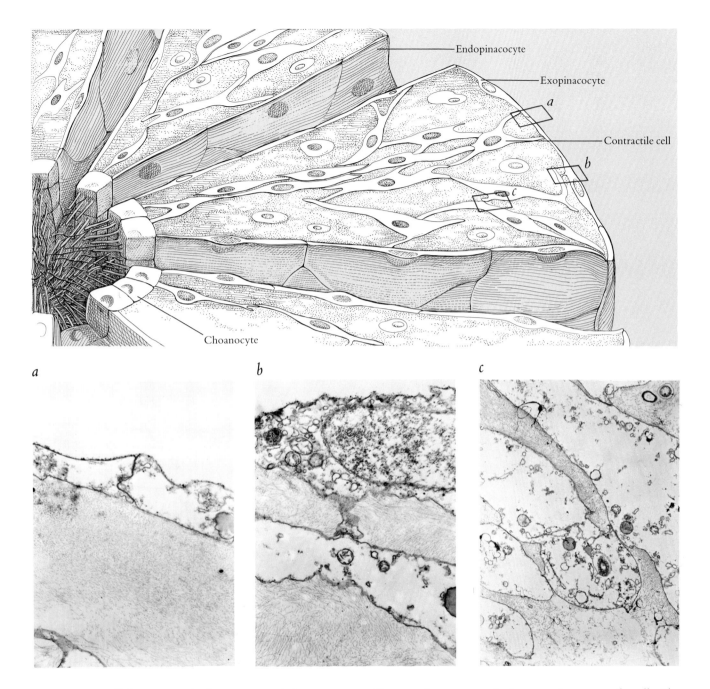

a

b

c

Figure 1: **Intercellular contacts** in the sponge may help to organize the filtering of nutrients from sea water; conceivably, then, they amount to a nervous system. In the gross anatomy of the sponge (*top*) no such system is explicit. The surface consists of flattened cells called exopinacocytes and others called endopinacocytes; they overlie networks of contractile connective-tissue cells, which occupy a matrix of large molecules, specifically glycoproteins and collagen. Still other cells called choanocytes beat water with their flagella.

Electron microscopy reveals the connections among the cells. The surface cells make contacts among themselves (*a*); the surface cells make contacts with the underlying contractile cells (*b*); the contractile cells make contacts among themselves (*c*). The micrographs were made by Max Pavans de Ceccatty of the Université Claude Bernard in Lyon; they show tissue from the thick-walled marine sponge (the common bath sponge) *Hippospongia* at an enlargement of approximately 9,000 diameters.

cell makes with other nerve cells. The second part of the book is an overview of the mammalian central nervous system in which the brain and the spinal cord are presented topologically and the basic connectedness — a broad-scale mammalian wiring diagram, if you will — is constructed. The third part superimposes on this topology some actual neuroanatomy.

Interneuronal Communication

When did nerve cells first appear in the course of evolution? A number of biologists have been trying to answer that question — one that earlier workers were hopeful they had settled. As a result, much of the certainty about the answer has evaporated, not that the early ideas are false, but rather, as a recent investigator has written, that they are not sufficiently true. The

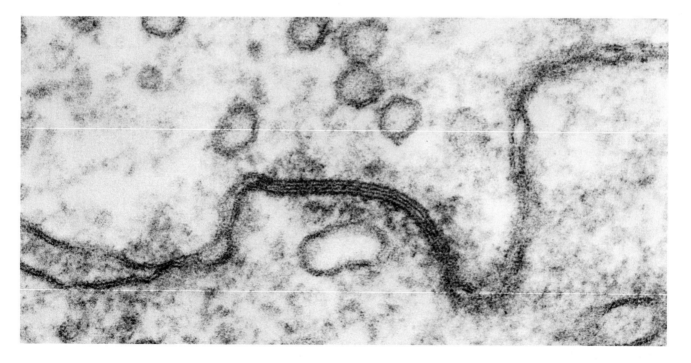

Figure 2: **Gap junction** in the nervous system of a vertebrate resembles, if only superficially, the intercellular contacts found in the sponge. In this example the junction links two neurons in the ciliary ganglion behind the eyeball of a chicken; thus it links two of the neurons that govern the contraction of the pupil of the eye. In general gap junctions enable ions and small molecules to pass from one cell to another through a lattice of channels spanning the distance between the surface membrane of the cells. Along the length of the junction that distance is only two nanometers (2×10^{-9} meter). The neuronal membrane itself is about seven nanometers thick. The electron micrograph was made by Thomas S. Reese and Milton W. Brightman of the National Institutes of Health.

problem is that nerve cells seem to have sneaked into phylogeny: they are much like other cells, with attributes all cells share. For one thing, all cells are irritable: almost any stimulus—mechanical prodding, heat or cold, electricity—can trigger a local change in the membrane forming the envelope of the cell, so that the membrane's permeability to various ions is altered. In this way, currents of ions are made to flow through the membrane; thus the concentration of ions on each side of the membrane changes, and with it the voltage difference (the bioelectric potential) across the membrane. In the second place, all cells are conductive: a local alteration in permeability can advance along the membrane, so that an altered bioelectric potential spreads over the surface of the cell. Although nerve cells, or neurons, have developed these attributes notably well—neurons are exquisitely irritable and exquisitely conductive—the universality of their most characteristic properties makes investigations into neural phylogeny extremely problematic.

Consider the sponge. It is thought to be the most primitive multicellular organism alive on the earth today. The sponge has no organized system of cells specialized for communication: it has no nervous system. Indeed, it hardly seems to have biological systems at all. Yet the sponge has several modes of contractility that give it a certain amount of responsiveness to its environment. When a sponge is touched, the surface of the colony may exhibit local, rhythmic pulsations. The local oscula (the openings through which the sponge expels water) may contract. The colony may curl up.

How is all that possible without a nervous system? Beginning with C. F. A. Pantin at Cambridge University and continuing with Max Pavans de Ceccatty at the Université Claude Bernard in Lyon, a school of investigators has examined the fine structure of sponges, in part by electron microscopy (Figure 1). The effort establishes that the surface of a sponge consists of cells that form plates resembling flagstones. One might take them to be analogous to a vertebrate's epidermis. Under the flattened cells are other, spindle-shaped cells. The spindle-shaped cells are contractile, like a vertebrate's muscle tissue. It is difficult to be certain that the images recorded by the electron microscope accurately represent the structure of a living animal. In fact, it is difficult to place untroubled faith in any histological technique. After all, the tissue under investigation must be killed and then subjected to chemical treatment before its microscopic structure can be observed. Still, the surface cells in a sponge appear to have processes (filamentous extensions of the cell body) that descend to contractile cells and touch them, it seems, at specialized regions: membrane-to-membrane appositions with little or no space intervening. It also appears that the contractile cells communicate among themselves at similar specialized regions. In the vertebrate nervous system, certain membrane appositions look very much the same (Figure 2). They are called gap junctions, and indeed, in spite of appearances, some substances applied by investigators (notably the enzyme horseradish peroxidase) can work their way between the two facing membranes. The gap junctions in the vertebrate are known to be sites of electrotonic transmission, a form of intercellular communication in which the bioelectric potential across one neuron's membrane is brought to bear on the membrane of the next by the passage of currents of ions from the one cell to the other through channels spanning the junction. (Gap junctions are typically two nanometers, or 2×10^{-7} centimeter, wide.) It could readily be proposed that the membrane appositions among the cells of a sponge serve a similar function.

Even if not, there is a second (though less likely) possibility. The electron microscope shows that both the surface cells and the contractile cells of the sponge include saclike organelles. Each is some 140 nanometers (1.4×10^{-5} centimeter) in diameter. In the cells of a vertebrate such sacs, or vesicles, are common. For example, they serve as secretory vesicles: they sequester a substance the cells have produced — say, the saliva synthesized by the cells of a salivary gland. In neurons they sequester neurotransmitter: a substance the neuron releases that mediates a chemical form of intercellular communication. The most typical arrangement is shown in Figure 3. There the vesicles in a neuron are shown to cluster at strategic sites where the membrane of the cell, viewed at low magnification, appears to be thicker and denser than elsewhere. Actually the membrane is unexceptional; high-power electron microscopy establishes that the density is a membrane undercoating. Evidently the density marks an "active zone" where vesicles can attach themselves to the membrane and come open at the point of attachment, releasing their chemical contents into extracellular space. The sequence agrees with the physiological finding, made in the 1950's, that neurotransmitter is released in quantal "squirts." After such a release, the transmitter molecules promptly make contact with the specialized receptor molecules that stud a neighboring vertebrate neuron's membrane (or the membrane of a muscle cell). Indeed, a density along a second, postsynaptic neuron's membrane (or a complicated furrowing in a muscle cell's membrane) is often nearby. The interaction of the transmitter and its receptors can open channels through the postsynaptic membrane, permitting ionic currents to flow and leading, therefore, to bioelectric activity on the part of the postsynaptic cell. All things considered, it appears that some structural bases for both electrical and chemical communication in a vertebrate neuron's style are teasingly present even in a sponge. Nevertheless, a sponge has no neurons — or else all its cells are neurons.

The One-Neuron Nervous System

Among the investigators who inquired into the phylogeny of the nervous system well before the most recent efforts, George Parker of Yale University is prominent. He published his findings in 1919. Parker was seeking the primeval reflex arc. Its putative descendants had been identified in the vertebrate: they are pathways composed of one or more neurons through which the excitation caused by a sensory stimulus to some part of the body can be conducted to muscle tissue and thus can make muscle contract. In Parker's time, reflex arcs were often taken to be the simplest pattern by which nature

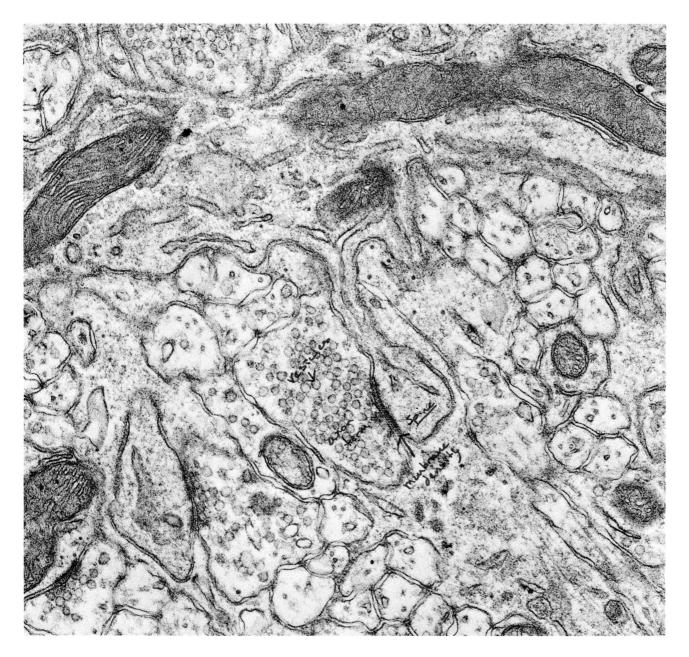

Figure 3: **Synapse** is the characteristic substrate for interneuronal communication in vertebrates and higher invertebrates; it is a site where the electrical activity of a neuron brings on the release of a neurotransmitter: a chemical messenger substance. This synapse is fairly typical. A dendrite crosses the top of the field of view: the two long, dark gray structures inside it are mitochondria cut lengthwise. At the middle of the field the dendrite emits a downward branch called a dendritic spine. The left side of the spine makes contact with an axon, cut in transverse section. The axon is the presynaptic part of the synapse: the part that releases transmitter. It is filled with round synaptic vesicles (chambers that store the transmitter). The dendrite, across a cleft of some 20 nanometers, is the postsynaptic part of the synapse. There the binding of transmitter molecules to receptor molecules induces electrical activity on the part of the postsynaptic cell. The synaptic membrane appears to be darker, thicker, and more distinct than cell membrane elsewhere. The distinctness is due to a density in the underlying cytoplasm, which forms a membrane undercoating. The electron micrograph was made by Sanford L. Palay of the Harvard Medical School. It shows tissue from the cerebellar cortex of a rat at a magnification of 54,000 diameters.

organized cells into a nervous system; hence the nervous system was thought to have originated when some organism first came to have a cell, or a chain of cells, to mediate between environmental stimuli and the organism's responsive movements. The evolution of the nervous system would then demand reflex arcs in increasing number and complexity.

Parker's search for the primeval arc was made possible by a staining technique the Italian physician Camillo Golgi had reported in the early 1870's. According to one account (that of a talkative laboratory assistant), Golgi had thought to stain the meninges: the membranous tissues that surround and cushion the central nervous system. He had not been successful at first. But when he passed a block of neural tissue that included meninges through a sequence of treatments, exposing it first to potassium dichromate and then to silver nitrate, a number of the cells in the block were rendered a deep brown approaching black (Figure 4). They were pervaded by silver chromate, which suffused even the filamentous extensions given off by the blackened cell bodies. Here, then, were neurons in silhouette, with all their processes revealed. The meninges took up no stain. It later developed that Golgi's black reaction (*reazione nera*) impregnates cells other than neurons: it stains supportive cells in the central nervous system and epithelial and muscle cells in the periphery of the body. The technique has, however, this remarkable characteristic: it picks out, from every hundred neurons in a given block of tissue, only some zero to five. That is the only reason the stain has value. If all the neurons in the nervous system were to accept the treatment equally, a slice of neural tissue would simply be blackened overall. Mysterious as the Golgi technique remains (there is still no sure explanation of its fickle selectivity), it was the greatest single blessing to befall the early studies of the nervous system's structure.

George Parker employed the Golgi stain on the tissues of many primitive multicellular organisms. He, too, saw neurons — or, at least, among the cells that form the epithelial layer in the tentacles surrounding the mouth of certain sea anemones, he saw an occasional cell that stood out in black (Figure 5*a*). At the base of each such cell Parker could see the beginning of a filament that ramified into end branches as it approached a muscle fiber. He could not be certain the two made contact, but he assumed they communicated. Surely he was correct; his findings can now be viewed as a somewhat artistic version of more recent discoveries. Still, the circuitry is simple: the entire line of conduction consists of a single cell. It is a one-neuron nervous system, and what it will do in response to a stimulus is as predictable as a doorbell. What is plain about more advanced nervous systems is that the behavior they make possible is predictable least of all.

Obviously something in phylogeny must intervene in the doorbell mechanism. Accordingly, Parker examined the action of Golgi's stain on somewhat more complex organisms. In certain jellyfishes he found an array of neurons in the epithelial layer similar to the one he had found before. Under the epithelium, however, he now found further neurons composing a widely distributed plexus (Figure 5*b*). The circuitry therefore gains some sophistica-

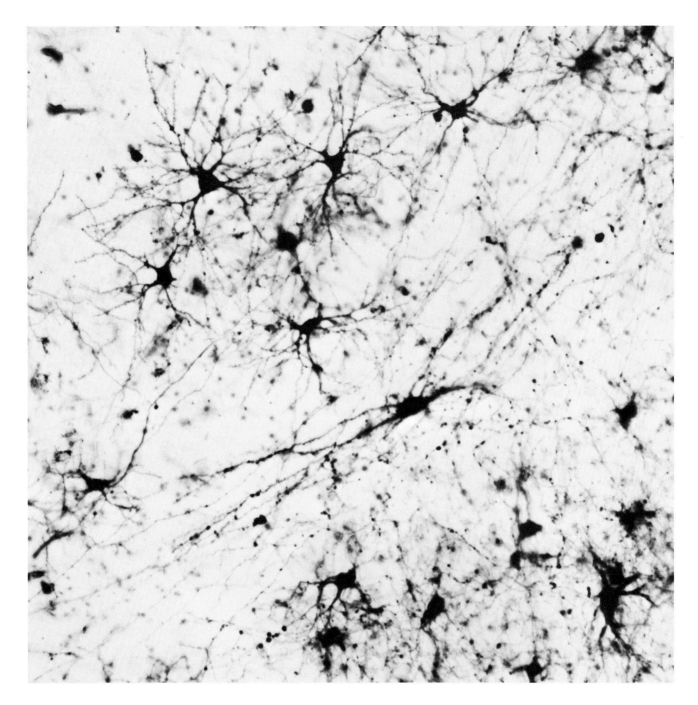

Figure 4: **Golgi technique** for staining brain tissue inaugurated the modern era of neuroanatomical investigation. Discovered by the Italian physician Camillo Golgi in the early 1870's, it blackens a sample of neurons, selecting, it seems, at random. The rest of the tissue it renders transparent. The blackened neurons are seen emitting filamentous extensions, namely axons and dendrites; the technique reveals their distribution. Before the advent of the Golgi tech-nique investigators seeking to study neuronal extensions could do little more than attempt to work them free of their prison of neuro-pil. The tissue is from the brain of a cat, in particular the thalamus. The field of view straddles the border between two thalamic cell groups, the lateral anterior nucleus (*upper left*) and the ventral ante-rior nucleus (*lower right*). The preparation was made by Enrique Ramón-Moliner of the University of Sherbrooke in Quebec.

tion: neurons in the epithelial layer make contact with a subepithelial net, and the cells of the net make contact in turn with contractile tissue in the depths of the animal. The arrangement, for the first time in evolution (as it is known from Parker's research), requires functional contact between a neuron and a neuron. In an indisputable nervous system such contact is called a synapse. The word, which was coined in 1897 by the founder of modern neurophysiology, the English physiologist Charles Sherrington, is a contraction from the Greek *syn,* meaning together, and *haptein,* meaning to clasp. A synapse is a clasping together of cells. The crucial fact about synaptic contact is that the neurons do not fuse — a truth that was established and forcefully defended by Santiago Ramón y Cajal, a Spanish contemporary of Sherrington and the founder of modern neuroanatomy. It came as the essential ingredient of the "neuron doctrine," in which the neuron is affirmed to be the anatomical, histological, embryological, and functional unit of the nervous system. In a

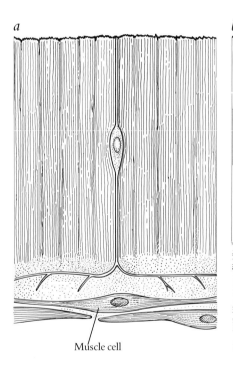
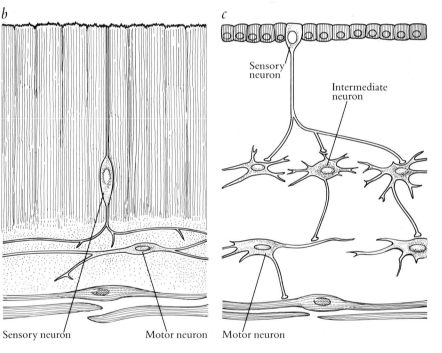

a

Muscle cell

b

Sensory neuron   Motor neuron

c

Sensory neuron

Intermediate neuron

Motor neuron

Figure 5: **Nervous system arose** by three stages of evolution, in the view of George Parker of Yale University, who studied Golgi-stained tissue from a progression of multicellular organisms and published his findings in 1919. In certain sea anemones he found a one-neuron nervous system (*a*). That is, the chains of conduction from sensory stimuli to motor responses are established by single cells. In certain jellyfishes he found a two-neuron nervous system (*b*). In it sensory neurons make contact with motor neurons, which in turn can cause muscle cells to contract. Finally, in certain jellyfishes and mollusks he found a three-neuron nervous system (*c*). There motor neurons are isolated from sensory neurons by a network of intermediate neurons.

word it is an individual, and all functional contacts between neurons are really confrontations of membrane with membrane, across a gap now called a synaptic cleft. The cleft is commonly 15 to 25 nanometers wide for a humoral synapse (one at which neurotransmitter is released), or about 10 times the width of an electrotonic, or gap-junction, synapse.

To summarize: Certain jellyfishes boast a two-neuron nervous system, in which sensory neurons (in these simple creatures the nerve cells in the epithelial surface layer of the body, in contact with the organism's ambient environment) communicate with motor neurons (nerve cells that make contact with effector cells, in this case contractile cells, and thus in essence muscle fibers). Does the arrangement remain predictable? Perhaps not. Imagine that the motor neurons communicate with one another, so that the input to any one of them includes not only messages from the ambient environment conveyed by sensory neurons but also messages from neighboring motor neurons. Imagine further that some messages are excitatory and make the motor neuron more likely to generate and transmit its own bioelectric activity, whereas others are inhibitory. Under these conditions there is a riddle to solve: predicting what a neuron will do in response to its inputs seems to be a matter of algebraically summing the excitatory and inhibitory messages that converge on it.

Then comes a third advance. It, too, is found in primitive marine organisms, such as certain jellyfishes and mollusks. In a way it is the final advance, because the nervous system of these jellyfishes and mollusks and the nervous system of man both consist in essence of only three classes of neurons. In mollusks as in man, most of the sensory neurons no longer communicate directly with motor neurons. Between the two a barrier of neurons has developed that have connections not only with motor neurons but also with one another (Figure 5*c*).

To be sure, this third and final step may already have been taken by all organisms that have subepithelial neurons. In the foregoing account of a two-neuron nervous system, all such cells were assumed to be motor neurons: cells that innervate effector tissues. In reality, only some of the many subepithelial cells may make those effector connections. The rest may be positioned in such a way that they get input from sensory neurons in the epithelium but can communicate only with others of their kind or with true motor neurons, not with effector tissue. Neither sensory nor motor, they are placed as go-betweens in the paths of sensory-to-motor conduction. In short, here, too, are intermediate neurons — the final step, as it were. Although a three-neuron organization is difficult to identify in a diffuse neuronal net, it is abundantly evident elsewhere, because in animals that are more highly developed than a jellyfish and whose bodies have become polarized so as to have a leading end (that is, a head), a tail end, and bilateral symmetry, the subepithelial neurons are concentrated into either sequences of ganglia (nests of neurons encapsulated by connective tissue) or a single, unsegmented central nervous system. The important point is the advent, shadowy though it is, of the great intermediate net: a barrier of intermediate neurons that interposes itself between sensory neurons and motor neurons quite early in evolution.

Chapter Two

The Neuron; Some Numbers

A stain representing a kind of counterpart to a Golgi preparation was developed in Munich in the 1880's, a time when investigators of the nervous system were mostly neurologists and psychiatrists driven by the hope that if the structure of the brain were known, its workings and disorders would soon be understood. Franz Nissl, a 24-year-old student later to become a distinguished clinical psychiatrist, recognized the need for sharper definition of neurons in slices of brain tissue. He devised a fitting method, one that revealed intraneuronal detail none of the earlier methods could show. He arrived at his procedure (Figure 6) in two steps: first by specifying alcohol as the fixative for brain tissue, and second by staining the neurons in the fixed tissue with magenta red, a dyestuff he later replaced, with steadily increasing success, by a curious mixture of methylene blue and soap (he specified shredded Venetian soap) and finally by aniline dyes, specifically thionine or toluidine blue. A century later, the need for Nissl's method persists. The method, however, can now be applied to tissue fixed in aldehydes (formaldehyde, glutaraldehyde, or both), and a variety of alkaline dyes can be used.

Axon and Dendrites

Figure 7 displays two Nissl-stained motor neurons from a human brain. The dye was cresyl violet. The appearance of the cells is characteristic of what the Nissl stain does. The cell bodies are distinct, and so are the beginnings of their processes: their filamentous extensions. But all of the latter soon disappear

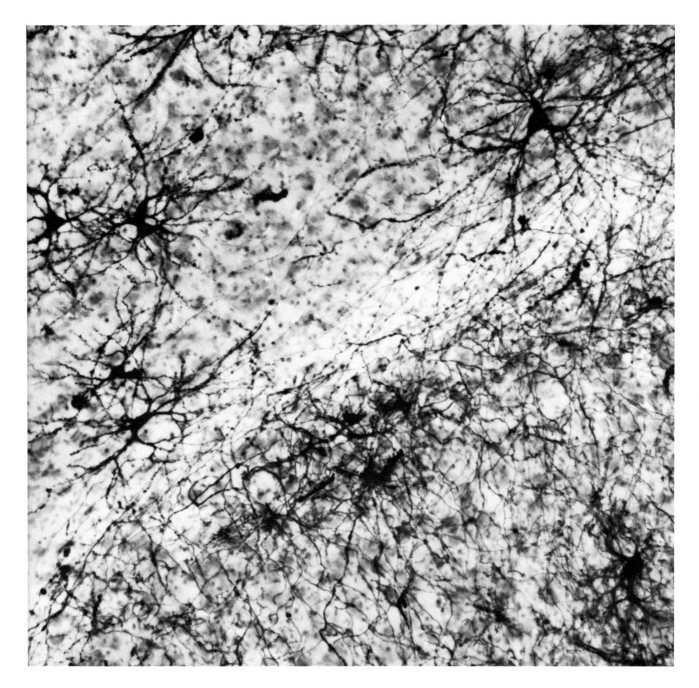

Figure 6: **Nissl technique** is a counterpart to the Golgi technique; discovered by the psychiatrist Franz Nissl in Munich sometime in the 1880's, it equably stains all neurons. In particular, a Nissl-stain dyestuff such as cresyl violet binds to Nissl substance: aggregations of ribosomes, the intracellular machines that make proteins. Ribosomes are notably abundant in neurons. In the illustration the tissue is counterstained: the Nissl technique and the Golgi technique have both been applied to the slice of brain tissue adjoining the slice shown in Figure 4. Again the staining was done by Enrique Ramón-Moliner. Golgi-stained neurons show up in black; Nissl-stained neurons are vaguer gray bodies. The narrow cell-poor zone between the lateral anterior nucleus and the ventral anterior nucleus runs diagonally across the field of view. The preparation establishes that the Golgi stain marks no more than some five percent of the neurons in a given sample of neural tissue. The Nissl technique finds its greatest utility as a means of surveying tissue architecture.

from sight, in what Santiago Ramón y Cajal once called "the dismal fog." Still, the Nissl stain makes possible some valuable observations. Note that both of the neurons in Figure 7 are filled with patchlike, dark-staining masses. The masses sometimes resemble stripes; thus they inspired the name tigroid substance. They are now called Nissl substance or Nissl bodies. According to current understanding, they consist largely of stacks of flattened caverns known as endoplasmic reticulum, on whose membranous walls are mounted ribosomes, the machines that assemble amino acids into proteins by

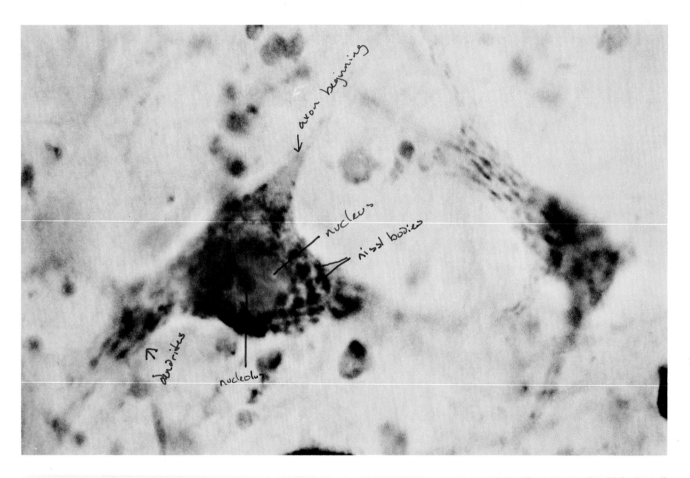

Figure 7: **Two Nissl-stained neurons** from a human brain demonstrate the most reliable distinction between axons and dendrites, namely that ribosomes are lacking in axons. In general, a neuron has only one axon. It is a smooth, cylindrical fiber with which the cell sends signals to other cells. Here an axon emerges from the top of the cell body at the left; its emergence, the axon hillock, is a conical region whose even gray tone in this micrograph shows that it harbors no Nissl substance. In contrast, a typical neuron has many dendrites. They are gnarled, irregular filaments with which the cell gathers signals. Here two dendrites emerge from the cell body at the left; four or five emerge from the cell body at the right. The dendrites are filled, like their parent cell bodies, with dark-staining masses of Nissl substance. The cells have additional dendrites, which are out of the plane of the section. The cells are motor neurons from the oculomotor nucleus; their axons join the oculomotor nerve to extend from the brain to a muscle that rotates the eye.

means of the coded instructions borne by strands of ribonucleic acid (RNA) that leave the nucleus of the cell. (The Nissl-stain dyestuffs combine with acid groups such as those in RNA. As it happens, ribosomes themselves are two-thirds RNA.) Ribosomes mounted on endoplasmic reticulum are present in every cell, but only in neurons do they aggregate so impressively.

An examination of Figure 7 will show that elongated islands of Nissl substance enter two of the neuronal extensions exposed at the plane of the cut through the cell at the left of the figure but fail to enter the third. By that criterion two varieties of neuronal process are distinguished. The first has Nissl substance at the beginning of its length; a typical neuron incorporates several such extensions. The second lacks Nissl substance. Given a Nissl preparation there is no more to be said. Examine, however, the drawings of neurons in Figure 8. The drawings are based on Golgi preparations. Here the processes are revealed in their full extent. Most of them — the ones whose beginnings are filled with Nissl bodies — turn out to be short; those as long as two millimeters can rightly be thought of as giants. These processes, distinguished most reliably (though not infallibly) by the Nissl substance in them, are known as dendrites, the diminutive of the Greek word *dendron,* meaning tree. The name is apt. The Golgi technique reveals that dendrites tend to arborize: they bifurcate repeatedly into ever thinner branches. Sometimes the result is a dense, shrublike tangle of ramifications. In other cases the density of arborization is less extreme. Even in the smallest details of a dendrite's overall shape, the treelike appearance persists, because dendrites are often gnarled: they have excrescences on their surface, like galls on the trunk of an oak. The most pronounced of the excrescences are called dendritic spines.

The remaining process emitted by the neuron at the left in Figure 7 — the one free of Nissl substance — is an axon. The name is the Greek word for axis. Nearly every neuron has only one such process, in contrast to a multiplicity of dendrites. Figure 7 shows the beginning of the axon to be a conical region whose absence of Nissl substance gives it a glassy appearance. This region is called the axon hillock. The axon itself is smooth and cylindrical throughout its length: the axon has no excrescences. In contrast to dendrites, axons can reach impressive lengths: as long as a meter in the human nervous system. Surely that helps to explain the pervasiveness of ribosomal aggregates — Nissl bodies — in neurons. Consider a neuronal cell body 100 micrometers (a tenth of a millimeter) in diameter. It is among the very largest in the human central nervous system; even a cell body half that size is quite large as neurons go. Let the cell body emit an axon tens of centimeters long. The axon is several thousand times longer than the cell body from which it arises. Yet since the axon lacks ribosomes, its need for various molecules must be met by the parent cell body. The axonal membrane, for example, must call chronically for maintenance, like a long bridge that must constantly be repainted. It is known that if an axon is severed from the parent cell body, it will die. It also is known that molecules synthesized by ribosomes in the cell body flow toward the ends of the axon. Some of these molecules (including enzymes soluble in cytoplasm) move no more than a few millimeters per day. Other molecules, or rather molecular assemblages (for the most part assemblages of protein and lipid that amount to prefabricated parcels of cell membrane), move a hundred times faster. Axons (and dendrites, for that matter) contain filamentous proteins. The thinner filaments are threads no more than 10 nanometers in diameter; they tend to be roughly coaxial with the axon (or the dendrite) in which they are arrayed. They make crosslinks with one another, thus forming a tensile internal skeleton. Perhaps they support the axon. The thicker filaments are microtubules. They, too, are longitudinal, but are as much as 30 nanometers across. Their disruption by drugs such as colchicine inhibits the swift form of transport. It is thought that the fast-moving material travels on the surface of the tubules rather than inside them.

The arborization of an axon is often limited to a short end stretch far from the parent cell body, where the process ramifies into what is called a terminal arbor. This pattern, however, is far from universal. Sometimes an axon ends in a single tip, without having ramified at all. Sometimes it gives off side branches fairly close to the parent cell body, and sometimes it gives off branches throughout its length. All such side branches, whose end stretches may likewise vary from single tips to prodigious terminal arbors, are known as axon collaterals. They have a tendency to leave the main trunk of the axon

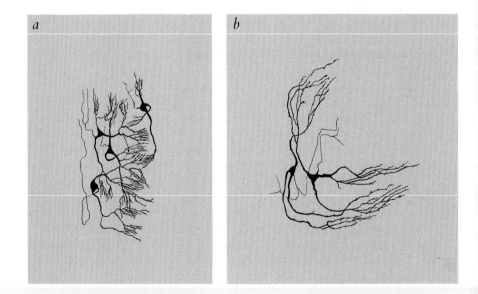

Figure 8: **Variety among neurons** is suggested by these camera-lucida drawings of neuronal constellations, all from the brainstem of the cat. At one site, the nucleus reticularis lateralis (*a*), the dendrites are short and bushy, and end in signal-gathering "pools." The axons, rather thinner than the dendrites, run upward. At a second site, near the hypoglossal nucleus (*b*), the dendrites are long and gently curved, with rather few branchings. The axons again are thinner, and tend toward the right. At a third site, the raphe nuclei (*c*), the dendrites form dense plexuses, in this case on the surface of a bifurcating blood vessel. The

at a right angle, and at each division point the diameter of the main trunk diminishes. Axon bifurcations are too infrequent, however, to produce the appearance of rapid tapering, which is typical of dendrites. The endings of an axon are commonly marked by terminal swellings. Ever since Cajal described them, the swellings have been called *boutons terminaux,* or terminal buds (Cajal is most frequently quoted from the French translation, *Histologie du Système Nerveux,* of the volumes he wrote in Spanish on the structure of the nervous system). Under the electron microscope, the boutons are nearly always found to contain synaptic vesicles, the organelles that store the neurotransmitter with which the cell communicates with other neurons or with effector cells in the periphery of the body.

Signal Transmission

A note on neuron physiology: According to the classical conception the path of electrical activity in a neuron leads from its dendrites to its axon, with the neuron's cell body (in the great majority of cases) interposed between the two. The first part of this path — the spread of an excitatory or an inhibitory signal

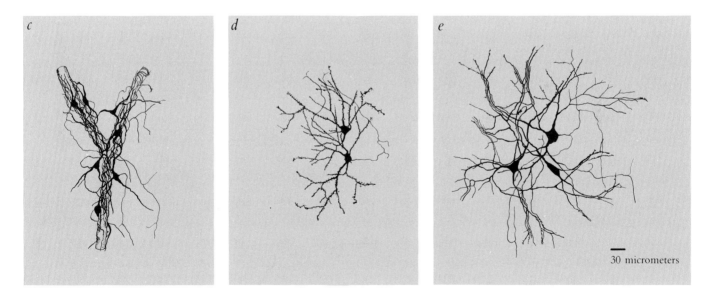

c *d* *e*

30 micrometers

axons turn downward. At a fourth site, the nucleus reticularis gigantocellularis of a newborn cat (*d*), the dendrites project in all directions and are covered with dendritic spines. The axons tend to bifurcate. When a cat is five months old (*e*), the dendrites of the neurons in the nucleus reticularis gigantocellularis are lacking most of their spines. Moreover, the dendrites tend by then to run in small, dense packets. The cells are now impressively large: their cell bodies can measure more than 30 micrometers across. The drawings were made by Arnold Scheibel at U.C.L.A.

along the membrane investing the dendrites and the cell body—is decremental. That is to say, the altered bioelectric potential diminishes in intensity as it spreads along the membrane (Figure 9). Ultimately the altered potential arrives at the axon hillock, where it contributes to the algebraic sum of the signals converging on the axon. Thus the shape of the neuron and the positions of synapses on it make the cell unique in the way it integrates data. Now begins the second part of the conduction path. Electron microscopy shows that the cell membrane just beyond the axon hillock takes on a granular undercoating throughout a short length of the axon known as the initial axon segment. Doubtless this special structure has something to do with a special kind of bioelectric activity: the initial axon segment is the site at which, if the arriving excitation is sufficiently greater than the arriving inhibition, a spike of bioelectric voltage called an impulse or action potential (Figure 10) is generated. The impulse invariably has the same electrical rise and fall and magnitude; it exists or it does not, and so it is described as all-or-none. If it is generated, it travels without decrement along the axonal membrane, because this type of bioelectric signal is self-renewing. On arriving at the axon terminals, it initiates the release of neurotransmitter, in most cases at a recognizable synapse, with specialized receptors on the membrane of a second neuron at the other side of a cleft some 20 nanometers wide. In the classical conception

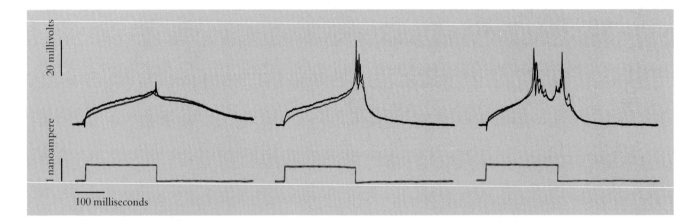

Figure 9: **Decremental signal conduction** is characteristic of dendrites, at least in the classical conception of how neurons process information. The electrical recordings displayed in this illustration were made with two microelectrodes, one positioned in the cell body of a neuron (a Purkinje cell) in the cerebellum of a rat, the other positioned some distance up a dendrite of the cell. In each of three experiments the first electrode injected square-shaped pulses of current (*gray*); it also measured the resulting dome-shaped change in the cell body's voltage (*black*). The change was conducted along the dendrite (in a direction antidromic to the physiological direction) and so had a lower height in the second electrode's record (*color*). At some point, the altered voltage opened membrane channels for calcium ions, enabling the dendrite to generate a "calcium spike." The spike (or set of spikes) protrudes above the dome. The spike was conducted back to the cell body; thus its measured intensity is lower in the latter. In essence, the recordings are a double demonstration of the decremental ("passive") conduction of signals by a dendrite. In contrast, the calcium spikes demonstrate the dendrite's "active" electrical properties, which defy the classical understanding of dendrites as purely passive. The experiments were done by Rodolfo R. Llinás and his colleagues at the New York University School of Medicine.

of interneuronal communication, the synaptic contact occurs on one of the second neuron's dendrites (dendritic spines are sites of predilection for synapses) or on the membrane of the postsynaptic cell body. In either case, the receipt of neurotransmitter initiates electrical activity in the postsynaptic cell — activity that will spread decrementally toward the second cell's axon hillock.

This, then, is the classical conception: in Cajal's phrase the nervous system is dynamically polarized, so that axons send signals to dendrites (or to a postsynaptic cell body). Neurons, however, are far more varied than that. Axons can transmit signals to axons. Dendrites can transmit signals to dendrites. Most surprisingly — in that it constitutes not a short circuit but a reversal of "dynamic polarization" — dendrites can transmit signals to axons. In sum, every possible mode of transmission between neuronal processes now seems to have a place in the organization of the brain and the spinal cord.

Axons signaling axons. The discovery of such a synapse is often achieved by inference. It can happen, for example, when an investigator examining an electron micrograph observes that a serial set of synapses is established by the terminals of three neuronal processes. The first and the second contain synaptic vesicles; the third does not. The investigator decides that the first and the second are the terminals of axons; hence the axoaxonal synapse. The problem is that synaptic vesicles do not invariably specify an axon. Dendrites, too, can be presynaptic. Other cases are less equivocal. For example, an axon may synapse on what is clearly an initial axon segment (Figure 11). Thus the path of signal conduction excludes much of the postsynaptic cell, namely its dendrites and cell body. What might this shortcut accomplish? The morphology of such a synapse is often of the type that tends to be correlated with inhibition. The zone of synaptic contact is rather small, the density at the membranes is not pronounced, and the synaptic vesicles in the presynaptic terminal are flattened, not round. Moreover, the insertion of a microelectrode into the postsynaptic cell often shows that the cell undergoes intervals of powerful inhibition. It seems a reasonable surmise that an axoaxonal synapse is always inhibitory, and in fact, neural circuits are known in which an axoaxonal synapse vetoes the output of the postsynaptic cell: it transmits an inhibition so potent that the postsynaptic axon is temporarily rendered incapable of conducting the impulses generated by the postsynaptic cell itself. One does well to be cautious, however. In a number of invertebrate species, conduction paths formed by giant neurons have been intensively studied by neurophysiologists. In the squid, for example, a path formed by three giant neurons enables the animal to propel itself from danger by jetting water out of its funnel. Each of the synapses in such a path is apparently axoaxonal, and some of the synapses are known to be chemical, not electrotonic. Yet some of the chemical synapses are demonstrably excitatory: the arrival of an action potential at the presynaptic terminal leads to the generation of an action potential in the axon next in the sequence.

Dendrites signaling dendrites. Such contacts have been encountered in many parts of the brain. One notable place is the olfactory bulb (Figure 12). Another is the retina. Indeed, it has been maintained that the retina processes visual data by dendrodendritic synapses almost exclusively. The retinal neurons called horizontal cells furnish, in any case, an extreme example of a neuron's reliance on dendrodendritic synapses. The horizontal cell has an axon, or at least one of its numerous processes is notably thinner (one micrometer) and notably longer (several hundred micrometers) than the others the neuron emits. The axon branches extensively as it nears the end of its course, so that the cell has two dense bushes of dendritelike ramifications, one near the cell body, the other some distance away. Each gets signals from retinal photoreceptors (the rods and cones of the eye), and each transmits signals to the dendrites of bipolar cells, the retinal neurons next in line to process visual data. Thus each bush dispatches its output through dendrodendritic synapses. The axon has no role in the transmission of visual data: it carries no bioelectric activity from one bush to the other. It appears, therefore, to be no more than a metabolic pipe enabling a single neuronal cell body to sustain two integrative apparatuses: in effect two independent microcomputers. In a dendrodendritic synapse the path of conduction excludes a presynaptic axon, and with it the all-or-none site of the presynaptic cell. This suggests that no all-or-none action potential is involved in the signal conduction. Instead, the varying electric activity — the so-called graded potential — conventionally associated with a dendrite might give impetus for the release of neurotransmitter. Presumably the release is quantal: a given synaptic vesicle contains a specific amount of transmitter, and the number of vesicles tapped for their content at a presynaptic dendritic terminal might vary with the strength of the arriving bioelectric activity. On the other hand, cases are emerging in which patches of dendritic membrane prove capable of generating spikelike signals.

Dendrites signaling axons. The best instance discovered so far is in the substantia gelatinosa, a district of the spinal cord first described in the 18th century by the Italian anatomist Luigi Rolando. Examining freshly cut spinal cord, Rolando saw that a part of the face of the cut was notably gelatinous: notably lacking in opacity. The Nissl stain would later show that the substantia gelatinosa is composed of small and very small neurons: the smallest in the spinal cord. Still later, the microelectrode would show that some of the neurons — the larger among them; the smallest ones cannot yet be probed — respond more or less selectively to nociceptive stimuli affecting the periphery of the body. They respond, in other words, not to touch or to moderate variations in temperature but to extremes of mechanical irritation and temperature that threaten harm to the body's tissues and indeed are perceived as painful. Then the electron microscope revealed the dendroaxonal contacts. They seem, as a rule, to be paired with the reciprocal connection: an "orthodox" axodendritic synapse. Perhaps they prolong the transmission of a signal (a nociceptive signal?) by feeding excitation back into the presynaptic terminal. Perhaps they damp the transmission by feeding back inhibition. Perhaps they perform a complex mixture of both.

One should not despair; the doctrine of dynamic polarization must apply broad-scale. After all, a given region of the brain or the spinal cord plainly has inputs and outputs. They travel on long nerve fibers that indisputably are axons, and they are coded as trains of action potentials, which are self-renewing signals. But then, only a self-renewing signal could travel more than a few millimeters along a neuronal process; a signal of smaller magnitude would be decrementally conducted, and so would die away. Inside a given region things are not that simple. A given site on a given neuron can prove to be presynaptic, postsynaptic, or both. It can prove, moreover, to be active (capable of generating spikelike bioelectric signals) or passive (capable only of conducting signals decrementally). Under these circumstances the best strat-

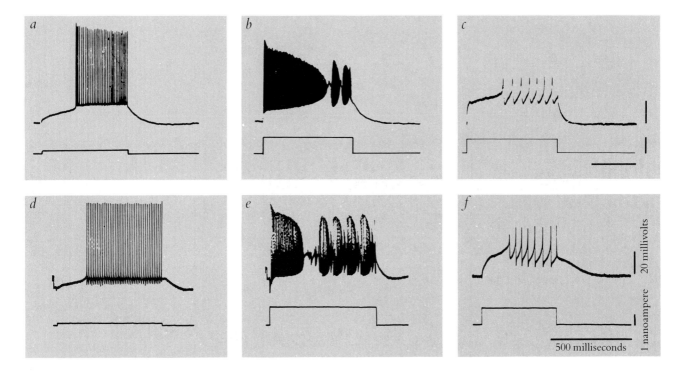

Figure 10: **Self-renewing signal conduction** is characteristic of axons, which are called on to carry signals over distances as great as several tens of centimeters. In the experiment documented at the top of this illustration the axon of a Purkinje cell from the cerebellum of a reptile (a turtle) was induced to "fire" (*a*) by the injection of electric current (*bottom trace*) into the neuron's cell body. The result was a volley of action potentials (*top trace*): a series of self-renewing, spikelike changes in the voltage across the axonal membrane. Greater current (*b*) yielded a pattern of oscillating voltage, recorded in the cell body. The administration of the blowfish poison tetrodotoxin (*c*), which eliminates action potentials by blocking sodium conductance across the neuronal membrane, suggested the source of the oscillation: the action potentials were being modulated by calcium spikes generated in the dendrites of the cell. The experiment was done by Jorn Hounsgaard at the New York University School of Medicine. Across the bottom of the illustration a similar set of recordings was made in a Purkinje cell from a mammal (a guinea pig). Current injected into the cell body again yielded action potentials (*d*); greater current yielded voltage oscillation (*e*); the administration of tetrodotoxin exposed dendritic calcium spikes (*f*). The experiment was done by Rodolfo Llinás and Mutsuyuki Sugimori at New York University. Neurons are revealing a multiplicity of conductances to sodium, potassium, and calcium ions, but across virtually all of evolution trains of action potentials based on inflows of sodium ions and outflows of potassium ions are the currency for axonal signal conduction.

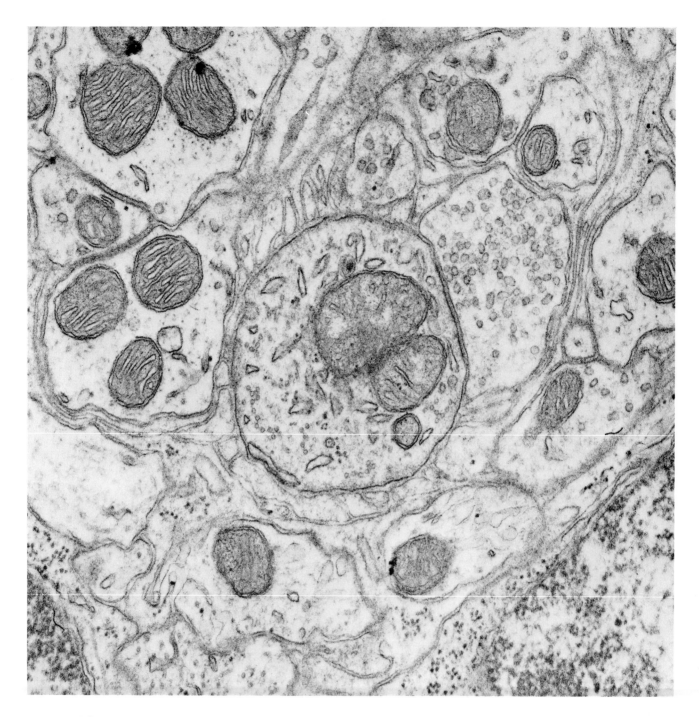

Figure 11 (left): **Axoaxonal synapse** subverts the classical concept that axons always transmit signals to dendrites or to cell bodies. The large, more or less circular region bounded by cell membrane at the center of the field of view is an axon cut in cross section. In particular, it is the initial segment of the axon of a Purkinje cell from the cerebellum of a rat. It includes an assortment of intracellular struc-

tures, ranging from mitochondria to neurofilaments and occasional ribosomes. Its microtubules are in groups, a characteristic of the initial axon segment. At the right the axon is abutted by an axon terminal: that of a cerebellar basket cell. The latter is filled with synaptic vesicles. The vesicles are flattened, which betokens an inhibitory synapse. Cross sections through other basket-cell axons

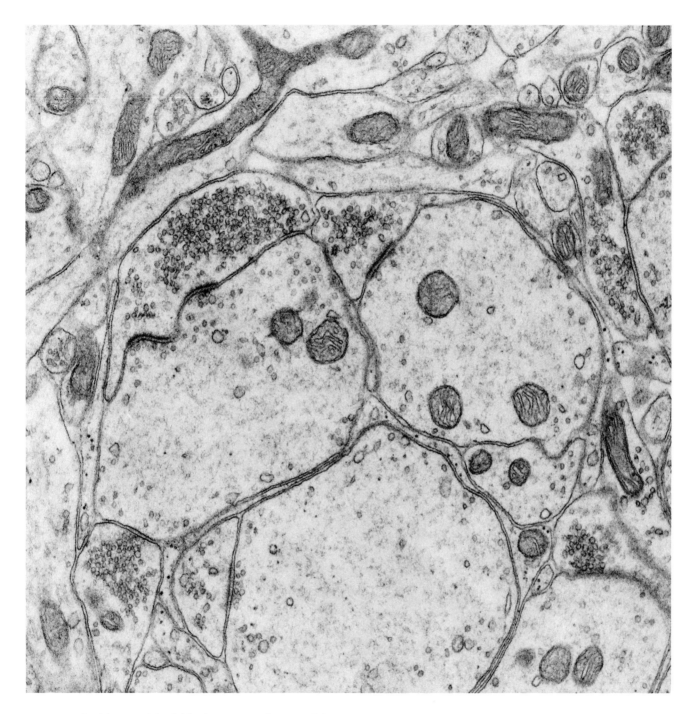

occupy much of the rest of the field. The micrograph was made by Sanford Palay at Harvard at a magnification of 52,000 diameters.

Figure 12 (right): **Dendrodendritic synapses** further subvert the classical concept of interneuronal communication. The micrograph shows tissue from the olfactory bulb of a rat at an enlargement of 27,000 diameters. Three large dendrites cut in cross section dominate the field of view. The one at the upper left establishes reciprocal synapses with a smaller dendrite above it. That is, the cells trade information. The smaller dendrite is packed with synaptic vesicles. The micrograph was made by Thomas Reese and Milton Brightman at the National Institutes of Health.

egy may be simply to identify a neuronal process as an axon or a dendrite by morphological criteria, including, for example, the pattern of branching or the presence or absence of Nissl substance. The functional properties of neural processes could then be studied independently. What proportion of synapses might turn out to be "orthodox" axodendritic synapses? It is of little help to know. In the retina the synapses are often "unorthodox." Yet one cannot conceive of the retina as exotic. It is certainly not inefficient. Presumably the retinal circuitry reflects an extreme need for miniaturization. In the cerebral cortex the synaptic arrangements are far more "conventional." The majority of synapses are probably axodendritic, and most of the rest are probably axosomatic (they convey signals from an axon to a postsynaptic cell body). Yet the cerebral cortex appears to serve the newest functions of the brain. In the human brain it is the neural substrate for language. The extreme variety of neuronal microcircuits suggests that evolution is open-minded — that a design is workable if it advances the brain's computational abilities.

One final heterodoxy. Axons have been discovered that fail to release neurotransmitter at recognizable synapses. For example, axons containing

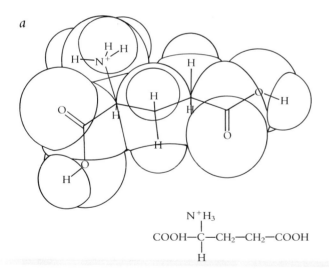

a

$$N^+H_3$$
$$COOH-\underset{\underset{H}{|}}{\overset{\overset{|}{}}{C}}-CH_2-CH_2-COOH$$

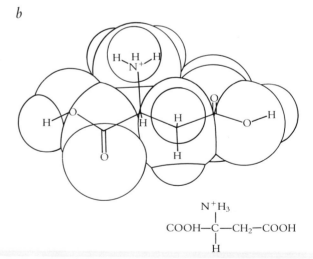

b

$$N^+H_3$$
$$COOH-\underset{\underset{H}{|}}{\overset{\overset{|}{}}{C}}-CH_2-COOH$$

Figure 13: **Amino acid neurotransmitters,** or more precisely the amino acids now thought to serve neurons as chemical messenger substances, are four in number. Glutamate (*a*), aspartate (*b*), and glycine (*c*) are constituents of protein. Gamma-aminobutyric acid, or GABA (*d*), results when a carboxyl group (COOH) is removed from glutamate. The four are displayed as models generated by a computer from X-ray diffraction data that specify the positions of the atoms in a crystal of the substance. In essence, each model depicts an

the neurotransmitter serotonin have been found to enter the cerebral cortex of the rat. The axons have swellings, or varicosities, that contain synaptic vesicles. Yet a great number of the swellings have no presynaptic density. Moreover, the swellings tend to lie where no postsynaptic membrane is nearby. The swellings might simply release their serotonin into extracellular space. That hardly seems to be a way to send a private message. It seems more like throwing leaflets from a rooftop. On the other hand, the arrangement has the advantage that neurons throughout a volume of brain tissue could be affected by a release of neurotransmitter. Indeed, the function of such non-synaptic axon terminals might be not the transmission of discretely ordered information but the mediation of widespread changes in the functional state of the cerebral cortex. Moreover, it is possible that even a seemingly aimless arrangement (an arrangement lacking recognizable synapses) affects only certain neurons — say the ones with a particular type of receptor arrayed inconspicuously on their surface. It should be said that the motor axons entering smooth muscle tissue also fail to make recognizable synapses. In smooth muscle (the contractile tissue in the walls of hollow viscera), the

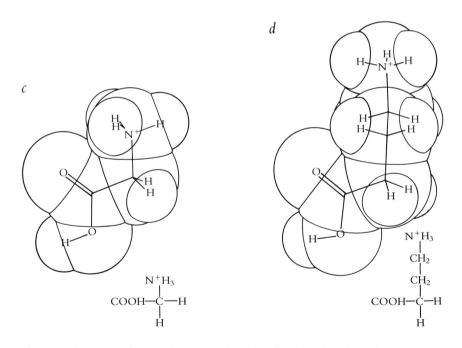

electronic shape. (Simpler stick figures are also shown.) Under physiological conditions the shapes are doubtless different. For example, at the pH characteristic of cytoplasm, glutamate and aspartate have a net negative charge owing to the loss of a hydrogen ion from each carboxyl group. The models (and the ones in the next two illustrations) were produced by David Barry with the PROPHET Computer System, operated for the National Institutes of Health by Bolt, Beranek & Newman, Inc., in Cambridge, Massachusetts.

endings of axons are scattered, perhaps at strategic sites in the matrix of muscle fibers, and when a given smooth-muscle fiber is made to contract by the receipt of neurotransmitter, its response can be communicated to neighboring muscle fibers through gap junctions among the fibers. In contrast, the muscle fibers composing striated muscle tissue each make private contact with an axon at the elaborate membrane specialization known as a motor end plate or neuromuscular junction. It should also be said that neurons may turn out to have many modes of communication that bypass synapses altogether. After all, cellular mechanisms for expelling molecules and cellular mechanisms for absorbing them are ubiquitous. Perhaps such transfers produce slow metabolic modulations in their target cells.

Neurotransmitters; Neuropeptides

A note on neuron chemistry: The chemical substances that best typify neurons are neurotransmitters: the substances neurons release to signal other cells. Their identity can be elusive. Ideally the neuropharmacologist seeks to establish that the stimulation of a particular group of neurons causes them to release from their presynaptic terminals a particular chemical that affects particular postsynaptic cells in the way observed in nature. In the periphery of

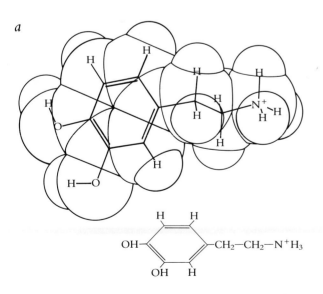

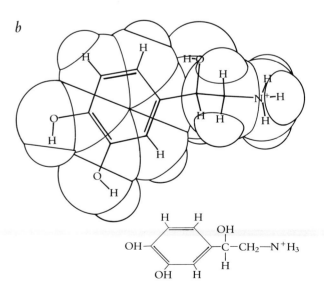

Figure 14: **Monoamine neurotransmitters** (that is, the ones well established today as being neurotransmitters) are four in number. They all result when enzymes in a neuron edit an amino acid. Dopamine (*a*), norepinephrine (*b*), and epinephrine (*c*) emerge in a

the body the project is feasible; in fact a crucial success was reported in 1921. Otto Loewi, a German pharmacologist, perfused the heart of a frog; the heart continued to beat. A length of the vagus nerve remained attached to the organ. He stimulated the nerve electrically; the beating slowed. He collected the perfusate and applied it to the heart of a second frog. It, too, slowed its beating. The perfusate eventually proved to contain acetylcholine; the vagus nerve had released it. In the brain and the spinal cord the project has never fully succeeded. Presynaptic terminals are measured in micrometers (thousandths of a millimeter); the presynaptic membrane has a surface area of no more than perhaps two square micrometers; the terminals lie in a welter of neural circuitry; the arrival of a presynaptic action potential induces each terminal to tap perhaps a few hundred synaptic vesicles, each containing no more than a few tens of thousands of transmitter molecules.

One seeks, therefore, to establish circumstantial evidence. If neurons must synthesize the putative neurotransmitter instead of simply capturing it from the extracellular environment, they ought to include the machinery, say the enzymes, that work the synthesis. The putative neurotransmitter ought to be present in presynaptic terminals. Electrical stimulation ought to bring on its release. The application of the putative neurotransmitter to postsynaptic neurons (say by bathing tissue slices in it) ought to duplicate the effect of natural neural events: for example, a transmitter might change the permeabil-

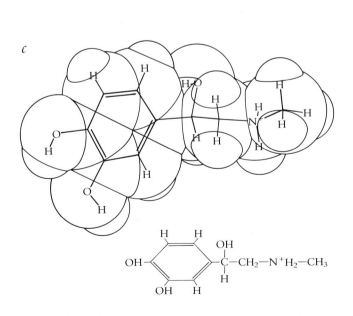

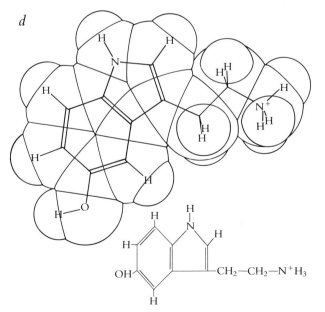

series of chemical steps from the amino acid tyrosine. Each is a catecholamine: a monoamine that incorporates a six-carbon ring. Serotonin (*d*) derives from the amino acid tryptophan. It is an indoleamine: it incorporates a six-carbon ring and a five-atom ring.

ity of the postsynaptic membrane to certain types of ion. There ought to be a mechanism by which the putative neurotransmitter is inactivated. Presynaptic reuptake will do, or alternatively the catalysis of the substance by extracellular enzymes. Otherwise a synaptic transmission would never end. Drugs known to affect a stage in the cycle of a transmitter — its synthesis, its storage in synaptic vesicles, its release from presynaptic terminals, its interaction with postsynaptic receptors, its inactivation — ought to modify the efficacy of the transmission: the drugs should predictably be agonists or antagonists.

Nine substances found in the vertebrate brain and spinal cord are canonical neurotransmitters: it is agreed that the circumstantial evidence is comparatively conclusive. Remarkably, four of them — glutamate, aspartate, glycine, and gamma-aminobutyric acid, or GABA — are amino acids (Figure 13). Indeed, all but GABA are dietary amino acids: they are molecules found in protein. Thus they are part of an animal's diet. The synthesis of GABA requires merely the decarboxylation of glutamate; that is, the removal of a carboxyl group (COOH). Another four — dopamine, norepinephrine, epinephrine, and serotonin — are monoamines (Figure 14). That is, they are derived from amino acids by no more than minor editing: the addition of hydroxyl groups (OH), the removal of a carboxyl group, the addition of a methyl group (CH_3). Dopamine, norepinephrine, and epinephrine are de-

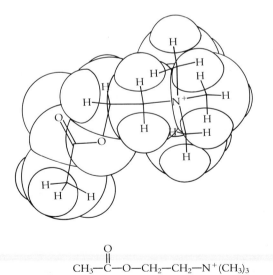

$$CH_3-\overset{\overset{\displaystyle O}{\|}}{C}-O-CH_2-CH_2-N^+(CH_3)_3$$

Figure 15: **Acetylcholine** is the ninth substance well established as being a neurotransmitter. Indeed, it was the first known neurotransmitter. It results from the joining of an acetyl group (CH_3CO) to choline, a constituent of lipids. Like the other eight, it is a fairly simple molecule produced in a small number of chemical steps from precursors available in what the animal eats.

rived from the dietary amino acid tyrosine; a six-carbon ring in their structure places them all in the class of molecules called catecholamines. Serotonin is derived from the dietary amino acid tryptophan; the presence of a six-carbon ring linked to a five-atom ring of carbon and nitrogen atoms marks it as an indoleamine. The ninth canonical neurotransmitter is acetylcholine (Figure 15). It results from the joining of choline to an acetyl group (CH_3CO). The choline is a problem: the brain cannot produce it. Choline, however, is a notable constituent of lipids in the diet. The liver can release it or make it de novo. Thus the pattern is unbroken: all nine canonical neurotransmitters are simple molecules made (or liberated) in a small number of chemical steps by enzymes acting on substrates readily available in what the animal eats. This suits them well for high-volume use and rapid replenishment. In that regard it may be relevant that the very simplest canonical neurotransmitters, the amino acid ones, seem to account for synaptic transmission from the majority of synapses in the central nervous system. A crude assay of brain tissue suggests this is the case. The amino acid neurotransmitters occur in concentrations of micromoles (10^{-6} mole) per gram of tissue. That corresponds to 10^{18} molecules per gram. The catecholamine neurotransmitters occur in nanomoles (10^{-9} mole) per gram. The simplest assumption consonant with the disparity is that the brain has a thousand synapses employing an amino acid transmitter for every synapse employing a monoamine.

In the 1930's the English pharmacologist Henry Dale proposed that a given neuron might employ the same neurotransmitter at all of its synapses. At the time acetylcholine and norepinephrine were known to be transmitters. Hence if one or the other could be identified at any one of a neuron's presynaptic terminals, the substance could be trusted to be the transmitter at other terminals less accessible to the investigator. This is not to say that the action of a neuron must always be the same at each of the neuron's synapses. It depends on the interaction between the transmitter and its postsynaptic receptor. The nervous system of the sea snail *Aplysia* offers a spectacular example. In the abdominal ganglion of *Aplysia,* workers including Eric R. Kandel and his colleagues at Columbia University can repeatedly identify more than 50 large neurons. Such identifications are one of the reasons why invertebrates are valued by neuroscientists. No one examining a more advanced species has much hope of finding large neurons that make precisely the same connections in animal after animal. Among the identified neurons the one designated *L*10 contacts the ones designated *L*2, *L*3, *L*4, *L*6, and *R*15. It inhibits all but the last. That one it excites. Acetylcholine applied to the surface of *L*2, *L*3, *L*4, and *L*6 proves to be inhibitory. Applied to the surface of *R*15 it proves to be the opposite.

Dale's principle is also being updated by recent discoveries suggesting that certain peptides (short amino acid chains) serve as intercellular messengers in the brain (Figure 16). The peptides tend to be found throughout the central nervous system. Receptors that bind them tend to be similarly widespread. In one place or another the concentration of any one of them may far exceed its background level. Elsewhere it may be notably lacking. The level is low: the

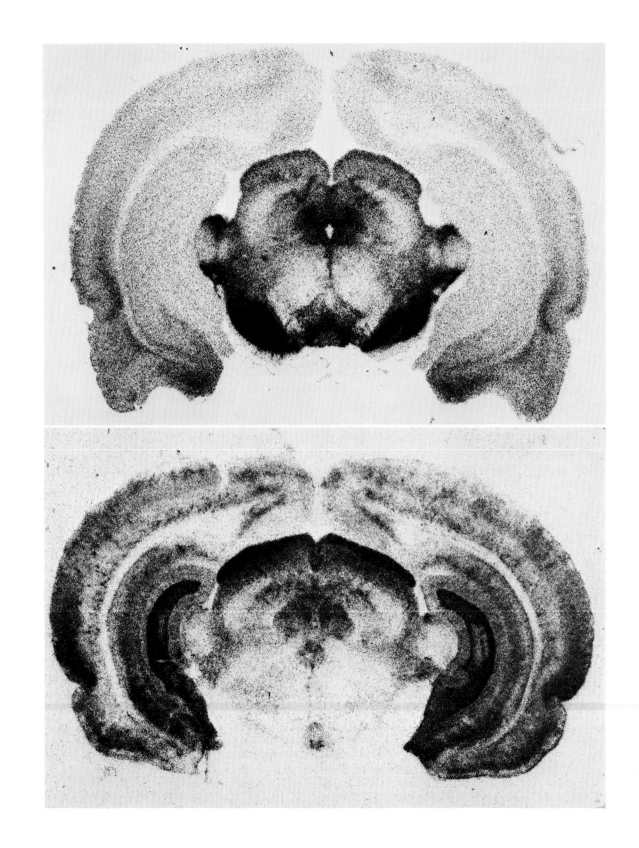

concentration of a peptide in the brain is typically measured in tens or hundreds of picomoles (10^{-12} mole) per gram. Moreover, a close look at the brain often places the peptide inside only a scattering of neurons; thus it is hard to ascertain whether the electrical stimulation of the neurons containing the peptide causes it to be released. On the other hand, the application of the peptide to slices of brain tissue affects the activity of many neurons. Three such "neuropeptides" — substance P, vasoactive intestinal peptide, and cholecystokinin octapeptide — showed up first in the mammalian gut. Then they showed up in the brain: they are now found, for example, in neurons in the cerebral cortex. Conversely, the peptide somatostatin first showed up in the brain: it was purified in minute quantity from literally tons of brain samples on the basis of its ability to suppress the secretion of growth hormone in the anterior lobe of the pituitary gland. Somatostatin now turns out to be present almost throughout the nervous system, from the cerebral cortex to peripheral ganglia. In addition it is found in cells that line the intestine and in certain cells in the pancreas. The peptides known as endorphins showed up both in the brain and in a gland. Specifically, neurons in the brain and cells in the anterior lobe of the pituitary proved to synthesize a protein, pro-opiomelanocortin, that incorporates several messenger peptides, including beta-endorphin, a putative neurotransmitter, and corticotropin, a hormone. (Released from the anterior lobe, it stimulates the cortex of the adrenal gland.) Neurons at a number of sites in the brain have receptors that bind opiates such as morphine, and some — not all — of the sites are known to participate in the perception of pain. The endorphins, occurring naturally in the brain, can bind to these receptors. So can the enkephalins, a pair of pentapeptides. The

Figure 16: **Substance *P* and its receptors** exemplify recent discoveries that a number of peptides (short amino acid chains) are active in the brain, perhaps as neurotransmitters. They are collectively called neuropeptides. Substance *P* is a neuropeptide consisting of 10 amino acids. Like several other neuropeptides it was found first in the gut and then in the brain: in neuronal cell bodies, axons, and axon terminals. Neurons with substance-*P* receptors on their surface have also been encountered. In these low-power micrographs, which show transverse slices of the brain of a rat, the distribution of substance *P* (*top*) was demonstrated with an immunological technique. An antibody to substance *P* was labeled with the radioactive isotope iodine 125 and applied to brain slices. The slices were then coated with photographic emulsion, in which the radioactivity laid down a visible pattern by transforming silver halide into black metallic grains. The micrograph shows the emulsion, not the underlying tissue. The distribution of substance-*P* receptors (*bottom*) was demonstrated in a similar way by labeling substance *P* with iodine 125 and applying it to tissue slices, so that it, and its label, could bind to receptors there. Curiously, the broad-scale distribution of substance *P* appears to correlate poorly with that of substance-*P* receptors. For example, the substantia nigra, at the base of each slice about two centimeters to each side of the midline, is rich in substance *P* but lacking in receptors. Perhaps a class of receptors with low affinity for substance *P* escaped detection. The distribution of substance *P* was determined by Stafford McLean of the National Institutes of Mental Health; the distribution of substance-*P* receptors was determined, again at the N.I.M.H., by Richard B. Rothman, Miles Herkenham, and Candace B. Pert.

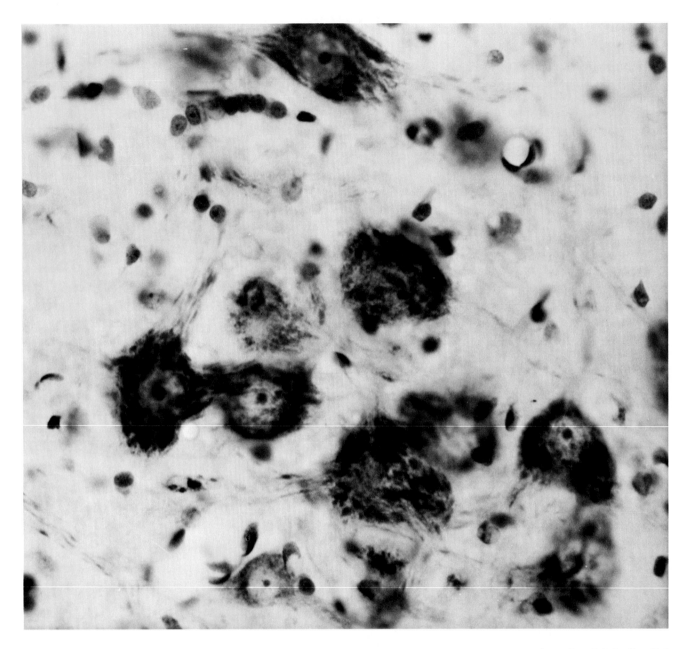

Figure 17: **"The dismal fog"** is the expression the Spanish neuroanatomist Santiago Ramón y Cajal employed to signify his dismay at the sight of neuronal processes vanishing as they emerge from their parent cell bodies in tissue stained for cell bodies. Here, in Nissl-stained tissue from the brain of a rat (in particular the motor nucleus of the trigeminal nerve), dendrites emerge from several neuronal cell bodies. The dendrites are invaded by elongated strands of Nissl substance, which enable their early trajectories to be traced. Then, however, the dendrites disappear. Even so, the dismal fog is far from featureless. It is populated by the nuclei of nonneuronal cells called glia. The largest, lightest-staining spots are the nuclei of glial cells called astrocytes; darker spots are the nuclei of glial cells called oligodendroglia; the darkest, angular spots are the nuclei of glial cells called microglia. To give examples: some closely spaced glial nuclei form an eyebrow-shaped crescent at the upper left. Three round, rather dark-staining bodies form the middle of the crescent; they are the nuclei of oligodendroglia. The larger, lighter-staining body abutting the leftmost of the three is the nucleus of an astrocyte; the very dark pellet just past the right end of the crescent is the nucleus of a microglial cell. The small white circle at the upper right is a blood vessel. It is lined by two dark crescents: the nuclei of vascular endothelial cells.

enkephalins are beginning to turn up in longer peptides, including one called dynorphin.

The updating of Dale's principle suggested by the study of neuropeptides comes about because the peptides are sometimes found in neurons already known to employ one of the canonical neurotransmitters. Some cells include both vasoactive intestinal peptide and acetylcholine. Others include cholecystokinin and dopamine. Still others include substance *P* and serotonin. A neuron may therefore release a mixture of chemical messengers; their actions doubtless differ. In particular, the canonical neurotransmitters open ion-conductance channels in the postsynaptic membrane. Thus they mediate rather directly between bioelectric activity on the part of the presynaptic cell and bioelectric activity on the part of the postsynaptic cell. The monoamine neurotransmitters have a further mode of action: they seem to alter the metabolic state of the postsynaptic cell. Neuropeptides, too, do both. In addition some of them, including the endorphins, are implicated in a curious mode of action. Here the arriving neuropeptide opens no postsynaptic channels and initiates no metabolic changes. And yet somehow it impedes the ability of the postsynaptic cell to respond to the arrival of canonical neurotransmitters, excitatory and inhibitory alike. To use a term favored by Floyd E. Bloom of the Scripps Clinic in California, it temporarily "disenables" the postsynaptic cell. The prospect arises that a mixture of messengers crossing a synaptic cleft and arriving at a postsynaptic membrane entails a complex course of events. The prospect is further complicated by the knowledge that neurons quite typically get input from a variety of brain structures, and that alone implies a variety of chemical messengers. In the cerebellum, for instance, the neurons called Purkinje cells are known to have receptors for norepinephrine and receptors for GABA. Other cerebellar neurons (ones that influence Purkinje cells) are known to have receptors for GABA and receptors for serotonin. Does the finding of a peptide in the intestine and in the brain seem like a humbling joke? It may simply reflect the usefulness of certain molecules as messenger substances. Evolution has employed them in many places. Does the number of substances—now in the dozens—suspected to be neurotransmitters seem like an excess? It may simply reflect the variety and the subtlety inherent in intercellular communication.

Glial Cells

Now let us peer into the dismal fog that surrounds a Nissl-stained neuron (Figure 17). It is far from featureless; one sees dark spots within it. For the most part they are the nuclei of glial cells, or glue cells in literal translation: cells that provide support to neurons throughout the central nervous system. Glial cells are thought to be 10 times more numerous than neurons. Yet the cell body in which each glial-cell nucleus lies embedded is invisible in Nissl preparations because it contains too few ribosomes to bind much of the Nissl dyestuff.

The largest but lightest-staining spots in the dismal fog are called open-faced nuclei; each belongs to a cell body of irregular shape that may look like a stylized star in the histological preparations that reveal it because its jagged sides sometimes taper to points (Figure 18). In addition (and perhaps more characteristically), the cell has numerous processes that radiate outward like a starburst. For either reason, the name astrocyte (from the Greek *astron,* or star) is descriptive. Astrocytes form the greater part of the matrix or scaffolding in which neurons are embedded. The astrocytes near the surface of the central nervous system have an additional function. They send processes to the surface, where the aggregation of their end feet forms a limiting membrane: a glial capsule that constitutes the outer wall of the brain and the spinal cord. The surface of the capsule is just under the pia mater, the innermost of the meningeal coverings of the central nervous system. In fact the glial capsule and the inner layer of the pia mater fuse: they form what is called the pial-glial membrane. The membrane is ubiquitous: its covering of the central nervous system is complete and unbroken. Indeed, wherever a blood vessel seems to invade the central nervous system, it never truly does so, because the pial-glial membrane funnels in around it. In this way, blood vessels are kept from making physical contact with neurons.

A second type of glial cell is characterized in Nissl preparations by a far more darkly staining nucleus, a round one in which the nucleic acids tend to aggregate more compactly. It is the oligodendroglial cell (Figure 19). The name means the glue cell with few processes. It does in fact have fewer than an astrocyte. Still, it has dozens; the electron microscope reveals them. Oligodendroglia coat axons in the brain and the spinal cord with an investment of lipid and protein called the myelin sheath (Figure 20). In particular, the membrane that forms the surface of an oligodendroglial cell compacts on itself to make as many as 40 veil-like extrusions, and each extrusion — in essence a doubled cell membrane — wraps around an axon. As the axon grows thicker in the developing central nervous system, more wraps are added. Thus the thicker the axon (the thickest ones in a mammal are from 12 to 14 micrometers in diameter, myelin included), the thicker its myelin sheath. There is, on the other hand, a cutoff diameter below which axons get no sheath. The cutoff seems to lie at about half a micrometer. When the myelination of an axon is complete, the axon is enveloped by lipoprotein except at the axon hillock, the initial axon segment, and the axon terminals. Moreover, the axon lacks myelin at a series of short gaps throughout its length where the sheath provided by one oligodendroglia ends and that of another begins. The gaps are known as nodes of Ranvier. They are the only places beyond the initial axon segment where ions can enter or leave a myelinated axon. The conduction of an impulse in a myelinated axon must therefore be discontinuous: it cannot be construed as simply the onrushing of an altered bioelectric potential. It can occur only because each node of Ranvier, like the initial axon segment, is an all-or-none site, complete with a granular undercoating, at which the impulse is regenerated. The impulse jumps from node to node, and in consequence its conduction is far faster than is possible in a process lacking myelin. The impulse is said to undergo saltatory conduction, meaning "moving by leaps." Small wonder that long-distance neural communication lines —those spanning centimeters rather than millimeters—almost always are established in vertebrate animals by myelinated axons.

The last variety of glial cell in the central nervous system is the microglia. Its nucleus is rarely round or even ovoid; it often is angular. It is the darkest among the glial nuclei that can be seen in the dismal fog. Microglial cells seem not to originate inside the embryonic tissues that become the central nervous system. Instead they are thought to arrive in the company of ingrowing blood vessels. In any event, microglia are the only cells in the central nervous system that can become militant. That is to say, they respond to a

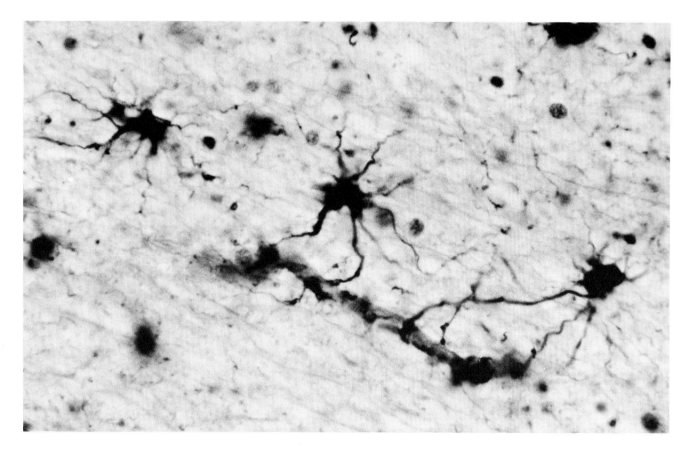

Figure 18: **Astrocytes** are the largest glial cells; their angular cell bodies emit a wealth of processes, which radiate outward like a starburst. In this micrograph, tissue from the axonal "cable basement" under the cerebral cortex of a human brain has been stained by the Cajal gold sublimate method, which is specific for astrocytes. Several astrocytes can be seen. Two of them extend their processes toward a small blood vessel crossing the bottom center of the image. There the end feet of the astrocytic processes contribute to a membranous glial capsule that keeps the vessel from making contact with neural tissue. Astrocytes serve, it seems, to establish neural compartments. Indeed, the end feet of astrocytic processes close off the surface of the brain and spinal cord.

pathological process by changing into phagocytes: cells that ingest microbes and the products of tissue breakdown.

How Many Neurons?

Since the cell bodies of glial cells are invisible in Nissl preparations, the Nissl technique can do no more than display the distribution of neuronal cell bodies

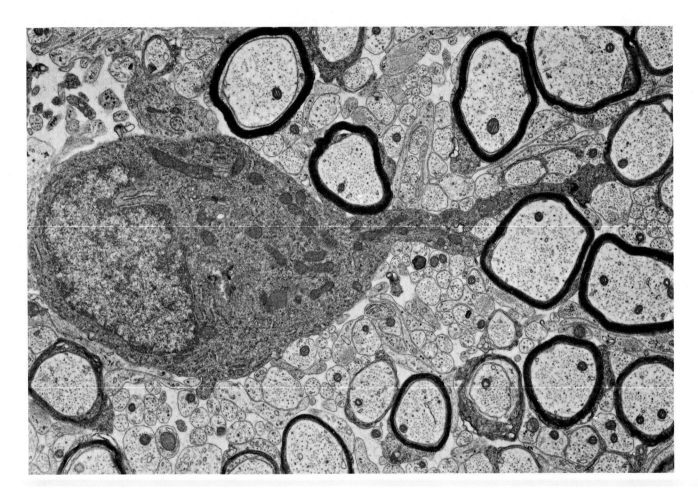

Figure 19 (left): **Oligodendroglia** invest the axons of neurons in the brain and spinal cord with a sheath of the fatty insulation called myelin. This electron micrograph was made in the spinal cord of a newborn cat at a magnification of 12,200 diameters. The cell body of an oligodendroglial cell is at the left. Its nucleus, which fills almost half the cell body, is at the extreme left. Toward the right the cell emits an extension, or process, that contacts two axons, cut in cross section. An oligodendroglial cell emits many such extensions and so may contact 40 axons or more, providing each with a sheath that covers part of the length of the axon. Oligodendroglia along the rest of the length of the axon contribute the other sheath segments. In this image a multitude of smaller axons fills much of the rest of the field; some would have increased in size and received a myelin sheath as the animal grew. The micrograph (and the one shown in Figure

in a section of tissue. But by that shortcoming, or rather by that virtue, it provides a survey of the cytoarchitecture of the brain and the spinal cord, and most basically, it permits a simple count of neurons per unit volume. How many neurons occupy the human central nervous system? True sensory neurons lie not in the central nervous system but in ganglia that flank the brain and the spinal cord; hence the answer must be an accounting of intermediate neurons and motor neurons. It often used to be said that the answer is 10^{10}. It is an attractive number, easy to remember and easy to state. Yet there

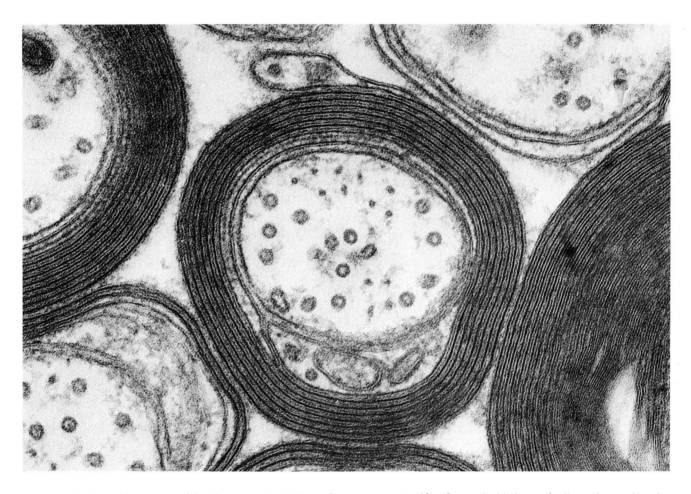

20) was made by Cedric S. Raine of the Albert Einstein College of Medicine of Yeshiva University.

Figure 20 (right): **Close view of myelin** shows details of how oligodendroglia make the myelin sheath. An axon is at the center of the field. On top of it is an oligodendroglial process, cut, like the axon, in cross section. Toward its right-hand side the process com-pacts on itself to form a double layer of cell membrane; then the double layer wraps repeatedly around the axon. In this instance the wrapping is clockwise. At the end of the innermost wrap the process expands again, producing a final cytoplasm-filled chamber. The axon itself includes a number of microtubules. The electron micrograph displays tissue from the spinal cord of a dog at a magnification of 163,000 diameters.

are classes of neurons so small and so densely crowded together that it is difficult or even impossible to judge their number. One such class is the granule cell. There are so many granule cells in just one part of the human brain, the cerebellum, that the estimate of 10^{10} neurons in the entire central nervous system becomes quite suspect. The total could easily be an order of magnitude higher — perhaps two orders of magnitude.

Assume, then, that the total is 10^{12}. How many are motor neurons? An estimate of the axons leaving the central nervous system to animate muscle fibers implies an answer of two or three million, which is disconcertingly few, because only through motor neurons can the workings of the nervous system find expression in bodily movements. Two or three million! The figure suggests that motor neurons are at a premium, and hence that a great number of influences must converge on them; it suggests, in other words, that a typical motor neuron must receive synapses from a multitude of axons emitted by a multitude of neurons in the great intermediate net. The facts agree. A typical motor neuron has perhaps 10,000 *boutons terminaux* on its surface. About 8,000 are on its dendrites and 2,000 are on its cell body. This is not to say that 10,000 intermediate neurons impinge on the motor neuron; the intermediate neurons tend to make multiple synaptic contacts when they communicate with a cell. Even so, being one among very few, the average motor neuron must be heavily impinged on; a neuron count of 10^{12} in the central nervous system implies as many as half a million neurons of the great intermediate net for every one motor neuron. Charles Sherrington had good reason to refer to the motor neuron, and in particular its axon, as the nervous system's "final common path."

One last conclusion remains to be drawn from the numbers we have cited: With the exception of a mere few million motor neurons, the entire human brain and spinal cord are a great intermediate net. And when the great intermediate net comes to include 99.9997 percent of all the neurons in the central nervous system, the term loses much of its meaning: it comes to represent the very complexity one must face when one tries to comprehend the nervous system. The term remains useful only as a reminder that most of the brain's neurons are, strictly speaking, neither sensory nor motor. Strictly speaking, they are intercalated between the true sensory side of the organization and the true motor side. They are the components of a computational network.

Chapter Three

Anatomical Divisions

The brain and the spinal cord of every vertebrate animal first appear in the embryo as no more than a tube formed by an epithelium only one cell thick. The forward part of the tube becomes enclosed inside the cranium. Long before that, however, it shows a series of three bulbous swellings called the primary brain vesicles (Figure 21). From back to front they are the rhombencephalon, or hindbrain; the mesencephalon, or midbrain; and the prosencephalon, or forebrain. In each case, the Greek name derives from the suffix *-encephalon,* meaning "within the head." Of the three primary vesicles the forebrain is the most productive in higher vertebrates, in terms of both further subdivision and further differentiation. The major event in its ontogenesis is the formation of a chamber on its left and right side. These become the cerebral hemispheres, also called the telencephalon or endbrain, which in lower vertebrates such as fishes are of modest size but in higher forms are enormous. Between the hemispheres lies the unpaired central part of the forebrain, from which the hemispheres diverge. It is called the diencephalon, which literally means "between-brain." Concurrent with these developments, the prosencephalon in a slightly more ventral position grows a further pair of lateral diverticula.* They are the optic vesicles. Even sightless animals

---

*The word lateral amounts to a navigational aid. There are several others. Throughout this book they have the following definitions. The word median (from the Latin *medium,* or middle) signifies a position at the midplane of the central nervous system, and hence at the midline of a slice through the nervous system. The word medial signifies a position toward the midplane. Thus a structure is medial only with reference to some other structure. The

have them, but in animals that can see they elongate toward the surface of the head. Ultimately they become the two retinas, connected to the base of the forebrain by their stalks, the optic nerves. Lastly, the ventral wall of the primary prosencephalon develops an unpaired midline diverticulum that differentiates to form the posterior lobe, or neurohypophysis, of the pituitary, or hypophyseal, complex.

Caudal Divisions

Figure 22 suggests the outcome of all these events; it is a schematic diagram that holds, by and large, for all mammals, and it shows the mammalian central nervous system broken up into several divisions. Many of its boundaries are more conceptual than biological, because every neural structure is continuous with its neighbors. Still, dividing lines, even arbitrary ones, are welcome. At the left of the figure is the first and most caudal subdivision of the central nervous system, the spinal cord, drawn with extreme foreshortening. Then, at no certain level — the transition is not abrupt — one's attention is transferred to the fully formed rhombencephalon, the caudalmost part of the brain. We shall often call it the hindbrain even though that straightforward English name is seldom used; the preferred name for the division, like the preferred names for all the great subdivisions of the brain, is the Greek one. "Rhombencephalon," then, was coined by affixing the prefix *rhomb-* to the ubiquitous stem *-encephalon;* "rhomb" refers to a progressive widening of the hindbrain, which reaches a maximum width at about the middle of its length, and tapers above and below. The organization of this brain division is remarkably consistent throughout the vertebrate orders. Its caudal half — the part immediately continuous with the spinal cord — is called the myelencephalon, from the Greek *myelon,* or marrow. Alternatively it is called the medulla oblongata, Latin for "the extended marrow." Both names have the same basis. Early anatomists described the spinal cord as the medulla spinalis, the spinal marrow. After all, the spinal cord is soft, whitish tissue and it is encased in bone: the bone of the vertebral column. The caudal half of the rhombencephalon was named by extension of this logic.

---

word lateral (from the Latin *latus,* or width) signifies a position away from the midplane. Again the term is relative. The word rostral (from the Latin *rostrum,* or snout) means "toward the end of the organism nearest the nose." Anterior is a synonym. The word caudal (from the Latin *cauda,* or tail) means "toward the tail end of the organism." Posterior is a synonym. The word dorsal (from the Latin *dorsum,* or back) means "toward the back of the organism." The word ventral (from the Latin *venter,* or belly) means "toward the front." In giving these definitions we are suppressing a complication that becomes important in the comparative anatomy of the brain. Basically, some animals walk on four legs, so that the spinal cord trails out horizontally behind the brain, whereas others walk on two legs, so that the spinal cord descends vertically under the brain, and this difference bedevils all attempts to establish a nomenclature that is totally unambiguous.

The rostral half of the rhombencephalon is called the metencephalon. Perhaps the name derives from *meta* and signifies "that which follows the myelencephalon." In any case, the metencephalon can be further divided. Its ventral part is the pons district, so named because it bulges outward there to form the pons Varolii, the bridge of Varolio. (Costanzo Varolio was an Italian anatomist of the 16th century.) Its dorsal part is an appendage called the cerebellum, the "little brain." In fact the size of the appendage varies greatly in different species: some fishes have an impressive cerebellum whereas most amphibians have a tiny one. The ancestry of the cerebellum suggests it was initially an auxiliary to the vestibular system but that other sensory systems later claimed its attention, too. Finally almost all the senses came to do so. Yet this cataloging of cerebellar input begs the more important question: How do the efferent, or outgoing, connections of the structure serve the needs of a living animal? One line of evidence is immediately available. When a person with cerebellar pathology is asked to bring his finger to the tip of his nose, his effort is decomposed: he jerks about, and as the finger approaches its target the jerkiness grows worse. This motor impairment is called ataxia — literally, loss of taxis, or order, in bodily motion. It is the only form of deficit that can be found in the patient. There is no sensory loss. Evidently, then, the cerebellum is a mechanism that integrates messages from all or most of the senses, and then brings that integral to bear on the organism's movements.

Rostral to the rhombencephalon is the mesencephalon, or midbrain. The English term is often used. In a mammal the midbrain develops two dorsal pairs of protrusions that together form a region of four hills known as the lamina quadrigemina, the tectum mesencephali, or simply the tectum, meaning roof. The more caudal pair are the inferior colliculi, from *colliculus,* or little hill; they are part of the central conduction paths for hearing. The rostral pair, the superior colliculi, are part of the paths for vision. Other than the colliculi, the mesencephalon gives little outward reason for subdivision; in fact, the mesencephalon is a rather short stretch in the human brain. The dorsal midbrain of vertebrates more primitive than the mammals has only a single pair of hills. Each hill corresponds to a superior colliculus, in the sense that its function is visual, not auditory. Accordingly, the hills are called the optic lobes or optic tectum. The functional homolog to an inferior colliculus in these nonmammalian forms occupies a deeper position and raises no bulge at the surface.

Rostral to the mesencephalon is the central, unpaired division of the prosencephalon, namely the diencephalon. Its dorsal two-thirds is the thalamus (where "thalamus" derives from the Greek for chamber). The thalamus will emerge as a crucial way station, a final checkpoint that intercepts messages to the cerebral cortex from all of the senses (except, it seems, olfaction). It is tempting to call any such interruption a relay. What happens at a break in neural circuitry, however, is far more than what happens in an athletic relay, where each runner simply hands a baton to the next and the baton arrives unmodified at the end of the course. In the central nervous system, the "relay" is quite different. At each synaptic interruption in a sensory pathway

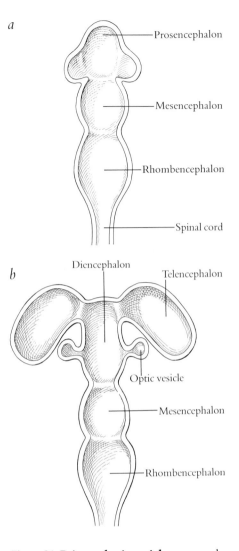

Figure 21: **Primary brain vesicles** are an early sign that the brain is taking form in the embryo of a vertebrate. They are a set of three bulbous swellings at the forward end of the neural tube: the precursor of the brain and the spinal cord. The swellings, from back to front, are the prospective rhombencephalon, or hindbrain; the prospective mesencephalon, or midbrain; and the prospective prosencephalon, or forebrain. In a human embryo the primary brain vesicles are apparent before the fifth week of gestation (*a*). Then, in the fifth week, the diencephalon, or central chamber of the forebrain, begins to develop side chambers: the telencephalon, or cerebral hemispheres (*b*).

the input is transformed: the code in which the message arrived is fundamentally changed. Presumably the data could not be "understood" at other levels; translation is needed, and the synaptic relays are better spoken of as processing stations.

Many such stations are found in the thalamus. Each is called a nucleus, a term that may be confusing. In a cytological context, the term refers, of course, to the nucleus of a cell. In neuroanatomical nomenclature, however, the term indicates a multitude of neuronal cell bodies lying in proximity to one another, and thereby forming a cluster that is more or less clearly delineated from neighboring structures in properly stained sections of the brain or the spinal cord (Figure 23). The ventral nucleus of the thalamus is a large cell

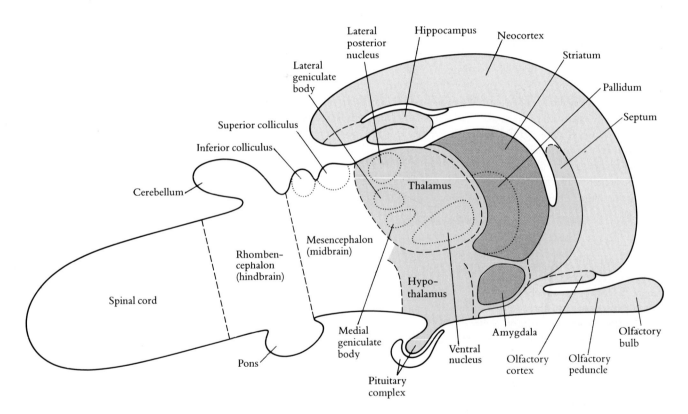

Figure 22: **Large-scale divisions** of the central nervous system arise from the neural tube. Here the mammalian brain is pictured. The rhombencephalon, or hindbrain, includes a massive protrusion, the cerebellum, and at the other side of the hindbrain an elevation called the pons. The mesencephalon, or midbrain, includes two elevations, the inferior and superior colliculi. The prosencephalon, or forebrain, is more complex. It has an outer part, the cerebral hemisphere (*color*), and an inner part, the diencephalon (*gray*). Each has further divisions. The cerebral hemisphere includes a "rind," the cerebral cortex (*light color*), which incorporates the hippocampus, the neocortex, and the olfactory fields. Beneath them (*dark color*) are stationed the amygdala and the corpus striatum. (The latter has two divisions, the striatum and the globus pallidus.) Meanwhile, the diencephalon includes the thalamus and the hypothalamus. The latter connects to the posterior lobe of the pituitary complex. The septum is best considered a diencephalic outpost. The scheme established in this illustration will serve as the basis for a sequence of diagrams throughout Part II of the book.

mass. Part of it serves the somatic sensory modality, specifically exteroception, comprising touch, pain, and temperature signals from the body surface, and proprioception, or perception of the body itself, comprising signals from muscles, tendons, and joint capsules and ligaments. Other thalamic nuclei serve other senses. The medial geniculate body (geniculate comes from *genu,* meaning knee) is a processing station for auditory sensation, whereas the lateral geniculate body is specialized for the processing of visual information. Figure 22 shows a further thalamic cell mass known as the nucleus lateralis posterior. This one resists any facile description; it cannot be characterized as solely a processing station for incoming sensory data. For now the best thing to say is that its position in the circuitry of the brain places it deep in the great intermediate net. The same must be acknowledged of many thalamic nuclei not shown in the illustration. In fact, the thalamic nuclei that are "merely" interposed in ascending sensory conduction paths make up only an eighth of the human thalamus.

The ventral district of the diencephalon is the hypothalamus, a part of the brain whose activity is expressed in the neural regulation of the viscera and of the endocrine glands. Like the thalamus it comprises a number of nuclei. One would estimate, however, that in the human brain its volume is no more than a tenth that of the thalamus. In the rostral direction the hypothalamus is continuous with the septum, a more or less triangular sheet of brain tissue best classified, despite its deceptive position, as a part of the diencephalon. In the ventral direction the hypothalamus becomes a narrow stalk. The stalk marks the alliance between the hypothalamus and the hypophysis, or pituitary complex. The stalk is thus a symbol of a way in which the hypothalamus governs the viscera. The stalk ends as the appendage called the posterior lobe of the pituitary. Sometimes called the neurohypophysis, it is a true part of the brain. It releases two hormones. The rest of the complex, namely the anterior lobe, or adenohypophysis (the prefix *adeno-* referring to gland), is not a part of the brain: it is an epithelial organ that develops from the roof of the embryonic oral cavity and applies itself closely to the posterior lobe, like a barnacle that clings to a piling. It releases several hormones. Regarding the name pituitary: it derives from a misconception on the part of the ancient anatomists who discovered the structure in unembalmed cadavers. The complex had decomposed, becoming a blob of mushy matter. Since it sat just above the roof of a side chamber to the nasal cavity, it was taken to be the master gland of mucus secretion. Thus it was called the *glandula pituitaria,* the mucus-producing gland; the Latin for mucus is *pitus.* The name survives in spite of the misconception.

Cerebral Hemisphere

The remaining subdivision of the forebrain is the telencephalon, or cerebrum, or cerebral hemisphere, or endbrain. In the brain of a mammal it is by far the largest part, and in many mammalian species its outer shell, the

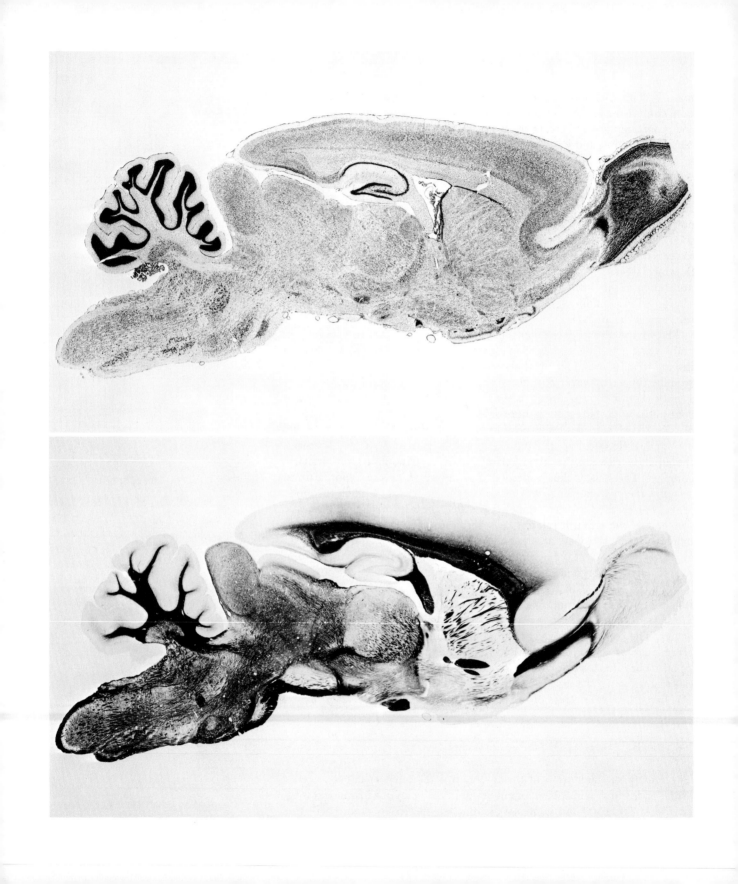

cerebral mantle or cerebral cortex (also called the pallium), is heavily furrowed into convolutions called gyri and fissures called sulci. The degree of furrowing is not indicative of a creature's phylogenetic status. Instead it appears to depend solely on the size of the species. Many small New World monkeys—for example the marmoset, and also the squirrel monkey—have brains whose surface is almost completely smooth. The sheep, the cow, and the horse, on the other hand, all boast respectable convolutions. So does man. Thus the human brain accommodates a cerebral cortex whose surface area is about 1.5 square feet. Every large mammal has a highly convoluted cortex; the whale's convolutions are perhaps the most extreme.

A matter of definition: The name cortex is bestowed on any neural structure that combines the following attributes. First, it is a sheet of gray matter*

---

*The term gray matter is best defined by reference to white matter, which is its opposite. White matter denotes districts of the central nervous system consisting of myriad axons. For the most part the axons are sheathed in myelin, a glistening, fatty substance highly

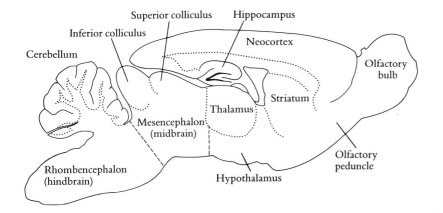

Figure 23: **Brain of a rat** looks much like the schematic mammalian brain displayed in Figure 22. Two adjoining slices are shown; they were stained by complementary techniques. In the Nissl-stained slice (*top*) each dot is a neuronal cell body; the dark-staining regions and bands are dense neuronal packings. The preparation establishes that the brainstem (the hindbrain and the midbrain) includes distinct neuronal communities, or nuclei. So does the diencephalon: the thalamus and hypothalamus. In contrast, the cerebral cortex and the cerebellar cortex have a layered cell architecture. In the Loyez-stained slice (*bottom*) only myelin is marked: the Loyez technique stains the fatty sheathing of axons. Accordingly, the dark-staining regions (including all of the brainstem) are regions dense in axons. The very darkest regions are axon bundles: the great communication channels of the central nervous system. For example, the dark band under the neocortex is in essence a neocortical cable basement. A number of smaller axon bundles traversing the corpus striatum validate the name of the structure: corpus striatum means "striped body." The map (*above*) identifies the anatomical structures visible in the stained slices.

at the surface of the brain; it is indeed the brain's rind or bark—the literal meaning of the term. Second, the neuronal cell bodies in a cortex are arranged in layers, so that under the microscope cells of one size and shape seem to occupy a common depth in the structure, and at different depths one finds different populations of cells. In a word, a cortex is laminated. Third, the outermost lamina contains axons and dendrites but few neuronal cell bodies. This zone is called the molecular or plexiform layer. Finally, and perhaps most characteristic, there is a tendency for the neurons in a cortex to have among their dendrites a long one that rises perpendicularly through the cortical laminations and into the plexiform layer, in which it ramifies. Such processes are called apical dendrites. In stained sections of the tissue they produce a palisadic appearance: a clear polarization of the dendritic field in a direction perpendicular to the surface of the brain. Only two loci wholly satisfy these conditions: the mantle of the cerebral hemisphere and the mantle of the cerebellum.

The mammalian cerebral cortex can be divided into a number of districts. It is convenient to begin at the base of the endbrain, where a structure juts forward composed entirely of cortex, though of varying cytoarchitecture. Its foremost, swollen end is the olfactory bulb; its shank is the olfactory stalk or olfactory peduncle. Only the portion under the rest of the cerebral hemisphere is the olfactory cortex proper. All three are notable for their primitive architecture: no more than three layers can be distinguished, including the plexiform layer, whereas in more advanced cerebral cortex one can distinguish six. The olfactory cortex is a common denominator in the brains of all vertebrates; it is often called paleocortex, Greek for "the old cortex." It forms the larger part of the cerebral cortex in a fish, whereas in reptiles and birds one finds a further field of cortex, also primitive in structure and appreciable in extent but more dorsal in position. Its function has proved embarrassingly difficult to determine. For that reason, it has tactfully been called general cortex.

A second portion of the mammalian cerebral cortex is of vast extent and structural complexity: in man and the other primates, it is estimated to contain no fewer than 70 percent of all the neurons in the central nervous system. This is the neocortex (Figure 24). It is the latest form of cortex to appear in evolution. We owe it to a branching: beyond the reptiles, one strain of animals elaborated on the reptilian pattern and became the birds, while another, more venturesome strain developed the neocortex as it became the mammals. From a strictly phylogenetic point of view, birds are thus the

---

reflective of light. Thus it is myelin that confers on white matter its eponymous white appearance; gray matter looks rather darker. Gray matter denotes districts of the central nervous system rich in neuronal cell bodies but poor in myelin-covered axons. The cell bodies are embedded in neuropil: a dense feltwork made up mostly of incoming axons and their terminal ramifications, along with the dendrites the local cells emit to meet the axons. Neither dendrites nor the thin end stretches of axonal ramifications are invested by myelin.

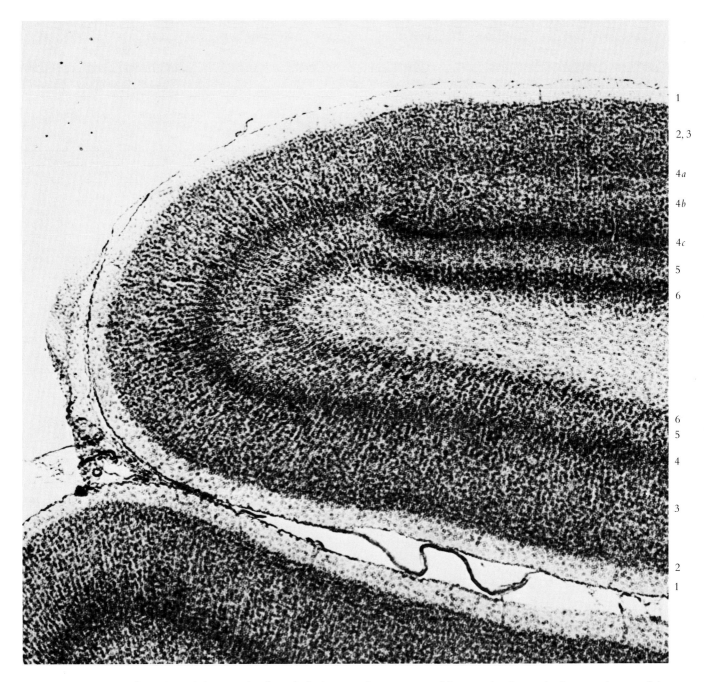

1

2, 3

4*a*

4*b*

4*c*

5

6

6
5

4

3

2
1

Figure 24: **Neocortex,** shown in a Nissl preparation from the brain of a macaque monkey, demonstrates three of the criteria distinguishing cortex from other neuronal organizations. The cortical tissue is at the surface of the brain; its neuronal cell bodies are organized into layers; and the outermost layer, called the plexiform layer, consists of closely packed dendrites and axons, with neuronal cell bodies more or less absent. In neocortex the plexiform layer is designated layer 1. The field of view includes a gyrus, or cerebral convolution. Most of the upper turn of the gyrus is primary visual cortex, the part of the neocortex where visual data arrive. Within its layered pattern three strata are dense in cell bodies. They are layer 6, sublayer 4*c*, and sublayer 4*a*. At the border of the primary visual cortex the sublayers abruptly coalesce, and layer 4 becomes unitary. The micrograph was made by David H. Hubel and his colleagues at the Harvard Medical School; the primary visual cortex of a human brain is shown in the micrographs in Figure 112.

logical end of the brain's traditional development. In contrast, mammals are deviants: no birds can be found in their ancestry. In one of the many radiations of mammalian evolution the primates appeared, an order in which the neocortex reaches its maximal development. We human beings are heir to all the consequences, perhaps including psychiatry.

A final district of the mammalian cerebral cortex is found at its medial edge, where the cortical sheet rolls inward and folds on itself to form a composite gyrus whose cross section is reminiscent of a rococo ornament. This remarkable structure is called the hippocampus — the sea horse — and in the human brain, it so strikingly resembles a sea horse, at least in the shape of its dorsal surface, that no other name seems conceivable. Hippocampal cortex is unique in that its neuronal cell bodies occupy only a single layer. (In olfactory cortex they occupy two layers; in neocortex they occupy five.) It is therefore called archicortex ("primitive cortex"). That name, however, is problematic. It suggests a phylogenetic sequence in which the hippocampus (and the olfactory cortex) arose before the neocortex. Yet the hippocampus cannot be placed in a scheme of evolutionary primacy; it is simply a characteristic feature of the edge of the cortical mantle. Specifically, the approach of the neocortex to its medial free edge is marked by a stepwise reduction in the number of laminations until a single cell-body layer remains. It should be said that the free edge of the cerebral mantle in reptiles and birds — that is to say, the free edge of the general cortex — also has a cytoarchitecture of only one cell-body layer. Hence the district is sometimes taken to be the homolog of the mammalian hippocampus. The extent of the homology remains a subject of debate. A true correspondence would require a similarity of function or a similarity of connections with other parts of the brain. The folding of the free edge of the cerebral mantle into a complex convolution is, in any case, peculiar to mammals.

In the depths of the mammalian cerebral hemisphere are further neuronal assemblages. One of them, the amygdaloid body, or amygdala (Greek for almond), is gray matter in which anatomists distinguish several nuclei. It lies immediately under the olfactory cortex. In fact, one of its nuclei (the cortical nucleus of the amygdala) fuses into the overlying olfactory cortex. The amygdala and the hippocampus are the main components of what is called the limbic system. It seems an odd alliance. For one thing, the hippocampus is cortex; the amygdala is not (except for the aforementioned cortical nucleus). Still, the hippocampus and the amygdala are allied (to give the most straightforward reason) by virtue of their placement in the circuitry of the brain. They stand out in the cerebral hemisphere because their axons descend most massively to the hypothalamus.

A final assemblage of neurons deep in the mammalian cerebral hemisphere is larger than the amygdala; indeed, it can impress one as being the solid core of the cerebrum. It is the corpus striatum: the striped or striated body. Clinical evidence reveals it is of crucial importance in the programming of complex bodily movements. In man, for example, the extensive destruction of tissue in the corpus striatum brings on motor automatisms. That is, it brings on complex movements, far more than mere tremors or muscle twitches, that begin without the patient's volition and are beyond his will to stop. The complexity of the movements may make them resemble a purposeful act: kicking or seizing, for instance. The name corpus striatum was coined several hundred years ago, when anatomists noted that the depth of the cerebral hemisphere is occupied by a large, gray mass crossed by slender, transverse white stripes. The stripes are now recognized to be bundles of myelinated axons. The corpus striatum is nonetheless composed of two great districts that are histologically distinct. One of them is a relatively large-celled inner zone called the pallidum or globus pallidus: the pale globe. The other one, darker looking, especially in a fresh (that is, an untreated) brain, is an outer zone whose cells are smaller and more densely packed. It is known as the striatum. In many mammalian species, including man, a plate of axons called the internal capsule cleaves the striatum into two anatomical divisions: the caudate nucleus and the putamen. "Caudate" refers to the trailing end of the cell mass: *cauda* is Latin for tail. "Putamen" is Latin for husk; in botanical usage it refers to structures such as cherry stones.

Chapter Four

Axon Tracing

The gross-anatomical distinctions made in the preceding chapter are helpful. Even so, they leave unanswered the first thing one asks about the organization of the central nervous system. What are the major pathways by which it conducts information?

Let us start with a more or less circumscribed part of the nervous system: a nucleus or a field of cortex. Fundamentally, it includes two classes of neurons. The neurons that make up one class each have a long axon with which they send signals out of the region: in neuroanatomical usage, they "project" to other regions, namely other nuclei or other fields of cortex. They are called projection neurons, or principal neurons, or (in honor of Camillo Golgi) Golgi type I cells. The neurons of the other class each have a shorter axon (or no axon, but only dendrites) and confine their connections to cells in their vicinity. They process information locally. They are called intrinsic neurons, or local-circuit neurons, or Golgi type II cells.

Let a thalamic "sensory relay nucleus" (the ventral nucleus, the medial geniculate body, or the lateral geniculate body) serve as a source of specifics. In a thalamic sensory relay nucleus, intrinsic neurons are relatively few: they amount to no more than a quarter the number of the projection neurons there. That proportion is quite unusual. In the brain overall, and especially in the brain of a primate, intrinsic neurons outnumber projection neurons by a ratio of at least three to one. (In the striatum they outnumber projection neurons by almost 20 to one.) The amount of data processing in a thalamic sensory relay nucleus must therefore be relatively modest. The transformation the nucleus performs on its incoming sensory data is nonetheless profound. Much of the synaptic contact inside the nucleus is in synaptic glomeruli: juxtapositions of numerous axon and dendrite terminals insulated by a glial capsule about 10 micrometers in diameter, which is formed by astrocyte membranes. The analogy to an electrician's junction box is irresistible. Such capsules are found elsewhere in the brain: notably the cerebellum. Within each thalamic glomerulus, an axon that enters the thalamus bearing sensory data passes signals synaptically to the dendrites of projection neurons. In turn, the projection neurons export data from the thalamus: they project to the neocortex. The sequence seems simple enough. The simplicity, however, is disrupted by a number of complications. Inside the glomerulus the arriving sensory axon signals not only projection neurons but also the dendrites of intrinsic neurons. In turn, those dendrites make dendrodendritic synapses with the projection neurons' dendrites. Outside the glomeruli the intrinsic neurons contact projection neurons in the more orthodox fashion of axon signaling dendrite. One imagines the intrinsic neurons help to determine which synapses interrupting sensory conduction lines will be open to impulse traffic and which will temporarily be closed.

The patterns of connection among inputs, intrinsic neurons, and projection neurons are extremely varied from place to place in the central nervous system (Figure 25). Still, it remains a fact that certain axons enter a nucleus or a field of cortex, often in circumscribed bundles, and that other axons leave it, often in circumscribed bundles. These axons establish the major conduction paths in the brain and the spinal cord. Tracing them is one task of this book. In practice the tracing begins with two questions. Given a part of the brain or the spinal cord, say a nucleus or a field of cortex, where do its axons go? The answer requires that the axons of its projection neurons be traced forward — that is, in the direction in which information is conducted along the axons toward their terminals. In brief, it requires anterograde (or orthograde) axon tracing. Conversely, given a part of the brain or the spinal cord, where do the axons that reach it begin? The answer requires that the axons synapsing on its neurons be traced backward to the projection neurons from which they arise. In brief, it requires retrograde tracing. A number of methods have been developed in efforts to meet each need. In general, the earliest methods, devised a century ago, were serendipitous discoveries. They were superseded a decade or two ago by methods capitalizing on the finding that an axon transports substances not only forward to its terminals but also backward to its parent cell body. The newer methods are now being superseded by still newer ones devised to capitalize on recent discoveries in molecular biology.

Retrograde Tracing

Consider the methods of retrograde tracing. The earliest way to identify the neurons sending their axons to a given neural structure was to destroy the structure. The axon terminals in the structure would also be destroyed, and throughout the nervous system the neuronal cell bodies emitting those axons

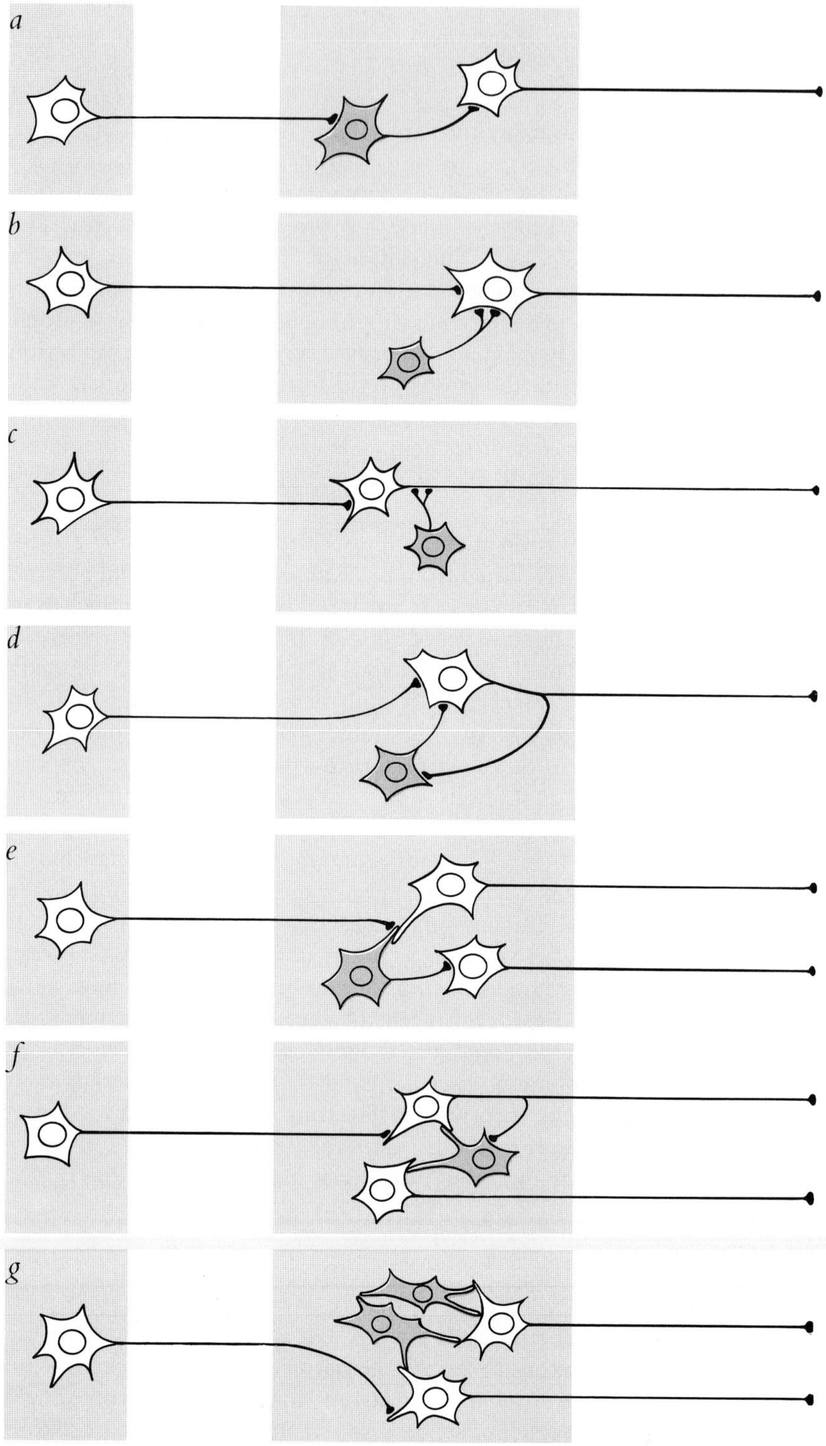

Figure 25: **Local circuits** among neurons in the central nervous system vary from place to place. This illustration gives some examples. In each a projection neuron exports signals from a nucleus at the left; it might equally well dispatch signals from cortex. Toward the center the projection-cell axon makes synaptic connections with cells in a target nucleus (or a cortical field). In *a* the axon contacts a local-circuit neuron (*color*): a nerve cell whose axon and dendrites ramify locally. In turn the local-circuit neuron contacts a projection neuron. In *b*, *c*, and *d* the local-circuit neuron receives no long-distance signals; it is a satellite of projection cells nearby. (In *d* it closes a local feedback loop.) In *e*, *f*, and *g* the local-circuit neurons act as bridges between projection neurons; they span what might be termed throughlines. (In *f* and *g* they lack an axon and transmit signals dendrodritically.) Synaptic complexes in the brain and spinal cord can be far more complex than the ones diagrammed. The illustration was devised by Pasko Rakic of the Yale University School of Medicine.

would undergo what is called the retrograde cell reaction. Such cells take on a typical appearance, which often can be recognized when the nervous system is sectioned and examined under a microscope two to three weeks after the lesion is made. In each such cell, the nucleus swells and becomes displaced from the center of the cell body to a position near the cell membrane. Meanwhile, most of the cell's Nissl substance disappears. (The process is called chromatolysis.) The most peripheral Nissl bodies—the ones just under the surface of the cell—persist the longest. Accordingly, the cell body becomes extraordinarily pale, but it keeps a dark edging.

The technique of destroying neural tissue and searching the rest of the nervous system for chromatolytic cell bodies was introduced in the 1880's. A different and far more effective technique appeared some 90 years later. Krister Kristensson, a Swedish neuropathologist, was studying the mechanism by which motor neurons are paralyzed by tetanus toxin. He had found that toxin labeled with radioactive iodine was absorbed by the axon endings in muscle tissue and transported in a direction opposite to the direction of axoplasmic flow. That is to say, it was transported up the axons and into the parent cell bodies, where he could demonstrate its presence by the ability of the radioactivity to fog the photographic emulsion with which he coated slices of neural tissue. Such transport is not astonishing. When a nerve in the periphery of the body is cut, the motor neurons that supply the motor contingent of the nerve show the retrograde cell reaction. They are trying to regrow their axons. In many cases they succeed, because in the peripheral nervous system the myelin that invests axons is the membrane of what are called Schwann cells, and Schwann cells, unlike oligodendroglia, maintain orderly positions after the death of the axons they envelop, providing tunnels through which regrowing axons can find their way. During the months that pass while the denervated muscle group is totally paralyzed (and therefore flaccid), its governing motor neurons remain in a state of chromatolysis. Then comes the first reinnervation of the muscle, and in a short time all signs of the retrograde cell reaction disappear. How does the cell body of a motor neuron in the central nervous system learn that its axon has reestablished motor end plates on the muscle? It must receive a signal: at the reestablished end plates the axon endings must take up a substance produced by the muscle —even an extremely atrophied muscle—and this substance must somehow send sign of its presence up the axon.

Kristensson found that bovine serum albumin, a large protein, was likewise absorbed by axon terminals and transported up the axon. But his most important success with retrograde axon transport involved horseradish peroxidase. HRP is one of a class of peroxidase enzymes found in various plants, and not in horseradish alone; it might equally well have been purified from the potato. It frees an oxygen atom from hydrogen peroxide, reducing the latter to water. Its ability to cross neural barriers had previously been exploited— to study gap junctions, for instance. Now it became the basis of a retrograde tracing technique (Figure 26). The technique begins with the injection of HRP into a given structure in the nervous system. The HRP is absorbed by the axon terminals there; then it travels up the axons toward the cell bodies that emit them. The HRP travels at a rate of 200 to 300 millimeters per day; hence the animal is sacrificed one or two days after the injection. The animal's brain is perfused with substances such as formaldehyde, glutaraldehyde, or both. The perfusate coagulates proteins, and so it fixes the tissue: it gives the tissue rigidity. The brain can thus be sectioned, typically into slices no more than 50 micrometers (a twentieth of a millimeter) thick. At such a thickness the brain of the rat, a common experimental animal, becomes a few hundred slices. Each of the slices is exposed to diaminobenzidine or, in more recent

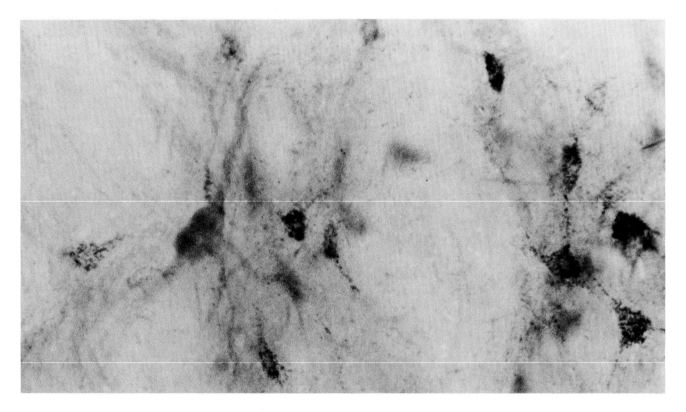

Figure 26: **Retrograde axon tracing** follows axons backward (that is, against the direction of signal conduction) from their terminals to the neuronal cell bodies from which the axons emerge. In this example of retrograde tracing the enzyme horseradish peroxidase (HRP) was injected in minute quantity (.1 microliter of a 10 percent solution) into the subthalamic nucleus of a living rat. The enzyme was absorbed by the axon terminals there and got transported up the axons toward their parent cell bodies. (The two-way transport of molecules is a property of axons.) The micrograph shows the globus pallidus. The pallidal neurons marked as origins of the pallidosubthalamic projection appear as cell bodies of medium size (from 20 to 25 micrometers in shortest diameter) containing a dark, granular pigment well into the dendrites of the cells. The pigment results from the oxidation of tetramethylbenzidine by oxygen liberated from hydrogen peroxide through the intervention of the HRP. To the left a larger neuron shows up in even tones of gray. It was rendered visible by subjecting the tissue to a second histochemical procedure, designed to demonstrate acetylcholinesterase, the enzyme that deactivates the neurotransmitter acetylcholine. The larger neuron is unlabeled by HRP. The tentative conclusion from several such experiments is that pallidal cholinergic neurons do not contribute to the pallidosubthalamic projection.

efforts, to tetramethylbenzidine. Then hydrogen peroxide is added. The hydrogen peroxide is reduced, the liberated oxygen combines with the benzidine compound to make a pigment, and by this relatively simple histochemical reaction the neuronal cell bodies containing the transported HRP stand out by dint of the colored stippling inside them.

Anterograde Tracing

How can axons be followed in the opposite direction—forward to their terminals instead of backward to their parent cell bodies? Again the early investigators destroyed parts of the living nervous system. In some experiments they destroyed cell bodies; in others they cut through a bundle of axons. Either way, the experimental intervention severed axons from the cell bodies that emitted them. The severed lengths of the axons would soon begin to disintegrate (the phenomenon is called anterograde or Wallerian degeneration, after the English physiologist Augustus Waller, who discovered it in the middle of the 19th century), and if the axons were myelinated, the myelin would disintegrate as well. This latter disintegration works a crucial change in the myelin's composition. Normal myelin incorporates quantities of unsaturated fatty acids. Such acids are capable of reducing osmium tetroxide to black metallic osmium. If normal neural tissue is placed, therefore, in a solution of osmium tetroxide, the myelin stains black. Suppose the tissue includes myelin sheaths that are disintegrating because an investigator has made a lesion somewhere in the nervous system. In addition, suppose the tissue is first placed in a solution of potassium dichromate, a powerful oxidant. It stays there for three weeks, and only then is it exposed to osmium tetroxide. Under these circumstances no normal myelin stains. The unsaturated fatty acids have all accepted oxygen from the potassium dichromate, and none remain to take it from the osmium tetroxide. The disintegrating myelin does, however, stain. Even after three weeks in potassium dichromate, it retains its ability to reduce osmium tetroxide to black metallic osmium. In all likelihood, its content of unsaturated fatty acids increases as it breaks down. Since the disintegrating sheaths are alone in turning black, they can be recognized and traced. The method was developed by the Italian physician Vittorio Marchi three decades after Waller's discovery.

Still later it became possible to mark degenerating axons instead of just their myelin sheaths. That represented an advance in the anterograde tracing of neural communication lines, because axons thinner than about half a micrometer could now be stained, and so could axon terminals, although both such structures lack myelin. The advanced techniques, which impregnate axons with silver, were developed in stages, beginning at the turn of this century when Cajal placed blocks—not sections—of fixed neural tissue in a bath of silver nitrate. After several days, he would transfer the blocks to a strong reducing agent: hydroquinone, for example. Nascent metallic silver would form in the tissue, and for an unknown reason it would selectively aggregate in axons. In the same year — 1901 — a second technique serving the same purpose was introduced by the German neuropathologist Max Bielschowsky. In his technique the tissue would be fixed and sectioned, and the sections would then be soaked in a solution of silver nitrate for a length of time varying between one hour and several days. The sections would next be transferred to a solution of the double salt silver-ammonia nitrate. It is an extremely labile substance. If it stands overnight, nascent silver will slowly precipitate out of solution. Mirrors used to be made by that method. A rather weak reducing agent such as formaldehyde can thus be substituted for the strong reducing agent that would otherwise be required. The silver techniques both of Cajal and of Bielschowsky impregnate normal axons; in this form, therefore, the deposition of silver has only limited utility as a tracing method. To make the Bielschowsky method selective for degenerating axons, an intermediate step is required; it was introduced in the 1940's. Immediately before the first of the two silver baths, the sections are placed in a sequence of mordants — tanning agents, in a rough analogy. The tanning selectively renders degenerating axons receptive to silver.

In the anterograde techniques the direction of the tracing is the direction of forward (or anterograde) axoplasmic transport; thus a technique might well begin by introducing a traceable substance into the cell bodies under investigation. Such a technique, called autoradiographic tracing, came into prominence in the 1970's; it employs amino acids labeled with tritium, the radioactive isotope of hydrogen (Figure 27). Tritiated amino acids are injected, then, into the neural structure whose outgoing connections are to be determined. The cells composing the structure absorb the amino acids from the extracellular medium. Often a cell's appetite for one amino acid is greater than its

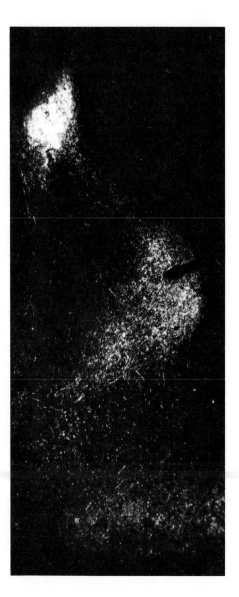

Figure 27: **Anterograde axon tracing** follows axons forward, in the direction of signal conduction, from their parent cell bodies to the terminals at which the axons send signals to other neurons. In this example the tracing was autoradiographic. The amino acid leucine was labeled with tritium (radioactive hydrogen) and injected into the internal segment of the globus pallidus of a cat. The leucine was absorbed by neuronal cell bodies there, which made it part of peptides and proteins and dispatched it down their axons. The axons emerge from the internal pallidal segment in a tract called the ansa lenticularis. Four days after the injection the brain was sectioned and the slices were coated with photographic emulsion. Then came six weeks in storage at $-20°C$. During that time the labeled axons in each slice recorded their position by releasing beta particles (energetic electrons), which reduce the silver halides in a photographic emulsion to grains of metallic silver, much as photic energy does in ordinary photography. The illustration, a dark-field micrograph, shows a section through the caudal thalamus; silver grains show up in white. The wide crescent of grains at center right marks the centrum medianum nucleus, a thalamic destination for the ansa lenticularis. The narrow black oval invading the nucleus from the right is a blood vessel in cross section; it extends some three-fourths of a millimeter into the nucleus. A denser, compact cloud of grains at top left marks the lateral habenular nucleus, a destination unexpected at the outset of the experiment, in 1974. The diffuse cloud toward the lower right is the ansa lenticularis itself, nearing the thalamus from below in what is called field H-1 of Forel. The experiment was done by Haring J. W. Nauta at Case Western Reserve University.

appetite for another. Still, certain amino acids are coveted: an infusion of tritiated leucine or proline almost always is effective. Within hours the neurons at the site of the injection are incorporating the labeled amino acids into the proteins they are making, and many of these proteins are transported down the axon. Some move one or two millimeters per day in the slow form of axoplasmic transport. Others move rapidly: on the order of 400 millimeters per day.

The subsequent treatment of the tissue begins with the fixing and sectioning of the brain. The sections are mounted on glass slides and dried; then, in a darkroom, they are dipped in photographic emulsion, dried again, and placed in light-tight boxes to be stored in a freezer for as long as 12 weeks. During that period, some of the atomic nuclei of the tritium atoms break down. The process is accompanied by the release of free electrons, or beta particles. The ones that fly out of the surface of each section are recorded in the overlying emulsion as grains of black metallic silver. Later, when the emulsion has been developed (in the photographic sense), the grains can be charted under the microscope. An alignment of grains suggests the presence of an axon through which radioactive molecules were passing when the animal was sacrificed; the fixation of the tissue coagulated all the protein in the axon and elsewhere and thereby locked the labels in place. A cloud of grains suggests a terminal arborization. A study of the patterns of grains from slide to slide permits the distribution of the axons arising from the cells at the injection site to be determined quite precisely.

New "Stains"

A crucial point about the axon-tracing techniques we have been describing is that they are all experimental. That is, they require an experiment: the choice of a region whose connections are to be studied, and then the making of a lesion or the injection of a traceable substance at the chosen site in a living animal. In brief, they require a local intervention in the brain. The newest techniques are often quite different. Many of them are complex, yet in a way they are throwbacks: like the Nissl technique, which marks nucleic acids, they reveal the distribution of something inherent in the brain. Thus they require no local intervention. In essence the newest techniques are stains. It is fair to say they derive from the hope that the neurons employing a particular neurotransmitter might be made to show themselves throughout the nervous system.*

---

*That hope has mostly been thwarted, in that the only simple way to mark a neurotransmitter is the histofluorescence technique. Devised in the 1960's by Bengt Falck of the University of Lund and Nils-Åke Hillarp of the Karolinska Institute, it demonstrates the presence of the monoamine neurotransmitters serotonin, dopamine, norepinephrine, and epinephrine in cell bodies, axons, and axon terminals at the surface of thinly sectioned neural tis-

At bottom the newest techniques exploit the nature of proteins. Notably, proteins are antigenic: if they invade the body of a vertebrate, they are met by defensive measures that constitute what is called the immune response. In one aspect of the response, plasma cells — the offspring of *B* lymphocytes, a type of white blood cell — secrete antibodies: molecules (specifically immunoglobulins) primed to bind to the invader. Each plasma cell secretes a particular antibody. The idea arises that antibodies could be primed to bind to a protein of interest to an investigator, and by that binding could mark its distribution in neural tissue. Thus a "staining" method develops. It is immunohistochemical (Figure 28). First a protein is purified from the brain of one species, say a goat. The protein can be a suspected neurotransmitter that has proved to be a peptide. The endorphin neuropeptides are prominent examples. It can be an enzyme that participates in the synthesis of a neurotransmitter — say choline acetyltransferase, which makes acetylcholine. It can be an enzyme that breaks down a neurotransmitter — say acetylcholinesterase. It can be an enzyme with a wholly different function. It can be a structural protein. Tubulin, a protein in microtubules, is an example. It can be a membrane protein: a receptor or part of an ion-conductance channel. In principle there is no difference; each is a chain of amino acids, and so is potentially antigenic. The protein is injected into the blood of a different species, say a rabbit. The immune system treats it as an invader and primes antibodies against it. The antibodies are collected. Then each antibody is given a label such as radioactive atoms or a fluorescent chemical group. Finally the antibodies are applied to sections of the brain of any species. There the antibodies bind to the antigenic protein intrinsic to the tissue.

Two problems can interfere with the project. In the first place, the immune response is diverse: it primes antibodies against different molecules on the surface of an invader (say the protein capsule of a virus), or even different parts of a molecule. This means the defenses of the body do not characteristically produce a pure strain of antibody, even in response to a single type of invader. In addition a given antibody can bind to different molecules, provided they share the sequence of amino acids against which the antibody is primed. (This broadening of the response is termed cross-reactivity.) In 1975 the problem was overcome, at least in part, when mouse lymphocytes were successfully fused with mouse myeloma (bone-marrow cancer) cells. The resulting hybrid cells — they are known as hybridomas — prove to have hybrid properties: like plasma cells, they secrete antibodies; like cancer cells, they are immortal in cell culture. As before, an animal is exposed to a protein purified

_____

sue. The technique rests on the happy circumstance that an indoleamine such as serotonin or a catecholamine such as dopamine, norepinephrine, or epinephrine combines with formaldehyde to yield a compound that fluoresces under ultraviolet light. Sections of the tissue are exposed to formaldehyde vapor. Serotonin fluoresces yellow; dopamine, norepinephrine, and epinephrine fluoresce green.

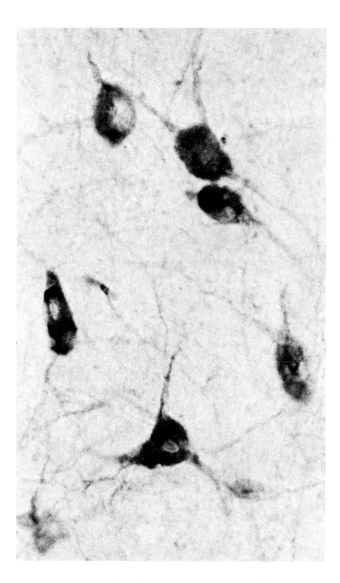

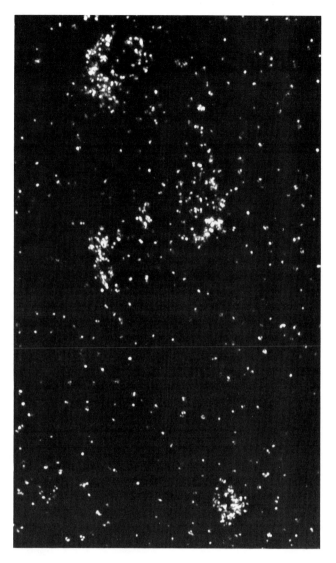

Figure 28: **Immunohistochemistry,** a new "stain" for neural tissue, exploits the immune response of vertebrate animals; in particular it uses antibodies. In its newest version the antibodies are monoclonal and monospecific: they are produced by a clone (the identical offspring of a single parent cell), and they bind to only one protein. The tissue shown is from the nucleus basalis, a part of the substantia innominata, at the base of the forebrain. It was exposed to a monoclonal antibody specific for the enzyme choline acetyltransferase, which makes the neurotransmitter acetylcholine. The antibody had been linked to a peroxidase, so that its binding sites in neural tissue could be marked by a pigment. Several neurons are darkly stained. Their cytoplasm includes choline acetyltransferase; evidently, then, their transmitter is acetylcholine. They are in fact the only known cholinergic neurons that project to the neocortex. The micrograph was made (with tissue from a rhesus monkey) by M. M. Mesulam and his colleagues at the Harvard Medical School.

Figure 29: **In situ hybridization,** a second new "stain," exploits the technology of recombinant DNA and genetic engineering. Here the stain is employed to locate neurons that synthesize adrenocorticotropin, or ACTH. The dark-field micrograph is of tissue from the arcuate nucleus of the hypothalamus of a rat. The tissue was exposed to a DNA engineered especially for the experiment. For one thing, the DNA binds to a particular messenger RNA: the one that specifies the structure of ACTH. In addition, the DNA incorporates tritium atoms, whose radioactivity produces metallic silver grains (*white dots*) in the photographic emulsion with which the tissue was coated. Clusters of dots mark neuronal cell bodies in which the genetic instructions for the making of ACTH are being expressed. ACTH, already known to be a hormone released by the anterior lobe of the pituitary gland, is now suspected of being a neurotransmitter, too. The "staining" was done by Josiah N. Wilcox of the College of Physicians and Surgeons of Columbia University.

from a different species. Lymphocytes proliferate, each producing a particular antibody. The lymphocytes are fused with myeloma cells; the fusion makes them immortal. The hybrid cells are then allowed each to give rise to a clone: a colony of identical offspring. The entire colony is devoted to the synthesis of a pure, or monoclonal, antibody.*

The second problem with immunohistochemistry is also inherent in the technique, which demonstrates the distribution of a protein in not only the cells that make it but also the cells that simply accumulate the substance: say target cells for the protein. Here, too, a solution has emerged. It takes the form of a very new "staining" technique; as this is being written, the technique is being refined. Called in situ hybridization (Figure 29), the technique relies on the central dogma of molecular biology, which affirms that a protein is made in a cell by ribosomes following instructions coded first in a gene in the nucleus of the cell and then by a messenger RNA dispatched from the nucleus to a ribosome. (In the language of molecular biology, the genetic material, DNA, is transcribed into messenger RNA, which is translated into protein.) Accordingly, in situ hybridization marks the distribution of an mRNA: the instruction tape for the protein, found only in the cells that actually synthesize the molecule. One begins with a collection, or "library," of mRNA's extracted from cells. Each is a single-stranded nucleic acid. A sequence of manipulations produces a corresponding double-strand DNA, each manufactured in quantity by a bacterial clone. A single clone's product is chosen; then the "staining" itself can begin. First the DNA is made radioactive. Next it is boiled, so that each double strand comes apart into single strands. The single strands are applied to slices of neural tissue. One strand from each pair is "coding": its sequence of nucleotides duplicates part of the messenger under study. It is useless as a marker. The other strand is "anticoding": it is the chemical complement of the messenger, and so the two can bind, producing an in situ hybrid: one strand is mRNA, the other is radioactive DNA. The slices are dipped in photographic emulsion and prepared for autoradiography.

The sequence is complicated. Nevertheless, it is a straightforward exercise in the new technologies of recombinant DNA and genetic engineering. Indeed, one moves almost too readily from a library of proteins to a library of

*An application of immunohistochemistry now promises to supersede autoradiography as a method of anterograde axon tracing. One begins by injecting into a chosen part of the brain or spinal cord a vegetable protein known as a lectin. The one now employed is purified from kidney beans. The lectin is absorbed by cell bodies and transported down their axons. Then, at the axon terminals, it becomes a marker when it binds to an antibody that has been primed against lectin and in addition has been linked to a peroxidase. (In effect the antibody is a tug that takes peroxidase to moorings the investigator has readied in the brain.) Lectin immunohistochemistry is the most sensitive anterograde tracing method yet devised; it reveals a wealth of detail that makes it rival a Golgi preparation. For example, it routinely reveals elaborate synaptic plexuses woven by axons around their target neurons. An example of lectin immunohistochemistry is displayed as the frontispiece to Part II.

monoclonal antibodies, or from a library of messenger RNA's to a library of DNA probes. One can make preparations of labeled neurons without knowing, or even guessing, what substance one has labeled. On the other hand, browsing in a library can be instructive in unexpected ways. Investigators at the Salk Institute and the Scripps Clinic led by Floyd Bloom and by J. Gregor Sutcliffe have undertaken what they term an "unconstrained" study of the mRNA's in neurons in the brain of the rat. They estimate the library of the mRNA's throughout the animal numbers from 50,000 to 100,000. Of these a given neuron has about 1,000. The number may seem small, but then, a neuron is a highly differentiated cell, one that has followed a particular developmental path among the many offered by the organism's genetic makeup. In effect it has renounced a multitude of possible careers and has correspondingly lost the capacity to synthesize a multitude of proteins. Among the 1,000 messengers, some 200 are found in roughly equal quantities in cells of the liver and the kidney. The proteins these messengers specify are equally useful there. Another 200 are found in the liver and the kidney, but in unequal quantities. The remaining 600 are unique to the neuron. This is not to say that the capacity to synthesize a mere 600 proteins is what distinguishes the brain from other organs. Neurons differ not only from liver or kidney cells but also from one another: they have distinctive shapes, distinctive connections, distinctive membrane channels and receptors. They have distinctive messenger libraries as well. Thus the number of messengers unique to the brain may be as great as 30,000. Some specify rather long proteins. Others are quite widely allocated among neurons. Still others are so abundant in certain neurons that they enable such cells to make a protein in great quantity. That leaves roughly 800 mRNA's. Each enables privileged neurons to make a short amino acid chain—a peptide—in small quantity. The 800 peptides are candidates for hitherto unknown neurotransmitters.

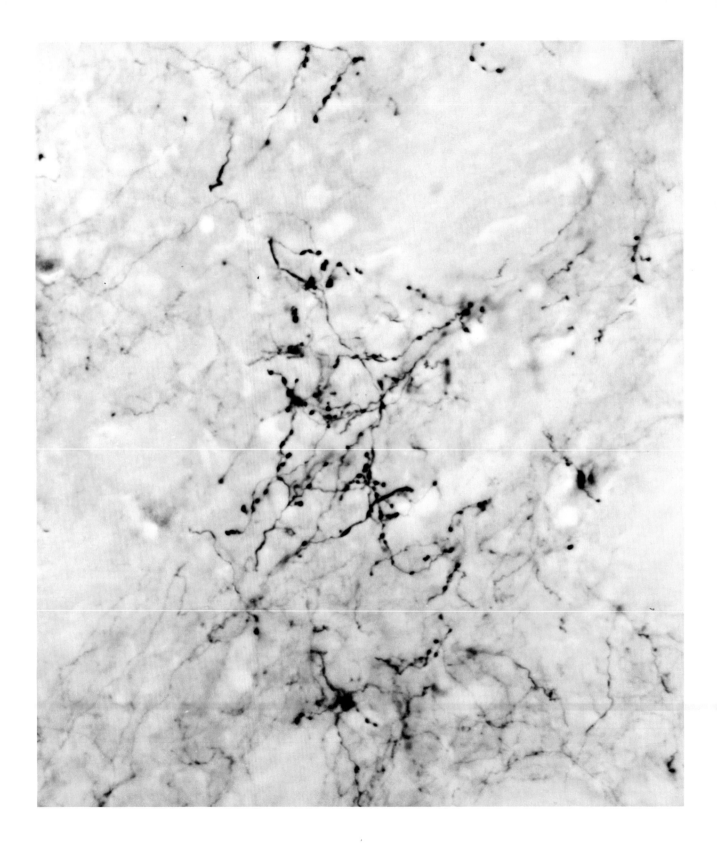

Part II

CONNECTIVITIES

Facing page: **Axon terminals** in the corpus striatum of a rat mark one of the chief conduction paths in the mammalian central nervous system, the paths to be described in this part of the book. To facilitate the staining of the terminals, the protein lectin was injected into the substantia nigra, at the base of the midbrain. Lectin is carried by axons in the anterograde direction; thus it was transported to the striatum, deep in the cerebral hemisphere, where its presence was demonstrated by immunohistochemistry (that is, by priming an antibody against it and labeling the antibody with a pigment). The experiment revealed two classes of nigrostriatal terminals. One, a fine plexus of axonal ramifications, pervades the field of view. The other, a network of fibers notable for large varicosities, or boutons, appears mostly toward the center. In a further immunohistochemical experiment an antibody was primed against the enzyme tyrosine hydroxylase, which initiates the synthesis of the neurotransmitter dopamine. The effort established that the fine plexus is dopaminergic. In man the incapacitation of the dopaminergic projection is thought to underlie Parkinson's disease. The experiments were done by Charles R. Gerfen and his colleagues at the National Institutes of Mental Health.

Chapter Five

Ascending Paths

A point from the foregoing description of axon-tracing techniques is worth repeating: the techniques demand the making of a lesion or the injection of a labeling substance at a chosen place in a living animal. This means the techniques cannot be used to study the human brain directly.

Can autopsy serve instead? The answer is, only rarely. In the first place, the human nervous system typically goes unfixed until as long as a day after death; it is hard for matters to be otherwise at the end of a human life. By that time, the postmortem decomposition (the so-called autolysis) of the tissue of the brain has altered both its chemical and morphological characteristics to such an extent that the chemical treatments required by the various axon-tracing techniques as a rule are unavailing. In the second place, the retrograde cell reaction brought on by a trauma or a disease is often followed in the living nervous system by the disappearance of the cell bodies themselves. The region they populated becomes filled instead by glia. It is estimated that unless a neuronal cell group has been depleted by 30 percent or more, no investigator who examines the region under a microscope is likely to notice anything unusual. Third, a pathological process that destroys neural tissue tends not to confine its damage to a circumscribed locus. So even if the tissue had promptly been fixed, the investigator might well find it impossible to sort out the degenerating axons that arise in a given structure from those arising in adjoining structures that also were damaged. Indeed, some degenerating axons might well arise quite far from the lesion. They were damaged along their trajectory.

To be sure, the investigator can hope to use with benefit a survey method

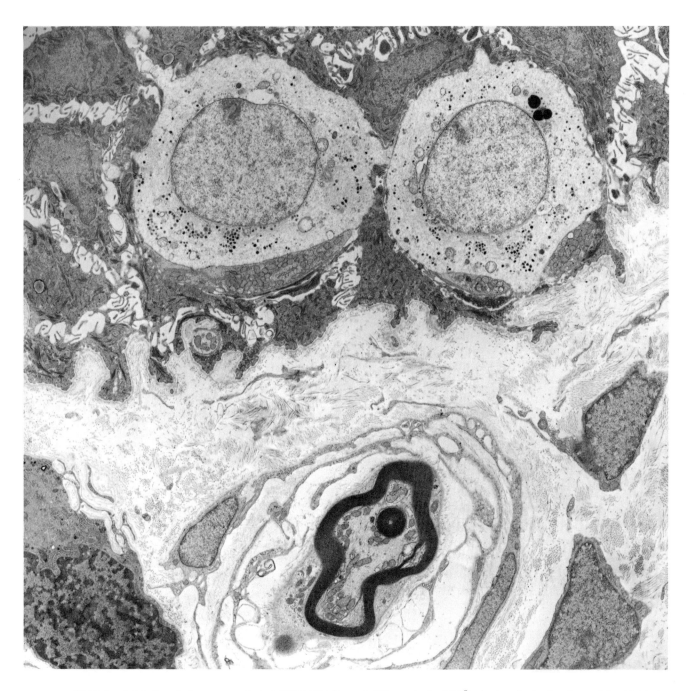

Figure 30: **Merkel's disks** are at the beginning of a sensory conduction path: they are receptors stationed in the skin, where they respond preferentially to a steady pressure applied to the body surface. Each disk associates itself with a specialized epithelial cell. Toward the top of the field of view two such cells, called Merkel cells, are side by side in the epidermis. The cell at the right includes three black spots of the skin pigment melanin. The cells are cupped from below by crescent-shaped axon terminals; these are Merkel's disks. Still lower in the field (in the dermis, the deep layer of the skin) is the irregular cross section of a myelinated axon some four micrometers in diameter. It is probably the parent of the terminals. The electron micrograph was made by Bryce L. Munger of the Hershey Medical Center of Pennsylvania State University; it shows skin from the finger of a man who had suffered a lesion cutting the ulnar nerve, in the arm. The regenerating axon has reestablished its alliance with Merkel cells.

such as the Nissl stain, which will reveal large-scale vagaries in the distribution of neuronal cell bodies in the nervous system. The yield of such efforts has been far from negligible. For example, the occlusion of an end artery that nourishes a particular part of the cerebral cortex causes a retrograde cell reaction in a particular part of the thalamus. The broad array of the thalamo-cortical connection in the human brain has been charted by this means. Conversely, the anterograde axon degeneration following a lesion in a particular part of the human cerebral cortex, the motor area, is known to result in a gradual reduction in the size and myelination of a particular axon bundle, the pyramidal tract. Further still, the axon tracing done in animals suggests a certain commonality in the principal features of the central nervous system across the various mammals. The connections you find in the rat you are very likely to find in the monkey, though not, perhaps, the other way around. The discoveries made at autopsy fit this basic pattern well. Indeed, in sporadic cases the silver-impregnation methods have been applied to the human brain and spinal cord to demonstrate detailed patterns of fiber degeneration. No surprises have developed. The fact, however, remains: the information to be gained by the investigator from the autopsied human brain is usually crude compared with the detailed information that emerges from studies done with

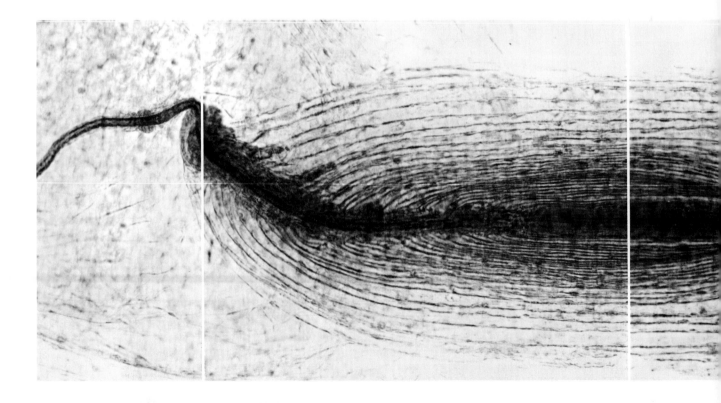

care in experimental animals. We are left to present a kind of hybrid. The anatomy is human, but the circuitry is that of a general mammal.

Somatic Sensory Endings; Reflex Connections

Our tracing of the circuitry in the mammalian central nervous system begins with an identification of sensory neurons like the ones George Parker found in the epithelial layer of the jellyfish. In the vertebrate their position is quite different. Only a single instance remains in which a vertebrate sensory neuron is also a receptor at the surface of the body: only the olfactory epithelial cells, in the lining of the roof of the nasal cavity, are exposed to the external environment. All the other sensory neurons are well below the surface; the ones for somatic sensation are in ganglia along the length of the spinal cord or in similar ganglia near the brain. (The name ganglion is reserved in vertebrates for an encapsulated cluster of neurons outside the central nervous system.) Each such neuron is pseudounipolar: it has an axon that divides into two branches. One branch enters the central nervous system. The other extends outward through the body as part of a peripheral nerve, on

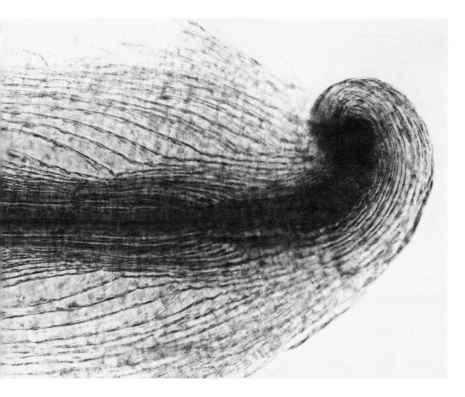

Figure 31: **Pacinian corpuscle** is the largest and most elaborate of the sensory receptors stationed in the skin. It is also the fastest to adapt, or stop responding, to a prolonged somatic sensory stimulus. Thus it is preferentially responsive to rapid vibratory compressions of the skin. Its onionlike, layered construction includes an outer zone of flattened cells and a core (*dark gray*) of specialized "lamellar cells." The example displayed in this montage is from the hind foot of a cat. It is some 700 micrometers (.7 millimeter) long. Before being photographed it was freed from surrounding tissue. An axon 10 micrometers in diameter enters from the left. About a third of the way toward the right, its myelination ends, and the lamellar core begins. The axon itself is the stimulus transducer; its elaborate encapsulation serves as a mechanical filter. The micrographs were made by Peter S. Spencer and Herbert H. Schaumburg of the Albert Einstein College of Medicine in New York.

a trajectory that will bring it to a striated muscle; to its sheath, a muscle fascia; to a joint capsule, a tendon, or a ligament; to periosteum, the sheath of connective tissue investing a bone; or to the skin. In the skin the endings of sensory axons are common. Some of them are simply the naked tips of axons;* these so-called free nerve endings appear in part to be nociceptive (they report tissue-damaging stimuli) and in part to be sensitive to temperature. Other, disk-shaped endings make contact with specialized epithelial cells (Figure 30). The endings, called Merkel's disks, respond preferentially to pressure applied to the skin. The role of the cells remains elusive. In one hypothesis, first advanced by Cajal, they are no more than a trophic influence: developing early in the embryo, they guide some of the sensory axons invading the skin.

The rest of the sensory endings in the skin are encapsulated endings: they are invested by bulbous coverings that are sometimes quite elaborate. The encapsulated endings are found in great variety. The ones called the end bulbs of Krause are thought to be cold receptors. They are stationed just under the epidermis, the surface layer of the skin. Each is a small, round aggregation of extremely flattened epithelial cells, which encase the tangled end branches of a single sensory axon. The endings called Meissner's corpuscles appear to be touch receptors. They are chiefly in hairless skin, just under the epidermis. For example, they are abundant and closely spaced in the skin at the fingertips. Each is an ovoid body about 100 micrometers long, consisting of layers of flattened cells. It receives from one to four sensory axons, which spiral through the layers, issuing varicose collaterals. The corpuscles of Vater-Pacini, also called Pacinian corpuscles (Figure 31), are doubtless vibration receptors. They are certainly the best studied among the encapsulated endings. Positioned deep in the dermis, the deep layer of the skin, they are large, ovoid bodies up to 2,000 micrometers (two millimeters) long and 1,500 micrometers across; each consists of as many as 100 onionlike laminations of flattened cells surrounding the naked tip of an axon. The whole of this elaborate encapsulation is no more than a high-pass mechanical filter: it best transmits rapid compressions and decompressions, so that each can cause the axon to generate one or two action potentials. In contrast, the capsule makes the axon relatively unresponsive to steady pressure. The axon tip itself is the element sensitive to mechanical stimuli: it alone transduces sensory stimuli into the bioelectric currency of the nervous system. The problem then arises of understanding how axon tips are rendered preferentially responsive to stimuli as different as touch, prolonged pressure, stretch, heat, and cold.

The endings of somatic sensory axons stationed deeper than the skin are equally complex and varied. Striated muscle tissue furnishes the most intricate example. Interpolated at intervals among the active muscle fibers—the

---

*In speaking simply of "axon tips" throughout these descriptions of somatic sensory endings we are neglecting the remarkable hypothesis, put forward by David Bodian of Johns Hopkins University, that the tips of the sensory axons emitted by pseudounipolar neurons are actually dendritic. We shall return to Bodian's hypothesis early in Part III.

ones that contribute to the force of a muscle's contraction — are less impressive striated muscle fibers, bound together in groups of two to 10 to form muscle spindles: fusiform organs, typically two to four millimeters long, arrayed in parallel with the active muscle fibers. They are found in all striated muscles but are especially common in the small muscles of the hand and the foot, where they can number 100 or more in a gram of muscle tissue. Each muscle spindle receives several somatic sensory axons. All but one of them terminate in small, dense, netlike endings (they are known as flower-spray endings) on the surface of spindle fibers. Their function is not well understood. The remaining axon is much thicker. It provides each spindle fiber

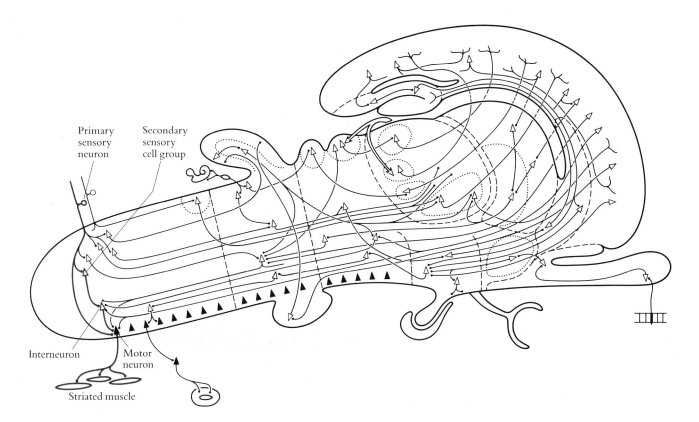

Figure 32: **Reflex connections** in the spinal cord appear in color in this diagram, the first of a total of 15 diagrams summarizing the broad-scale pattern of "wiring" established by axon bundles in the mammalian central nervous system. The anatomical divisions employed in the diagrams were established in Figure 22. At the upper left a primary sensory neuron flanking the spinal cord projects one branch of its axon through the periphery of the body, to end as a naked axon tip or in somatic sensory receptors such as Pacinian corpuscles or Merkel's disks. The second branch of the axon enters the spinal cord, where one of its collaterals arcs to a motor neuron (*solid triangle*). The synapse there is depicted by a dot at the end of the fiber. In turn the motor neuron animates striated muscle. Another collateral conveys signals to an intermediate neuron (*open triangle*) in a secondary sensory cell group. From there the path extends toward motor neurons. The path is interrupted; the neuron that actually synapses with motor neurons is called an interneuron. The paths directed more or less promptly from sensory receptors toward motor neurons might be called the local reflex channel.

with a two-branched collateral. One branch spirals upward around the fiber; the other spirals downward. They form the so-called annulospiral ending. Whenever a muscle is lengthened, by the force of gravity or by the activity of an opposing muscle group, so are its muscle spindles, and as this happens the coils of each spiral draw apart. The result is a volley of action potentials: an alarm to the nervous system that the muscle is being stretched. Remarkably, the fibers composing the muscle spindle receive a motor innervation from small motor neurons called gamma motor neurons. Thus the annulospiral ending is like a vine coiled around a trellis, and the trellis is adjustable. The adjustments are important. When a muscle contracts and shortens, its muscle spindles would develop slack unless they, too, were made to contract. The gamma motor system enables muscle spindles to ignore a muscle's contraction and maintain a position of readiness to report the next passive stretch.

Muscle spindles are not the only means by which the central nervous system monitors muscle tension, or more generally the body's arrayal in space. For one thing, joint capsules and the movement-limiting ligaments in joints include stretch receptors. At least in part, they take the form of dense end arbors of sensory axons. In addition, tendons (which anchor muscles to bones) include the stretch receptors known as Golgi tendon organs. Each consists of sprays of the tips of a single thick sensory axon that insert themselves among the slightly twining collagen strands composing a tendon. The stretching of a tendon will squeeze its tendon organs, and that will activate the organs. The organs, however, are unadjustable, so that unlike muscle spindles, they respond to increasing tension without regard to what caused it: a passive muscle stretch or an active muscle contraction.*

What becomes of the signals produced by somatic sensory endings when they enter the central nervous system? At the left of Figure 32, a representative somatic sensory neuron — we shall call it a primary sensory neuron — in a ganglion of pseudounipolar neurons flanking the spinal cord sends its axon into the cord, bearing reports of somatic sensory events such as a touch on the skin, the movement of a joint, or the contraction of a muscle. The messages it carries do not immediately reach motor neurons. Instead the primary sensory neuron makes its first synaptic contacts with intermediate neurons. There is, however, an exception. It is the monosynaptic reflex arc, also shown in Figure 32. Here a side branch from a primary somatic sensory axon bridges much of the width of the spinal cord and makes synaptic contact with a motor

---

*In the sensory end structures mentioned so far it appears to be the rule that the peripheral tip of the sensory axon, sometimes encapsulated, sometimes not, is the true receptor element. In other words, the task of transducing a mechanical or thermal stimulus into a neural signal falls on the sensory neuron itself. This is not universally the case in sensory systems. Several senses, such as hearing and taste, employ epithelial receptor cells at the ends of their sensory axons. In the case of hearing the cells transduce mechanical stimuli; in the case of taste they transduce chemical stimuli. The cells are known generically as neuroepithelial cells, and in fact they are almost neurons: although they lack dendrites and Nissl substance, they contain synaptic vesicles at the site of the synapse they make with a sensory axon.

neuron. Now that is really dismaying. Not too many pages ago, we suggested that motor neurons beyond the earliest episodes of neural evolution no longer were bothered with raw data; we suggested they were always offered informational digests by neurons of the great intermediate net. A monosynaptic reflex might therefore seem to be a primitive neural circuit. Yet it could also be fairly new. After all, air and land are the cruelest of environments; for a mountain goat, one misstep could be fatal. In contrast, a fish can make any number of similar faux pas and not be harmed at all. Plainly terrestrial life requires a high-security reflex system for maintaining balance. Specifically, a way is needed in which a muscle can signal to the appropriate motor neurons (and only the appropriate motor neurons) that it is being unduly stretched by the force of gravity. That appears to be the function of the monosynaptic arc. The arc begins with somatic sensory endings in striated muscles and in their tendons that are specialized for proprioception: the sense of the body's arrayal. Muscle spindles are an example; so are Golgi tendon organs. Their

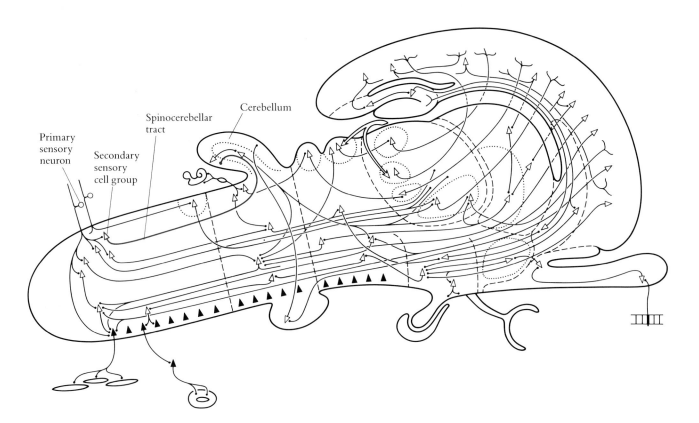

Figure 33: **Spinocerebellar channel** consists of axons projecting from secondary sensory cell groups into the cerebellum, which protrudes dorsally from the hindbrain. The figure shows one such axon (*color*); actually there are millions, which course toward the cerebellum in two more or less circumscribed axon bundles, or spinocerebellar tracts, on each side of the spinal cord.

reports of passive stretching can go directly to the motor neurons that animate the muscle. Suppose you happen to sway forward as you stand. Your hamstring muscles are passively stretched, and the muscle spindles in them send alarms to the spinal cord, eliciting the prompt contraction of those very muscles. If things were otherwise, you would not be able to stand. Suppose the correction overshoots, so that your body now begins to sway in the opposite direction. Similar alarms to a discrete set of motor neurons will arise from the quadriceps musculature.

Monosynaptic reflex arcs have not been found outside the domain of proprioception. Thus the short circuits between sensory input and motor output appear to be a small minority. The vast majority of mammalian primary sensory axons (including great numbers of proprioceptive axons) enter

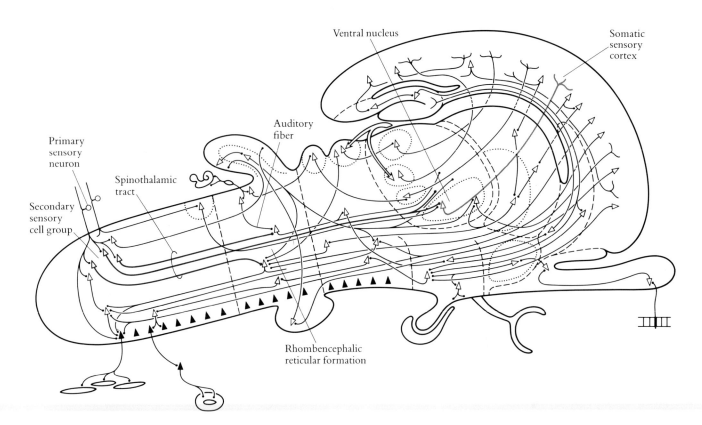

Figure 34: **Spinothalamic tract** consists of axons (*dark color*) ascending toward the forebrain from secondary sensory cell groups throughout the length of the spinal cord. The ones attaining the forebrain end in the ventral nucleus of the thalamus, which in turn projects, or sends axons (*light color*), to the primary somatic sensory cortex, a part of the neocortex. The others end in the core of the brainstem, which is called the reticular formation. Two such axons are shown. One of them synapses with a neuron that also accepts auditory input. The subsequent path toward the forebrain is therefore termed multimodal, nonspecific, or open. Tracts directed from secondary sensory cell groups toward the forebrain are known as lemnisci; the spinothalamic tract is sometimes called the paleolemniscus.

the great intermediate net and synapse with members of what we shall call a secondary sensory cell group—neurons first in line to receive primary sensory data. From there, many pathways are directed more or less promptly toward motor neurons. They might collectively be called a local reflex channel, if it is kept in mind that "local" can be misleading: many reflexes involve the entire length of the spinal cord but nonetheless are considered local because they remain inside it. The first link in the local reflex channel is a cell of a secondary sensory cell group. But often it, too, does not contact a motor neuron: it may synapse instead on still other cells of the great intermediate net, and only these latter neurons may contact a motor neuron. Neurons that synapse on motor neurons we shall refer to as interneurons. The term is somewhat arbitrary: it is difficult to say whether a neuron one happens to see

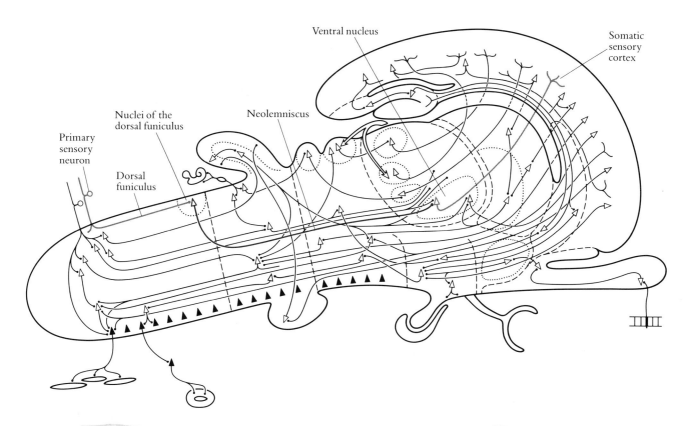

Figure 35: **Neolemniscus,** like the spinothalamic tract, ascends from the spinal cord toward the forebrain. It, too, directs its fibers (*dark color*) to the ventral nucleus of the thalamus. The fibers, however, are closed: almost all of them pass uninterrupted through the reticular formation. Then, too, the fibers arise in a specialized pair of secondary sensory cell groups: the nuclei of the dorsal funiculus, also called the dorsal-column nuclei, stationed at the transition from the spinal cord to the hindbrain. The primary sensory fibers climbing through the spinal cord to the nuclei of the dorsal funiculus form a circumscribed bundle: the dorsal funiculus, or dorsal column (*light color*). In more recent neuroanatomical terminology the neolemniscus is called the medial lemniscus.

is indeed the last link in a chain leading to a motor neuron. The term is more a physiological notion. At each synaptic interruption in a given conduction path there is a delay in transmission of half a millisecond or more. Such delays can be detected, and it can then be suspected that between an axon undergoing electrical stimulation and a motor neuron that is responding, an interneuron must be interposed. Alternatively, the latency might be so short that a direct connection is suspected.

Cerebellar Channel; Lemniscal Channel

What other channels originate in a secondary sensory cell group? Channel number two is the cerebellar channel: from secondary sensory cell groups in the brainstem and the spinal cord, one commonly finds axons ascending direct to the cerebellum. The axon that does so in Figure 33 originates in a secondary sensory cell group of the spinal cord and is therefore called a spinocerebellar fiber. ("Axon" and "fiber" are synonymous in neuroanatomical usage.) Many such fibers together compose a spinocerebellar tract, or bundle.*

Channel number three is the lemniscal channel. The word lemniscus is Latin for ribbon, and it refers here to fiber bundles that originate in secondary sensory cell groups and ascend toward the forebrain — in particular, toward the thalamus. In Figure 34 one such bundle is shown, ascending at the center of the spinal cord. In truth, it ascends near the spinal cord's lateral surface. (We should emphasize that a diagram such as Figure 34 cannot be topographically accurate.) The bundle is called the spinothalamic tract, yet only one of its three representative fibers is depicted as arriving at the thalamus. The others accompany it for some distance, but then they crash-land, so to speak: both are shown terminating on neurons in the core of the rhombencephalon, although one or the other might just as well have terminated somewhat farther rostrally, in the mesencephalon. The point is that of the so-called spinothalamic fibers, only a small proportion reach the thalamus. Even so, the tract is named for the minority, which terminate in the ventral nucleus. There the fibers synapse with thalamic neurons whose axons travel without interruption to a specific field of neocortex, a field known as the primary somatic sensory cortex.

Note that in this case the path from a primary sensory neuron to the

---

*Regarding synonyms for axon and dendrite: The word fiber refers to an axon or to a branch of an axon, whether or not it has a myelin sheath. Thus the terms fiber bundle and fiber system (as well as fasciculus and tract) denote axons that course through the brain or the spinal cord in a more or less well defined group. Dendrites are also fiberlike structures. Moreover, in certain places dendrites bundle together. Still, dendrites are not called fibers. For certain neurons it is proving difficult to distinguish dendrites from axons. In such cases the noncommittal term neurite is offered for all of the filamentous extensions arising from the cell body.

neocortex involves only two synaptic interruptions, or more precisely two transfers of information from axons to constellations of intrinsic neurons and projection neurons. The first such interruption is in the spinal cord, between a primary sensory fiber and neurons in a secondary sensory cell group. The second interruption is in the diencephalon, between a lemniscal fiber and neurons in the ventral nucleus of the thalamus. In sensory paths to the neocortex two synaptic interruptions appear to be the minimum; hence a two-synapse sensory line might well be called a throughline. It might also be called a closed or labeled line, because in general the sensory pathways of minimal interruption rigorously maintain the topology of the sensory periphery from which they come. A fingertip, for example, can detect two distinct stimuli when it is touched by the points of a pair of drafting dividers no more than two or three millimeters apart. This ability is called two-point discrimination. Its existence means that each point must stimulate a path of

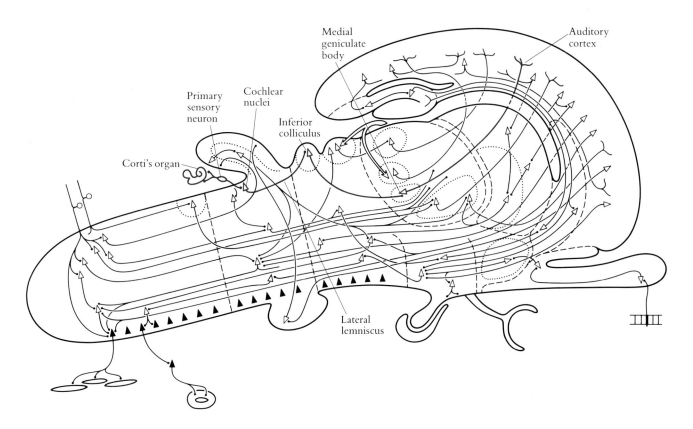

Figure 36: **Auditory pathway** (*color*) ascends from the ear to the neocortex. The path begins in Corti's organ, a sensory epithelium found in the inner ear. Then come the cochlear nuclei, a pair of specialized secondary sensory cell groups in the hindbrain. The cochlear nuclei emit the lateral lemniscus, which rises no farther than the midbrain: in particular, the inferior colliculus. From there the path attains the thalamus: in particular, the medial geniculate body. A final link projects to the primary auditory cortex.

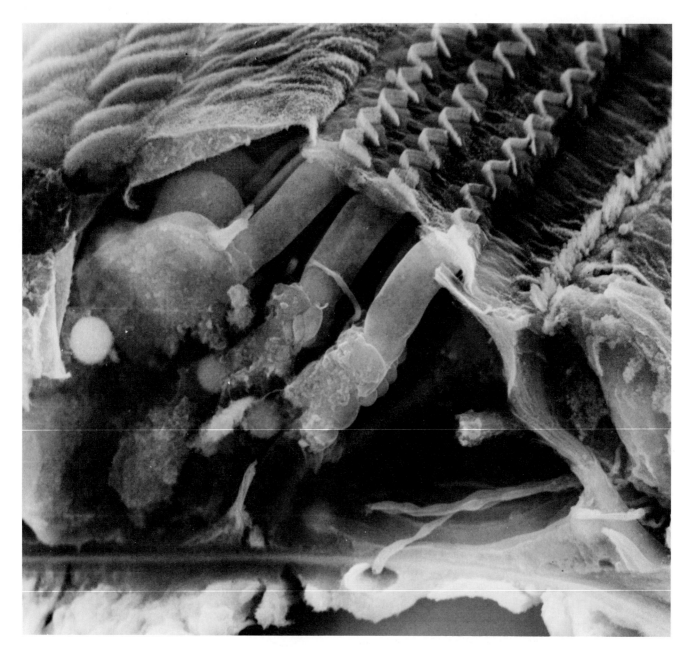

Figure 37: **Corti's organ,** the epithelial complex serving the sense of hearing, is shown in a cross section of tissue from the inner ear of a guinea pig. Three smooth tubular bodies occupy the center of the section. They are the hair cells of Corti's organ, or rather the outer hair cells of the organ. Each emits as many as a hundred stereocilia, or hairlike extensions, which contribute to three fringed rows on the surface of the organ, seen at the upper right. (The tectorial membrane, a gelatinous mass swathing the rows of stereocilia, has been removed from the tissue.) At the extreme right a more nearly linear fringe of stereocilia emerges from a single row of inner hair cells.

The hair cells are sensory transducers: each includes synaptic vesicles, which cluster at the base of the cell near the end of a sensory axon. Thus the hair cell converts auditory stimuli (a shearing force on the hairs) into neural signals, which it transfers to the nervous system. Here one sensory axon is plain: it is the filament curving over the surface of the outer hair cell at the front of the middle row. Other axons course horizontally at the lower right through a triangular space called the tunnel of Corti. The scanning electron micrograph was made at an enlargement of 2,150 diameters by Robert S. Kimura of the Massachusetts Eye and Ear Infirmary in Boston.

conduction that is sufficiently independent to permit what might be termed sensory resolution. Some cell in the somatic sensory cortex, if interrogated with a microelectrode, might reveal that its only interest is one square milli- meter of skin on the index finger. One of its close neighbors might be monitor of an adjoining square millimeter, and so on. In that way, the topology of the body surface can be faithfully maintained.

A conduction path diametrically opposed to a "labeled" path would be one in which the line becomes involved in the conduction of topologically mud- dled messages from a given sense, or even messages from several different senses. In fact this arrangement exists: one of the spinothalamic dropouts in Figure 34 ends in synaptic contact with a rhombencephalic neuron whose axon extends the line into the thalamus. Perhaps the arrangement constitutes a three-synapse line to the neocortex. At the extra interruption, however, the line accepts messages not only from the spinothalamic fiber but also (in this instance) from the auditory system. How can the thalamus know what has happened when an impulse arrives? The rhombencephalic neuron is called multimodal or nonspecific, and the conduction path might be called open- line: wherever there is a synaptic interruption the line is open to inputs from other neurons. The great majority of neurons in the core of the hindbrain and the midbrain are of this curious nonspecific nature. They sit with their dendrites — their cellular hands — spread across several millimeters, hoping, it seems, to catch any kind of message. They are typical of what is called the reticular formation, a place where few cell groups get homogeneous inputs. One might examine this situation and predict that nothing could come of it but noise. The situation nonetheless prevails in the brain of all vertebrates. One must therefore suspect that its existence corresponds to a particular need.

One contemplates more happily a second somatic sensory lemniscus rising from the spinal cord (Figure 35). It is sometimes called the neolemniscus because it was long thought to be the prerogative of animals that have a well-developed cerebral cortex. And indeed it is far more prominent in mam- mals than in nonmammalian species. The neolemniscus is more tightly orga- nized than the spinothalamic tract: almost all its fibers are labeled lines that ascend directly to the ventral nucleus of the thalamus from a pair of secondary sensory cell groups at the transition between the spinal cord and the medulla oblongata that are called the nuclei of the dorsal funiculus. One is not amazed to learn that two-point discrimination is prominently represented in the neolemniscus, far more so than in the spinothalamic tract, which in the parlance that dictates "neolemniscus" is called the paleolemniscus. As it happens, the neolemniscus was the first lemniscus to be discovered, and it is the eponym of all lemnisci: its discoverer, the German neurologist Johann Reil, described it as a ribbon. In more recent terminology, it is called the medial lemniscus because its position in the brainstem (the hindbrain and the midbrain) is medial to that of another lemniscus, the lateral lemniscus, which serves the sense of hearing.

We can summarize as follows. The medial lemniscus and the spinotha- lamic tract are fundamentally different systems of somatic sensory conduction to the forebrain. The neo- or medial lemniscus is essentially a set of labeled lines that preserves a map of the sensory receptor surface. The paleolemniscus or spinothalamic tract is in large part an open, polysynaptic system, some of whose lines nonetheless arrive at the thalamus. The idea persists that the labeled lines are more recent in phylogeny, but there is reason to be skeptical. Suppose a frog's attention is drawn to a small, dark speck that moves in front of its eyes. When such a speck is registered, a sequence of synapses in the retina dispatches a signal to neurons in the optic lobe. The further details of the circuitry have not yet been elucidated. It is certain, however, that the circuits engage motor neurons. After all, the frog propels itself (and flicks its tongue) in a motor program that is tailored to capture the morsel. It seems plain, moreover, that any one sensory conduction line in the visual system of the frog must monitor only a small part of the animal's visual field; otherwise fly catching could not succeed. Labeled lines of a similar sort must be needed by all free-ranging animals to find their way in a complex world. Surely, then, it is mistaken to think that polysynaptic pathways of the open-line variety are older. It appears instead that the two categories are contemporaries. Still, as terrestrial animals evolved, the closed-line systems that had always been there tended to augment markedly, whereas the open-line systems did so much less conspicuously. In the human brain the neolemniscus is large: it comprises perhaps a million fibers, which makes it the equal of an optic nerve. The spinothalamic tract is more difficult to assay; it is far less circumscribed on a cross section of the brainstem or spinal cord. It includes a multitude of fibers. The ones attaining the thalamus may number only in the thousands—perhaps only in the hundreds. The rest of the multitude have other destinations.*

Hearing; Vision; Olfaction

What about senses other than the somatic sense? The allegorical little structure that appears for diagrammatic convenience near the cerebellum in Figure 36 is the membranous labyrinth, a part of the inner ear. The anterior end of the labyrinth is the duct of the cochlea, a fluid-filled spiral canal that makes almost three complete turns in a bony casing, for a total length of almost three

---

*A list of destinations for spinothalamic fibers that do not attain the thalamus will gain meaning mostly in Part III of this book. Yet the list is worth giving. Many spinothalamic fibers actually end, as we have just seen, in the brainstem reticular formation. They are therefore spinoreticular. Others end in the inferior olivary nucleus, a part of the hindbrain. They are spino-olivary. Still others end in the nucleus of the solitary tract, a further part of the hindbrain. They are spinosolitary. A substantial number ascend to the midbrain—in particular, to the superior colliculus as the spinotectal tract and to the central gray substance of the mesencephalon as the spinoannular tract. In the spinal cord these various fiber systems all occupy the district of spinal white matter where true spinothalamic fibers were the first to be identified.

centimeters. Along the inside of the duct runs an epithelial complex, the spiral organ of Corti (Figure 37). It includes four or five rows of sensory cells—about 15,000 cells in all. Each cell sends some 50 or 100 stereocilia (hairlike extensions) into the lumen of the duct, not into fluid-filled space but into a delicate, almost jellylike membrane hinged to the wall of the duct. The cells lack dendrites and an axon, and so they are not neurons. On the other hand, they include vesicles identical to the ones found at the presynaptic terminals of a neuron. The vesicles tend to be crowded near the part of the membrane of the cell that confronts the tip of an axon. Plainly the "hair cells" of Corti's organ transduce sensory stimuli into neural signals. In particular, they transduce auditory vibrations, which produce a complex pattern of

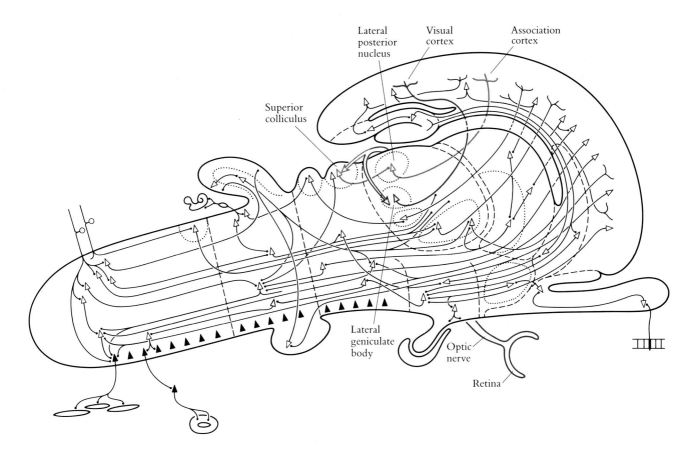

Figure 38: **Visual pathways** begin in the retina, which is part of the brain. (It arises as an evagination, or outpouching, of the embryonic forebrain.) From it a prominent visual path (*dark color*) leads to the primary visual cortex. The path employs a thalamic way station, the lateral geniculate body. A second path (*light color*), less prominent than the other in primates, including man, attains first the superior colliculus, a part of the midbrain; next the lateral posterior nucleus of the thalamus; and then a field of neocortex distinct from the primary visual cortex. Such fields, which lack "raw" sensory input (that is, input of straightforward sensory content), are termed association areas. For its part, the lateral posterior nucleus, which likewise lacks straightforward sensory input, cannot be termed a sensory "relay."

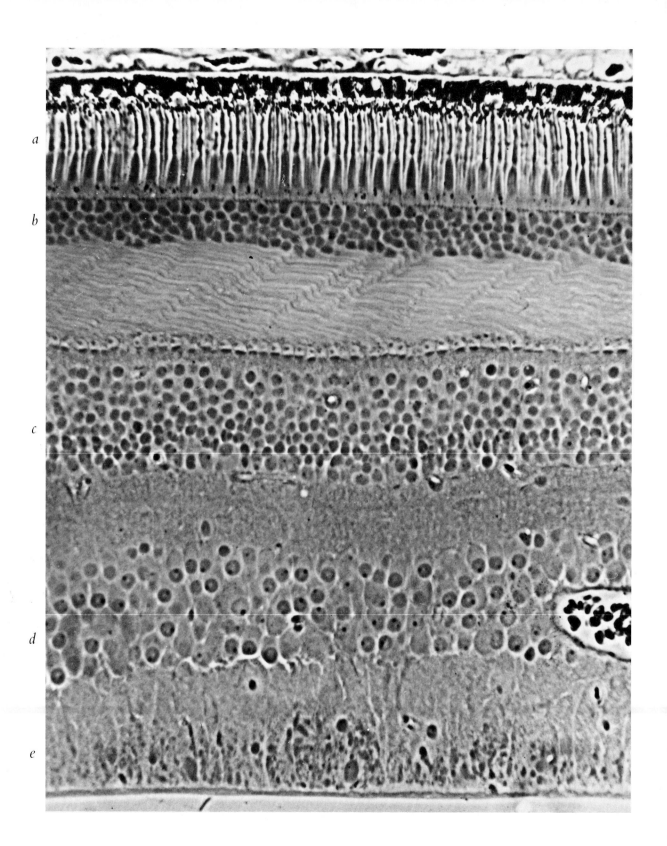

a

b

c

d

e

shearing forces on the hairs along the length of Corti's organ. Then the nervous system takes over. The axons arriving in Corti's organ number roughly 30,000. They are emitted by primary sensory neurons arrayed in the inner ear in the so-called spiral ganglion. Each such neuron is bipolar, not pseudounipolar: it emits an axon at each end of its fusiform cell body. One axon goes to the hair cells; it gets primary sensory data. The other enters the brain. There it passes the data to secondary sensory neurons of the cochlear nuclei, a pair of cell groups in the rhombencephalon specialized for the processing of auditory traffic. Figure 36 shows two such neurons; actually there are hundreds of thousands. From the cochlear nuclei a tract called the lateral lemniscus ascends toward the thalamus. It is remarkably unsuccessful, because few if any of its fibers get past the inferior colliculus. In this unbypassable way station in the mesencephalon (it is the only auditory way station shown in the figure, although several others, apparently more optional, are associated with the lateral lemniscus itself), axons originate that do attain the thalamus, where they terminate in the medial geniculate body. The neurons of the medial geniculate body project in turn (that is, they send their axons) to a specific part of the neocortex called the primary auditory cortex.

The visual system is quite different (Figure 38). For one thing, the receptor cells for vision, the rod cells and the cone cells, are inside the brain. They form a layer in the retina and are therefore part of the forebrain. Like the hair cells in Corti's organ, they lack dendrites and an axon; they are not quite neurons themselves. But they do have synaptic vesicles; they are sensory transducers. The rod or the cone of each receptor cell is filled to capacity by a stack of flattened membranous sacs. Doubtless the stack is the site at which the cell reacts to the arrival of photons (quanta of light) by producing neural signals. For its part, the retina includes not only the layer of rod cells and cone cells but also a complex neural circuitry (Figure 39). Specifically, it includes the retinal

Figure 39: **The retina** interposes several synapses in each conduction line for visual data. Fundamentally, it includes three layers of cell bodies and intervening layers in which cellular processes make synaptic contacts. First in the signal processing, but at the back of the eyeball, farthest from arriving light, are the visual receptors: the rods and cones of the retina (*a*). Their cell bodies occupy the outer nuclear layer (*b*). Then come neurons: the bipolar cells, the horizontal cells, and the amacrine cells of the retina. Their cell bodies occupy the inner nuclear layer (*c*). Last are the retinal ganglion cells, whose cell bodies have their own layer (*d*). Each emits an axon that joins with other such axons (*e*) just under the inner face of the retina to compose the optic nerve. The bipolar cells establish conduction lines from the rods and cones to the ganglion cells; the horizontal cells and the amacrine cells establish crosslinks among these conduction lines. The section, stained with osmium tetroxide, is from the human eye, some 1.25 millimeters from the center of the fovea (the place of greatest visual acuity); the preparation was made by B. B. Boycott and John E. Dowling of Harvard University. The distance across the neural circuitry, from the outer nuclear layer (*b*) to the zone of optic-nerve axons (*e*), is 400 micrometers. The layer of ganglion cells includes, at the right, a blood vessel cut in cross section. The vessel is filled with erythrocytes (red blood cells).

bipolar cells, a class of neurons to which the rod cells and cone cells transfer their output. Farther down the line, it includes the retinal ganglion cells, a class of neurons with which the bipolar cells communicate. The ganglion cells were named by early investigators in token of their resemblance to the nerve cells in true ganglia, outside the central nervous system. It is tempting to assign the bipolar cells the position of primary sensory neurons; the ganglion cells would then assume the position of a secondary sensory cell group. The retina, however, includes additional classes of neurons, the horizontal cells and the amacrine cells, which establish elaborate crosslinks among the basic conduction lines.

One thing is certain: the convergence of retinal conduction lines is prodigious. In the human eye the retina includes as many as 125 million rods, at a packing density as great as 160,000 per square millimeter of retinal surface, and 6.8 million cones, at a packing density as great as 150,000 per square millimeter. The data produced by this multitude cascade toward the ganglion cells, which number 1.2 million. The ganglion cells are projection neurons; they export data from the retina. Their axons assemble at the surface of the retina to form the optic nerve. Then, at the base of the brain, comes a rechanneling of axons in which the ones from the medial half of one eye's retina cross the midplane of the body to join the ones from the lateral half of the other eye's retina. It is a hemidecussation.* The result is the optic tract. (No hint of this partial crossing appears in Figure 38). Each optic tract distributes its axons to two great terminal areas. One is the superior colliculus. In all primates, however, the more important one, in terms of the number of axons, is the lateral geniculate body of the thalamus. The neurons of the lateral geniculate body project in turn to the neocortex. Specifically they project to an area at the posterior pole of the cerebral hemisphere, far removed from the auditory cortex, that is known as the primary visual cortex. It must be added that the superior colliculus projects to the thalamus, not to the lateral geniculate body but to the lateral posterior nucleus. The neurons of the lateral posterior nucleus project in turn to the neocortex. They project, however, not to the area in which axons from the lateral geniculate body terminate but to a nearby cortical expanse that is distinct from the visual cortex. The visual system apparently has two channels ascending from the retina to the cerebral cortex.

Olfaction (Figure 40) breaks whatever laws there seem to be that govern the organization of other sensory mechanisms. It differs from hearing and

---

*The term decussation derives from *deca,* the Roman numeral X. It refers to a crossing of fibers through the midplane to the opposite side of the brain or the spinal cord on their way to some remote contralateral (that is, opposite-sided) target. The fibers of the spinothalamic tract decussate in the spinal cord on their way to the brainstem, for instance. A second type of crossing, referred to as a commissure, is an exchange of fibers between two structures symmetrically positioned on the left and right side of the brain or the spinal cord. The largest commissure in the human brain is the corpus callosum, the great fiber plate interconnecting homotopic fields of neocortex on the two cerebral hemispheres.

vision in that it does not assign to nonneuronal cells the task of converting sensory stimuli into neural signals. The cells performing that task, the olfactory chemoreceptors, are primary sensory neurons (Figure 41). Stranger still, the olfactory chemoreceptors, which occupy a specialized epithelium amounting (in the human body) to five square centimeters of the surface area of the epithelial lining at the roof of the nasal cavity, are the only known instance, at least in the mammal, of primary sensory neurons at the surface of the body. They are therefore the only known instance of neurons in the mammal that sample the world directly. In the rabbit they number 100 million. The conduction lines for taste, which is also a chemical sense, obey a more typical pattern. (For taste the primary sensory neurons, found in ganglia near the brain, innervate nonneuronal receptor cells deployed in the epithelium lining the oral cavity.) Each olfactory chemoreceptor is perpendicular to the surface of the body. From the end nearer the surface comes a single

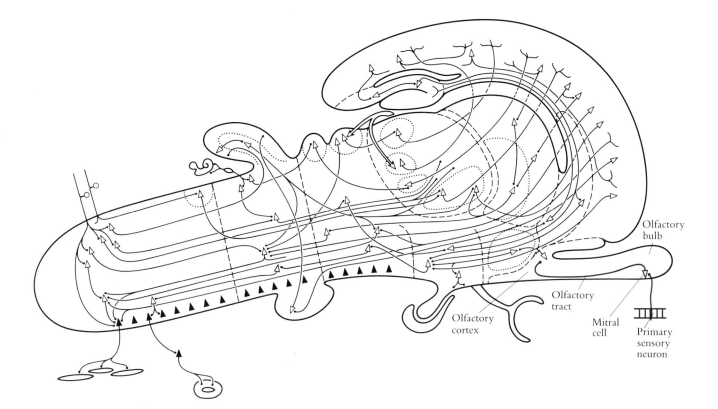

Figure 40: **Olfactory pathway** (*color*) breaks the rules that seem to govern other sensory paths. In olfaction the receptor cells and the primary sensory neurons (the first neurons to handle the sensory data) are one and the same: they are neurons exposed at the surface of the body in the olfactory epithelium, a specialized part of the mucosa of the nasal cavity. The axons the neurons emit project to cerebral cortex — specifically the olfactory bulb — without the mediation of a thalamic sensory relay nucleus. In turn, the neurons of the olfactory bulb produce an axon bundle, the olfactory tract, which projects to the primary olfactory cortex.

dendrite. It extends to the surface and even slightly above it, in a terminal swelling two to three micrometers in diameter. The swelling emits a number of cilia. From the deeper end of the cell comes a thin, unmyelinated axon. It is in fact among the thinnest in the nervous system: it is only .2 micrometer in diameter. Its destination is the olfactory bulb. This breaks the law that sensory conduction paths attain the cerebral cortex only after synaptic interruption in the thalamus. Moreover, it makes the olfactory bulb, a specialized part of the cerebral cortex, a recipient of primary sensory data. One is compelled to consider the olfactory bulb as a secondary sensory cell group. Among the neurons in the olfactory bulb that receive the primary data are the mitral cells. They bear that name because the shape of their cell body is reminiscent of a bishop's miter. They are a mere 50,000 in number on each side of the brain. The mitral cells give rise to axons that travel along the surface of the olfactory peduncle, where they compose the olfactory tract. At the base of the cerebral hemisphere, the axons synapse with cells of the primary olfactory cortex, also called the piriform (the pear-shaped) cortex in recognition of the shape it takes in animals such as the cat.

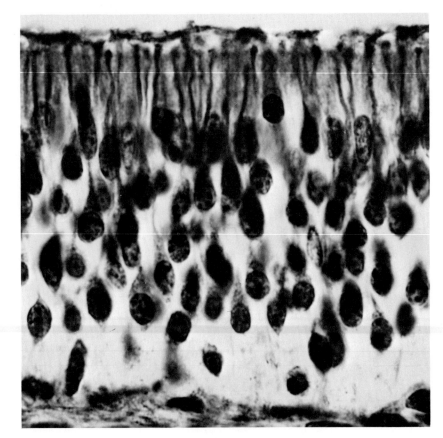

Figure 41: **Olfactory receptors** are shown in the olfactory epithelium of a mouse, in which they were stained by means of a method that impregnates neurons with silver. The olfactory receptors are the roundish cells throughout the lower two-thirds of the tissue. Each is less than 10 micrometers in diameter. (Cylindrical cells toward the top of the tissue are columnar supporting cells.) Each receptor cell is bipolar. From its lower end comes a very thin axon, not visible in this preparation. From its upper end comes a dendrite that climbs into a layer of mucus coating the tissue. There, at the surface of the body, the dendrite ends in a swelling. Scattered cells immediately above the base of the epithelium are basal cells, now recognized as precursor cells that differentiate into new olfactory receptors. The olfactory receptors are replaceable when they die at the body surface. The micrograph was made by P. P. C. Graziadei and G. A. Monti Graziadei of the Florida State University at Tallahassee.

Chapter Six

Neocortical Function

We have now traced the ascending fibers of four senses: hearing, vision, and olfaction in the paragraphs just above, and the somatic sense before that; and in each case the cerebral cortex has emerged as an end station of the ascent. The problem with further tracing is the complexity of the cerebral cortex: in the human brain, as we have noted, it is thought to contain no fewer than 70 percent of all the neurons in the central nervous system. What are they doing with their input? Two observations might be offered. First, the thalamocortical projections are reciprocated: the visual cortex projects back to the lateral geniculate body, from which it received its input; the auditory cortex projects back to the medial geniculate body; and the somatic sensory cortex projects back to the ventral nucleus. The reciprocating fibers synapse outside the thalamic glomeruli with the dendrites of both intrinsic neurons and projection neurons. The reciprocity undoubtedly signifies that the functional state of the cerebral cortex can influence how the sensory way stations of the thalamus screen the cortically directed flow of information. Second, the visual, the auditory, and the somatic sensory area embody only a first cortical step in sensory processing. Out from these primary sensory fields come fibers to adjoining areas that cannot unreservedly be termed sensory; they are a block away, so to speak, from the sensory input. And out from those areas come fibers that terminate in areas still farther away from the primary sensory fields. The areas of the neocortex at various synaptic removes from the primary sensory fields are called association areas, and in the human brain they compose by far the largest fraction of the cortical expanse: the visual cortex, the auditory cortex, and the somatic sensory cortex together account for no more than a quarter of the total. In association cortex more advanced stages of processing presumably are embodied. There are cortical regions, for example, that are converged on by inputs with antecedents in all of the primary sensory fields.

Visual Syndromes

In approaching the march of projections across the neocortical sheet, one's first thought is to study the clinical evidence. One finds it tantalizing, but frustrating, too. The clinician indeed encounters a range of behavioral abnormalities linked to the destruction of neocortical tissue, yet the site of the lesion that causes any one of them is often quite uncertain. A number of abnormalities may occur in combination. A "higher-order" abnormality may be counterfeited by a lesion affecting sensation, or motor ability, or a patient's motivation to deal candidly with physicians, or a patient's intelligence quite generally, as in dementia, which causes ideational paucity and emotional obtuseness. The lesion itself may be hard to specify. An autopsy may show simply the widespread brain damage attendant on atherosclerosis, or syphilis, or the rupture of a blood vessel, or a brain injury, or a combination of traumas. Often there is no autopsy; the patient is quite alive. One suspects that lesions in association cortex, where a wealth of inputs converge, might have more subtle consequences than lesions in a primary sensory field. Yet even the simplest of the neocortical dysfunctions have their complexities.

Take hemianopia. The essence of the condition is that a lesion destroying part of the primary visual cortex on one side of the brain (Figure 42) entails a loss of sight affecting the contralateral half of the patient's visual field. The locus of the loss in the patient's visual field is known as a scotoma. There is, however, a curious complication. It is typical of a patient with a slowly expanding lesion in the primary visual cortex that he first consults a physician when he finds himself repeatedly colliding with obstacles to the opposite side of his body. His complaint is that something must be wrong with the eye on that side. Yet his vision seems normal, he says. Evidently the patient with a lesion developing in the primary visual cortex perceives no patch of blackness. The missing part of the visual field simply loses its existence, just as a normal visual field simply does not include the part of the world that lies behind one's head. Indeed, the patient is so unaware of his scotoma that it fails to interfere with the continuity of a road, or a chessboard, or a regular pattern of wallpaper. A less predictable visual stimulus—a car on the road, or a chesspiece on the board, or the head of someone standing in front of the wall—disappears. One concludes that the neocortex is capable of making certain "reasonable" extrapolations to fill up perceptual gaps. Still, the primary visual cortex seems well characterized as the neocortical staging ground for sight.

Next consider agnosia, in essence the inability to recognize. The term derives from the Greek *gnosis,* or knowing. It is said that an agnosia can strip

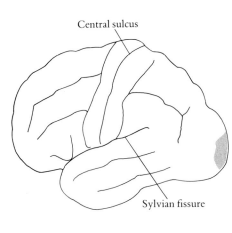

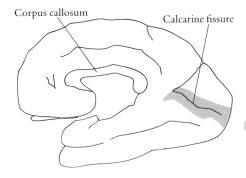

Figure 42: **Hemianopia,** the loss of sight from half of the visual field, results from a lesion destroying the primary visual cortex on the opposite, or contralateral, side of the brain. The condition is straightforward, as cortical syndromes go. Still, it has its curiosities. For one thing, a scotoma, or lost part of the visual field, is not perceived as a locus of blackness. It just ceases to exist—like the visual world behind your head. The figure shows the human cerebral hemisphere in a lateral view (*top*) and a medial view (*bottom*). The pattern of gyrification has been reduced to its fundamentals; the details are highly variable from one brain to another. The primary visual cortex, at the occipital (rearward) pole of the hemisphere, appears in color. Much of its full extent is hidden in the walls of the calcarine fissure.

the meaning from a single sense, say, vision, leaving the other senses intact, and encounters with certain patients suggest this is the case. You display an object, for instance, and ask the patient to touch it. This he can do. You ask the patient to describe it. This, too, he can do, at least to the extent of speaking about its shape or even its parts. Yet when you ask the patient to tell you what it is you are showing him, he proves unable to name it. Nor can he suggest a use for the object, or remember having seen such a thing before. If he handles the object, however, or hears its characteristic sound or smells its characteristic odor (if the object has such an attribute), the recognition is unlocked: he now knows quite well both its name and its employment. Agnosia results from a lesion beyond the primary sensory fields. A special form of agnosia is prosopagnosia. Here the lack of vision-based recognition applies specifically to the human faces that ought to be familiar to the patient. The patient's close relative enters the room; the patient fails to identify him. Then the visitor speaks, and the patient brightens up and begins an animated, knowing conversation. Pure prosopagnosia is rare. Nevertheless, the lesion that causes prosopagnosia is said to involve association cortex on the underside of the cerebral hemisphere near the primary visual cortex.

Linguistic Syndromes

Visual agnosia is unusual among the various cortical syndromes in that a hauntingly similar condition can be induced in experimental animals. The condition is known as psychic blindness; Heinrich Klüver of the University of Chicago induced it in rhesus monkeys. From each side of the brain of the monkeys he excised the temporal lobe. The excision included the association cortex on the underside of the cerebral hemisphere near the primary visual cortex. The monkeys showed no sensory deficit; in fact, they spent much of their time examining objects. Apparently, however, they did not know what they were seeing. A live snake (an object of terror for normal monkeys) aroused the same enthusiastic — one might say fearless — curiosity as a rubber ball. Indeed, the brain-damaged monkeys developed a predilection for putting things in their mouth, and the snake was no exception.

The cortical syndromes we shall now discuss have utterly no counterpart in any experimental animal. They affect behavior that is distinctively human. Consider two lesions (Figure 43). One of them destroys an area named for Pierre Paul Broca, the French surgeon, neurologist, and anthropologist who in 1861 published an article entitled "Perte de la Parole" ("The Loss of Speech") and thus became the first investigator in modern science to propose that damage to the human brain might be associated specifically with a disorder of language: an aphasia. He proposed, moreover, that such a lesion might be peculiar to the left cerebral hemisphere. (It is now known that language has its seat in the left cerebral hemisphere for almost every right-handed person and for all but perhaps a third of all left-handed people. In short, a right-sided localization for language is a neurological curiosity.)

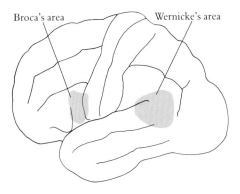

Figure 43: **Aphasias,** or disorders of linguistic competence, result from two distinct lesions. The disorder called Broca's aphasia results from a lesion of Broca's area: association cortex on the convexity of the cerebral hemisphere, almost always on the left side of the brain. The patient comprehends language, but can speak only haltingly, and in incomplete sentences. The disorder called Wernicke's aphasia results from a lesion of Wernicke's area: association cortex toward the rear of the convexity of the cerebral hemisphere, again on the left side of the brain. The patient cannot comprehend language, and so speaks fluently but nonsensically.

Broca's area is on the convexity of the cerebral hemisphere. It is an association field. In the wake of a lesion destroying the field, a person's speech is rendered slow, infrequent, effortful, and poorly articulated, in spite of the lack of paralysis, or even paresis (that is, weakness), in the musculature serving speech. Moreover, certain words are missing. They tend to be the syntactic scaffolding of a sentence: the articles, the prepositions, and to some extent the adjectives. The result is speech that might be termed telegraphic: the same words are missing that one would omit in sending a telegram. The telegraphy is apparent even when the patient attempts to repeat on request a phrase or a sentence that the diagnostician utters first. Remarkably, the patient's comprehension of written or spoken language appears to be normal. Then, too, the patient proves capable of humming a tune, and emotional stress may render him suddenly able to fluently curse.

The second lesion destroys an area named for Carl Wernicke, whose monograph, entitled *Der Aphasische Symptomencomplex* and subtitled (here we translate) "A Psychological Study on an Anatomical Basis," was published in 1874. In its pages, Wernicke, who was 26, proposed that lesions toward the back of the convexity of the cerebral hemisphere might have consequences for linguistic ability quite different from those of a more rostral lesion. In fact the signs of a lesion in Wernicke's area — association cortex near the primary auditory cortex — are in essence the reverse of the signs of a lesion in Broca's area. The patient's speech is fluent and rhythmic, if it is taken as simply a string of phonemes. The problem is that it lacks meaning. For one thing, single phonemes are replaced by others: the patient may say "snick" when one expects to hear "stick." The example was cited by Norman Geschwind of Harvard University. In addition, words in the patient's sentences tend to be replaced, typically with words of little specificity. Again an example was cited by Geschwind: "I was over in the other one," the patient observes in flowing, grammatical speech "and then after they had been in the department I was in this one." The patient's writing is much the same: letters and words are well formed, and the sentences are grammatical, but they are lacking in meaning. Perhaps the single most telling symptom of a lesion in Wernicke's area is that the patient proves incapable of comprehending language, either written or spoken.

It is plain to see why language has been posited to have two distinct embodiments on the left side of the brain: Broca's area, said to be motoric, and invoked for uttering language, and Wernicke's area, said to be sensory, and invoked for understanding it. The symptoms seem clear — one set for speaking and another for listening — and they seem to be entailed by cortical lesions in different places. (The symptom of fluent speech lacking in meaning that characterizes Wernicke's aphasia can be taken to reflect the function of Broca's area without guidance from Wernicke's area.) It is beginning to appear, however, that Broca's aphasics show a subtle impairment of linguistic comprehension — a "sensory" impairment that seems to invert the "motor" symptom of telegraphic speech. When Broca's aphasics hear that "the dog the man patted is brown," their understanding is likely to be good. The man does the patting; the dog is the recipient; the dog is brown. But tell them that "the man who was chased by the dog is tall," and matters are quite different. Did the man chase the dog, or was it the other way around? Which of the two was tall? Broca's aphasics cannot tell; a study by Edgar Zurif and his colleagues at Boston Veterans' Administration Hospital suggests that their success at answering such questions is at the level of chance.

Frontal-Lobe Syndrome

We have left for last in this sampling of neocortical dysfunctions the syndrome known to be correlated with extensive and bilateral lesions of the frontal association cortex (Figure 44). In many ways it is the most mysterious syndrome of all. Perhaps it is significant that the frontal association cortex is the part of the neocortex most remote, in position and in the number of intervening synapses, from the primary sensory fields. As we shall now see, the signs of the frontal-lobe syndrome are neither sensory nor motoric nor agnosic nor apraxic. (Apraxia signifies a loss of capacity for purposeful action. Implicit in this definition is the notion that it is one thing to flex the fingers spontaneously and quite another to flex them in the course of waving goodbye or responding to a request to demonstrate how to use a toothbrush.) Nor is the frontal-lobe syndrome linguistic (that is, aphasic).

To be sure, there are signs of the syndrome that might be termed quasi-motoric. In the hours that follow a traumatic frontal-lobe lesion, the patient, perhaps still unconscious, often shows a reflex called compulsive grasping, which is comparable to the closure of a newborn infant's hand around an object placed lightly in contact with the palm. In the infant such grasping disappears in a matter of months, and an adult never shows it, except as a sign of pathology. Then, too, there are signs of the frontal-lobe syndrome that might be termed quasi-sensory. They are discovered well after the trauma. For example, the patient shows impairment in correctly perceiving the vertical when his body is placed at a tilt. Moreover, if you show the patient an outline drawing of a human body and ask him to touch with his right hand the right hand of the figure, the patient's performance is defective: as often as not, he touches the figure's left hand. Finally, there are signs that are clinically valuable but have no obvious category. One such sign involves what might be called the programming of the gaze. In a normal person this programming seems to follow a well-ordered unconscious strategy. It is likely, for example, that when a normal person looks at a portrait, his gaze centers first on the face and then makes saccades, or eye-scans, to take in the limbs. The scans grow shorter and shorter; they come to concentrate on ever finer detail. (You know of yourself that when you contemplate a painting, you require a certain amount of time to "absorb" all the details.) In contrast, the eyes of a victim of the frontal-lobe syndrome tend to scan almost at random; thus the patient takes longer to interpret an image. It is as if the intact frontal association cortex could express, so to speak, its degree of dissatisfaction with

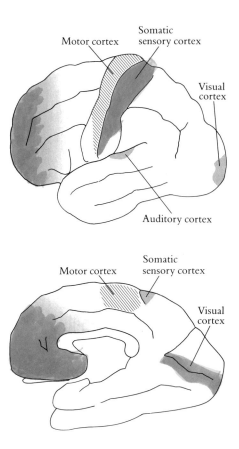

Figure 44: **Frontal-lobe syndrome,** a remarkable condition neither sensory nor motor nor linguistic, results from extensive damage to association cortex surrounding the frontal pole of the cerebral hemisphere. The patient shows changes in character: for example, he may become impulsive and flippant. Subtle tests suggest that his thought processes have lost their power to modulate his behavior. The frontal association cortex is the part of the neocortex most remote, in position and also synaptically, from the primary sensory fields, shown in gray in the illustration. (Motor cortex, outlined in hatching, will be discussed in Chapter 7.)

the information available after each scan of the world and could formulate a strategy by which to augment its knowledge through an additional pass.

Do the random saccades signify a sensory deficit in the neocortical evaluation of visual data? Or do they signify a motor deficit by which the neocortex is rendered unable to formulate what it is the eyes should do? In a way, there is little use wondering. All of the signs described in the preceding paragraph prove to be mild in the life of the patient. As a rule they escape his notice. The following signs are quite different. To begin with, a person with an extensive, bilateral frontal-lobe lesion often shows striking changes in character. He is indifferent to matters that ought to concern him. He is impetuous: he chooses an action as if its outcome had not entered his thoughts. Quite commonly, he shows a striking loss of social decorum. He recites off-color anecdotes in company that is certain not to appreciate them. At inappropriate times he offers puns and witticisms that strike him, at least, as funny. He seems compulsively flippant. Cases are known of corporate executives who rise at a business meeting, stride to a corner, and urinate. The associates and the family of such a person are dumbfounded.

Perhaps the most effective way to unmask an extensive lesion of the frontal association cortex employs the Wisconsin modification of the Weigl card-sorting test. The patient is given a deck of cards and asked to arrange them into stacks. Each card shows a type of geometric figure: either triangles, circles, squares, or rectangles. It shows one, two, three, or four of them, and it is printed in black, red, green, or blue. The patient is given no criterion for sorting. Instead he is assured that he will be told each time he places a card whether his choice is correct or not. At first this proves to be adequate; the patient has no initial difficulty in deducing a strategy from the signals he is given. Thus he creates four stacks on the basis of the shape of the figures, or their number, or their color. Then the diagnostician changes the criterion (from color to number, for instance), and the patient is required to identify and follow a new ordering system. Under such conditions the patient tends to maintain his original strategy in the face of an ever-mounting score of errors. According to Brenda Milner of the Montreal Neurological Institute, the patient may even "state spontaneously that 'it has to be the color, the form, or the number.'" Nevertheless he persists. His intelligence is intact: he can comprehend language, he can analyze a general instruction — "Please sort these cards" — into its conceptual content, and he can formulate strategy. Moreover, he can make an appropriate beginning (which the apraxic person often cannot) and his motions show no motor deficit. But once his program of action has started, it is likely to stagnate. It is as if the patient were unable to internalize signals of imminent error — including self-directed verbal commands — that would normally modulate the unfolding of behavior.

Chapter Seven

Descending Paths;
The Motor System

In 1870 Gustav Theodor Fritsch, an amateur investigator, and Eduard Hitzig, a doctor in private practice in Berlin, reported the results of experiments in which they applied electric current to the neocortex they exposed at the surface of the brain of a living dog. In some places the current elicited twitchings of striated musculature on the side of the body contralateral to the site of the stimulation. Often it was the foreleg or hind leg that moved. In other places the cortex was "silent." The place at which the required strength of electric current was minimal turned out to lie on the convexity of the cerebral hemisphere not far behind the frontal pole of the brain. The work provoked an enduring interest in the organization of the parts of the brain involved in effector, or motor, functions. After all, here was a motor cortex: a circumscribed place at the highest level of the brain that plainly involved itself in the governance of bodily movement. Perhaps a purely motoric organization could now be found throughout the brain and the spinal cord.

Thus began the quest for "the motor system," a vague term designating not only the motor neurons governing striated musculature but also the neural channels converging on motor neurons. The quest continues today, and one may ask whether it can ever be completed. Consider a band of neocortex not far from the visual cortex that is designated area 19 in a system of neocortical subdivision published by the German neurologist Korbinian Brodmann in 1909. When area 19 is stimulated electrically in an experimental animal, the eyes of the animal turn in unison to the contralateral side — that is to say, the gaze moves to an alignment directed away from the side of the brain receiving the current. It is tempting to call area 19 a motor area. Doing so, however, would be arbitrary. From another point of view area 19 is sensory: it is known to reprocess information that has passed through the visual cortex. A similar example, area 22, lies near the auditory cortex. The electrical stimulation of area 22 will cause the animal to turn its eyes to the contralateral side. Yet area 22 stands in synaptic relation to the auditory cortex much as area 19 does to the visual cortex. As a final example, consider an intervertebral ganglion. Even modest electrical stimulation of an intervertebral ganglion will cause a vigorous bodily movement—the contraction of a limb, perhaps. Yet the intervertebral ganglion contains only primary sensory neurons.

The point of these examples is that no line can be drawn between a sensory side and a motor side in the organization of the brain. To put it another way, utterly every neural structure is involved in the programming and guidance of an organism's behavior. Surely that is in essence the function of the nervous system, and the reason evolution has favored its development. Of course, some cell groups in the great intermediate net are situated in a way that encourages one to regard them as sensory structures. The lateral geniculate body of the thalamus is an example. Other cell groups, synaptically close to motor neurons, tempt one to call them motoric. It may be best, then, to explore the motor aspects of the central nervous system by beginning at the level of the motor neuron, which by anyone's definition is a part of the motor system. The strategy is to trace into the brain the lines that play on motor neurons. One is, of course, moving upstream: against the impulse traffic.

Local Motor Apparatuses

The first step upstream is in general very short: it begins in the spinal cord, in the hindbrain, or in the midbrain, where motor neurons are found (there are none in the forebrain), and it leads to a pool of cells that usually are smaller and usually are nearby. One could call them interneurons, but it is likely that only some of them contact motor neurons directly. The pool nonetheless provides the dominant input for a typical motor neuron. The sum of all motor neurons and their interneuronal pools we shall call "the lower motor system," and we shall divide it into functional subunits, each called a "local motor apparatus," in correspondence to the parts of the body: the arms, the legs, the eyes, and so on. The reason emerges from an experiment done almost three decades ago by the Hungarian neuroembryologist Gyorgi Székely in which two parts of the immature spinal cord were interchanged in developing chicken embryos. The part of the cord that would normally come to innervate the legs was exchanged with the part that would come to innervate the wings. One can never hope to do such a thing to a mammal. Perhaps the spinal cord of the mammal becomes dependent too early on an uninterrupted supply of blood. Still, the results in the chicken were impressive. When the animal was dropped a few feet, the spinal segments that would normally innervate the wings caused the legs to make fluttering movements. The wings made no fluttering movement at all.

The conclusion is in essence a tautology: the local motor apparatuses at particular places in the central nervous system fulfill specific requirements. In other words, the constellation of striated musculature in any one part of the body is sufficiently idiosyncratic in its repertoire of possible movements so that an idiosyncratic organization of motor neurons and interneurons is required for its governance. Perhaps the idiosyncratic organization is imposed on the nervous system by the peculiar ways in which the joints are designed. In the human body, for example, the hip joint is quite different from the shoulder joint. Both are ball-and-socket arrangements, but their limits of freedom are not at all alike. In any case, once a particular set of connectivities had become established for the chicken's caudal spinal cord, no fibers, reaching from the brain down into the cord, could extract from that organization a

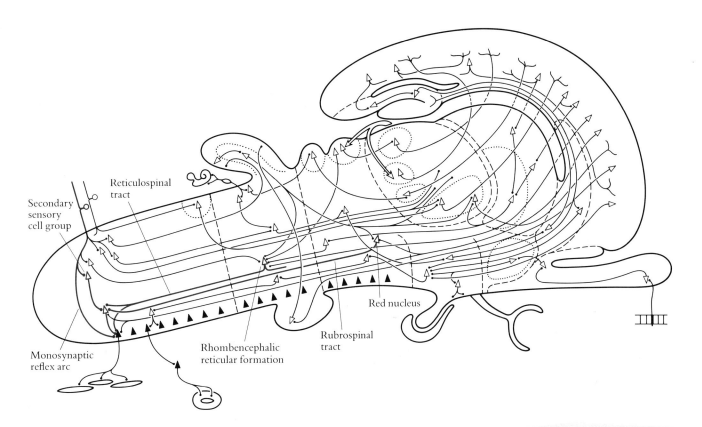

Figure 45: **Convergence on motor neurons** typifies the "motor system," a vague term denoting the motor side of the organization of the brain and spinal cord. Here the convergence is symbolized by four projections (*color*), which impinge, at the lower left, on a local motor apparatus: an alliance of motor neurons and interneurons. The apparatus is shown getting input from a monosynaptic reflex arc; from a secondary sensory cell group in the spinal cord; from the rhombencephalic reticular formation, by way of reticulospinal fibers; and from the red nucleus, a cell group in the midbrain, by way of the rubrospinal tract. A fifth projection, from neocortex, is described in Figure 47. Two sources of input not shown in this illustration are the vestibular nuclei, in the hindbrain, which emit two vestibulospinal tracts, and the superior colliculus, in the midbrain, which emits the tectospinal tract.

pattern of motor-neuronal discharge appropriate for the upper extremities. It becomes tempting to consider the lower motor system as a sort of file room in which blueprints are stored, each representing a possible movement of a particular part of the body. The brain, with its descending fiber systems, reaches down and selects the appropriate blueprint.

Encephalospinal Tracts

What, then, are the sources of the descending systems? Where is one led by a second step upstream? The answer is, everywhere: the projections converging on the local motor apparatuses of the spinal cord (deferring for now a discussion of the ones in the brainstem) originate in all the main divisions of

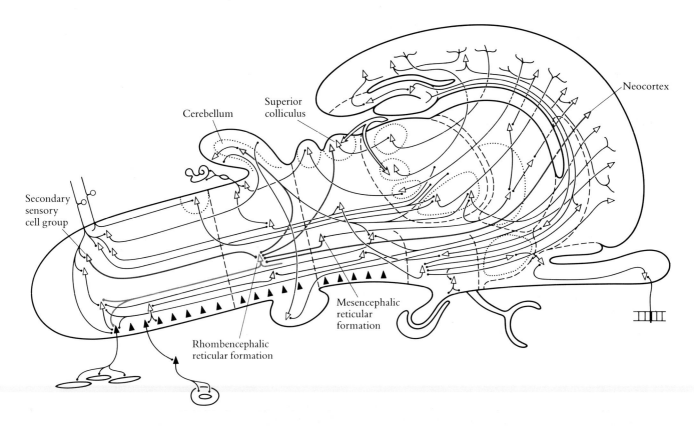

Figure 46: **Convergence on the reticular formation** is symbolized by five axons (*dark color*) that carry signals of widely varying provenance but all impinge on a single neuron in the reticular core of the hindbrain. One of the five—a spinothalamic "dropout"—arises in a secondary sensory cell group in the spinal cord; it carries somatic sensory data. A second axon arises in the superior colliculus; it carries visual data. A third axon arises in the cerebellum; a fourth in the mesencephalic reticular formation; a fifth in the neocortex. The axon of the rhombencephalic neuron (*light color*) projects both downward into the spinal cord and upward toward the thalamus.

the central nervous system. Figure 45 gives examples. In the spinal cord itself the projections originate in secondary sensory cell groups, and even, in the case of monosynaptic reflex arcs, as the collaterals of primary sensory fibers. In the rhombencephalon, the projections originate in the vestibular nuclei, a set of secondary sensory cell groups not shown in Figure 45 that receive primary sensory data from receptor cells in the inner ear: in particular the vestibular part of the membranous labyrinth. They also originate in roughly the medial two-thirds of the rhombencephalic reticular formation, a district known as the magnocellular reticular formation in recognition of its content of large and very large neuronal cell bodies. In the mesencephalon, the projections originate in the superior colliculus and also in a large cell mass called the red nucleus. Generally speaking, all four of these descending fiber systems (the vestibulospinal, the reticulospinal, the tectospinal, and the rubrospinal tracts) bear information — commands, if you wish — that have antecedents in wide regions of the brain. The vestibular nuclei get input not only from the vestibular labyrinth, by way of the vestibular nerve; they also get input from the cerebellum. Apparently this is a path by which the cerebellum can bring its influence to bear on bodily movements. The superior colliculus gets input not only from the optic nerve but also from large areas of the neocortex, including the visual cortex and much else. The red nucleus gets input from the cerebellum and from the motor cortex.

The reticular formation is notorious as a place of convergence for information of widespread antecedent. We suggested that earlier, when we were speaking of ascending conduction lines. We must also suggest it now, in the context of descent. A neuron representing a target of such convergence appears in Figure 46; it is modeled on neurons whose electrical activity was recorded by Giuseppe Moruzzi of the University of Pisa and others. It lies in the rhombencephalic reticular formation, and it responds to input from a secondary sensory cell group in the spinal cord. A flash of light, however, can provoke it equally well, since the news of a flash of light can reach the reticular formation by a path descending from the superior colliculus. Indeed, the cell can respond to signals from great expanses of the brain, including the cerebellum, the neocortex, and the mesencephalic reticular formation. Plainly the reticular formation must integrate this variety of afflux, ascending and descending in the brainstem, and in the wake of that integration it dispatches impulses over reticulospinal fibers that terminate on interneurons, or even, although infrequently, on motor neurons directly.*

---

*Perhaps it seems again that the reticular formation makes no sense, now that descending lines with heterogeneous afferents are seen to be part of its repertoire. Yet there is worse. Some of the neurons in the reticular formation have an axon with not only a descending branch that joins a reticulospinal tract, but also an ascending branch. Thus the ascending and descending lines that involve the reticular formation are sometimes intermingled. Figure 46 leaves undecided the destination of a representative ascending branch; it can go to many places, but the thalamus is often the terminus for fibers ascending in the brainstem.

Pyramidal System

It now remains to superimpose on the encephalospinal paths of the brainstem the descending paths that originate in the forebrain. We begin at the neocortex. All parts of the neocortex project to the thalamus, in a pattern that reciprocates the thalamocortical projections. All parts of the neocortex project to the striatum, the outer zone of the corpus striatum. Much of the neocortex projects to the superior colliculus; all parts of the neocortex project to the pons. Certain parts of the neocortex project to the hypothalamus; certain parts of the neocortex project to mesencephalic destinations: the red nucleus and the midbrain reticular formation. The remaining corticofugal fibers—the ones that extend beyond the pons—originate mostly in the motor cortex. Some of them go no farther than the rhombencephalon (the rhombencephalic reticular formation and certain rhombencephalic motor apparatuses); they are called the corticobulbar tract, in reference to their destination, the bulbus encephali, an early name for the medulla oblongata. The others attain all levels of the spinal cord: they are the corticospinal tract. Together the corticobulbar tract and the corticospinal tract compose the pyramidal tract (Figure 47). The name derives from a circumstance of gross anatomy. In the medulla oblongata the tract appears at the ventral surface of the brain and takes on a triangular cross section. The tract thus forms a prominence that is called the medullary pyramid.

It is remarkable in itself that fibers leaving the motor cortex reach into the spinal cord. It is remarkable, too, that an estimated five percent of the fibers synapse directly on motor neurons instead of making their connections in an interneuronal pool. Doubtless the privileged five percent help to account for the observation that of all the fields of the cerebral cortex the motor cortex requires the least degree of electrical stimulation to elicit bodily movement. The privileged five percent ensure that of all the cerebral cortex the motor cortex is closest to motor neurons, in that the fewest synapses intervene. Which among the motor neurons are only one synapse away? To put the question conversely, which among the spinal cord's motor neurons get some of their input direct from the motor cortex? The answer is found when a stroke (an intracerebral bleeding or an arterial blockage that damages the great mass of fibers connecting the cortex with subcortical stations) interrupts the corticospinal tract. The typical sign of the lesion is hemiplegia: a marked motor weakness on the side of the body opposite the site of the necrosis. It is a weakness, not a paralysis, because the trauma destroys no motor neurons. Indeed, the muscles nearest the midline of the body regain much of their missing strength in the weeks that follow the trauma. In the musculature of the extremities the impairment remains much greater. It is maximal and enduring in the musculature of the hand. The impairment itself is curious. If a patient convalescing from a stroke is asked to flex his thumb, the patient will make an effort, and the hand will move in flexion, often along with the wrist and the elbow. It is as if the functioning corticospinal tract had served not so much to elicit movement as to help to define it, like a sculptor (in John Eccles' simile) removing superfluous parts from a block of marble. After a stroke, the brain can still generate a command—"Flex!" But the sculptor is no longer there to eliminate the superfluous contractions.

Extrapyramidal System

The pyramidal tract is not the only neocortical projection implicated in motor function. In addition there is the projection to the striatum (Figure 48). The layout of that projection is loosely topologic: the somatic sensory cortex projects to a striatal district more or less distinct from the one receiving the visual projection, or the auditory projection, or the projections from the association areas or from the motor cortex. From the striatum a massive

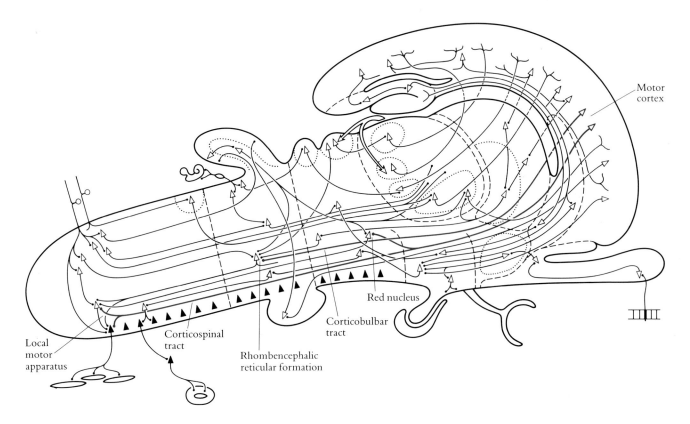

Figure 47: **Pyramidal tract** spans the central nervous system. Its source is the motor cortex, a part of the neocortex, from which it descends in great volume. It has two components: the corticobulbar tract, which projects to local motor apparatuses and the reticular formation in the rhombencephalon (the "bulbus encephali"), and the corticospinal tract, which projects to local motor apparatuses throughout the length of the spinal cord. (An additional destination is the red nucleus in the midbrain.) The pyramidal tract is notable for its proportion of privileged axons that circumvent interneurons and synapse directly with motor neurons.

projection converges on the globus pallidus, or pallidum, the inner zone of the corpus striatum. There are many fewer neurons in the globus pallidus than there are in the striatum, and so this system must be seen as a kind of funneling. From the globus pallidus the path continues downward as a fiber bundle called the ansa lenticularis. Or rather it continues downward except for the curious fact that a large part of the ansa lenticularis curves back on itself (ansa signifies a handle-shaped structure) and enters the rostral part of the ventral nucleus of the thalamus. We have said that the ventral nucleus receives the two great somatic sensory lemnisci, the medial lemniscus and the spinothalamic tract, and that it projects to the somatic sensory cortex. Only the caudal part of the ventral nucleus, however, is a somatic sensory way station. It is called the ventrobasal nucleus, or the ventral posterior nucleus. The rostral part of the ventral nucleus consists of the ventral anterior nucleus and the ventral lateral nucleus. It is called the V.A.-V.L. complex. It receives two fiber bundles, the ansa lenticularis and the cerebellum's upward projection, called the superior cerebellar peduncle or the brachium conjunctivum. It, too, projects to neocortex — not to any sensory area, but instead to the motor cortex.*

Lesions that disrupt this looping circuitry can cause havoc in bodily movement. In man, for instance, extensive destructions of the striatum bring on motor automatisms. The clinician sees various types. In some cases the automatism is no more than a slight exaggeration the patient uncontrollably shows in the course of an otherwise normal act. The act of walking yields an example. The walking itself may be normal, but the swing of the patient's arms may end in a slight flourish that seems at first to be an affectation. In other cases, as we have noted, the automatism resembles a complex act such as kicking or seizing. If the automatism is rapid (it can be explosively rapid), the disorder is called chorea, which means "dance." If, on the other hand, it is slow and wormlike in its unfolding, the disorder is called athetosis, which means "without position." The term apparently derives from a symptom of incipient athetosis: the patient cannot keep the weight of his body primarily on either leg, and so he is constantly shifting his stance.

Lesions affecting the neural lines that feed into the looping circuitry also cause motor havoc. Item: The subthalamic nucleus, a small, lens-shaped mass of gray matter in the caudal diencephalon, receives fibers from the globus pallidus and sends back a return projection. It is, in a word, a satellite of the pallidum. The destruction of the subthalamic nucleus causes hemiballism, an automatism of the contralateral arm and leg that resembles throwing and kicking respectively. Movements of the face and the trunk are unimpaired. Item: The substantia nigra, a cell group in the midbrain, receives fibers from

---

*Recent evidence places a neocortical way station in the path by suggesting that the part of the V.A.-V.L. complex receiving the ansa lenticularis projects not so much to the motor cortex in the strict sense (area 4 of Brodmann) as to cortex just anterior: the premotor cortex (areas 6 and 8). From the premotor cortex a massive projection attains the motor cortex.

the striatum and sends back a return projection. It is a satellite of the striatum. Many of its neurons include a black pigment; hence the cell group's name. The pigment is neuromelanin, a polymer formed from DOPA (dihydroxyphenylalanine), which is a precursor of the catecholamine neurotransmitters. The neurons employ dopamine as their striatal neurotransmitter. Extensive loss of the neurons causes Parkinson's disease. It is characterized by a muscular rigidity that greatly hampers movement and is betrayed by a masklike face. One also observes a peculiar tremor, of low frequency and almost rotatory, that affects the arms and hands. The tremor reminded early clinicians of the rubbing motion of the fingers by which a pharmacist would make pills; thus the symptom was described as pill-roller's tremor. Typically, however, the

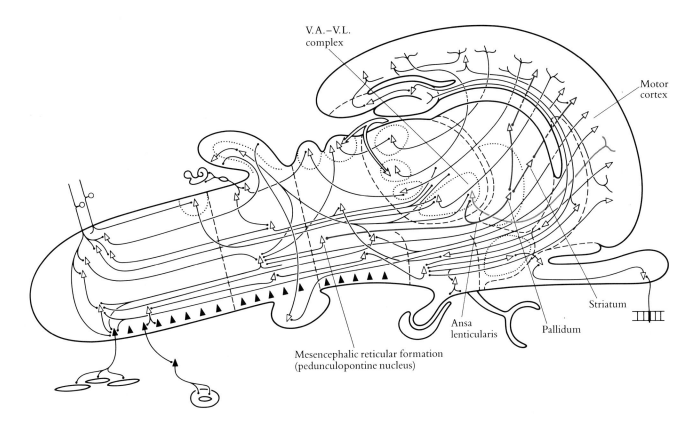

Figure 48: **Extrapyramidal motor system** begins (if one can speak of a beginning) with a descent from the neocortex distinct from the pyramidal tract's descent. Specifically, all parts of the neocortex project (*dark color*) to the striatum, the outer zone of the corpus striatum. The striatum then projects to the pallidum, or globus pallidus, the inner zone of the corpus striatum. The pallidum projects to a part of the mesencephalic reticular formation called the pedunculopontine nucleus. In large measure, however, the pallidal outflow —a bundle called the ansa lenticularis—curves dorsally to enter a pair of thalamic cell groups: the ventral anterior (V.A.) nucleus and the ventral lateral (V.L.) nucleus. The V.A.-V.L. complex projects (*light color*) to the motor cortex, by way of adjacent association cortex. Thus the extrapyramidal motor system serves chiefly to influence the source of the pyramidal tract. Not shown in the illustration are two other extrapyramidal cell groups, the subthalamic nucleus, in the diencephalon, and the substantia nigra, in the midbrain.

patient's foremost complaint is that he has difficulty initiating the movements he intends to make. He wants, for instance, to adjust his clothing, and though he knows quite well how to do it (as he may insist with chagrin), he somehow cannot start.

Clearly the corpus striatum can be considered an important influence on bodily movement. More broadly, it is one among a number of brain structures whose output seems to be channeled toward motor neurons. Yet the fact remains that the corpus striatum cannot directly affect motor neurons, nor even the interneuronal pools that act as motor-neuronal gatekeepers. We have just seen that the greater part of its outgoing tract, the ansa lenticularis,

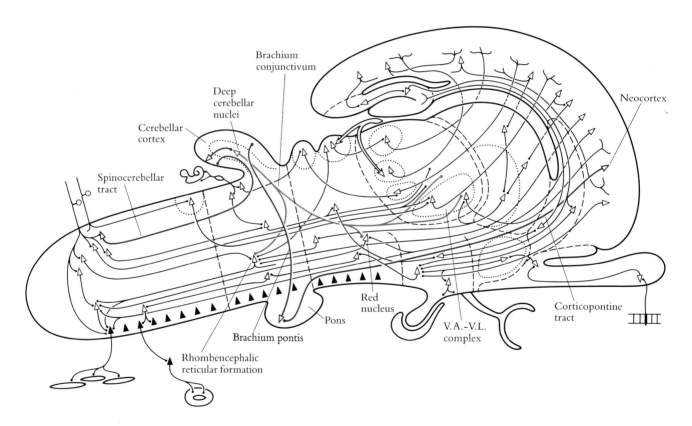

Figure 49: **Paths to the cerebellum** are diverse. Here two are diagrammed (*dark color*). One of them begins throughout the neocortex and is interrupted in the pons; hence it consists of two projections: the corticopontine tract and then the brachium pontis. The other is spinocerebellar. Additional paths to the cerebellum, not shown in the illustration, begin in the reticular formation; in the vestibular nuclei, which are part of the hindbrain; and in the vestibular sense organs of the inner ear. (The latter afferentation makes the cerebellum a recipient of primary sensory data.) The cerebellar afferents are shown ending in the cerebellar cortex, which projects to nuclei deep in the organ. In turn, the deep cerebellar nuclei project (*light color*), in a bundle called the brachium conjunctivum, to the red nucleus in the midbrain, to thalamic nuclei including the V.A.-V.L. complex, and to the rhombencephalic reticular formation. A further projection goes to the vestibular nuclei, as if to reaffirm the close association between the cerebellum and the vestibular sense.

turns upward and enters the ventral nucleus of the thalamus. The rest of the ansa lenticularis continues downward past that turning. It gets no farther than the caudal limit of the midbrain, where a single neuron in Figure 48 symbolizes the several thousand neurons composing the nucleus tegmenti pedunculopontinus, or, somewhat less forbiddingly, the pedunculopontine nucleus. It is a part of the mesencephalic reticular formation. From there on, the descending path grows vague. The reticular formation projects some of its fibers downward, but along no circumscribed neural highway.

As the lesions associated with chorea, athetosis, hemiballism, and Parkinson's disease were located in the brain, the corpus striatum became known, with the subthalamic nucleus and the substantia nigra, as the extrapyramidal motor system. The disorders themselves became known as the extrapyramidal dyskinesias. It was plain that the corpus striatum and its satellites have much to do with bodily movement, yet it seemed that none of those structures contributes fibers to the brain's most prominent descending bundle, the pyramidal tract. It still appears they do not, but the adjective "extrapyramidal" is tarnished all the same. As Rolf Hassler, a German neuroanatomist and neurologist, noted some decades ago, the main target of the extrapyramidal system, acting through the intermediary of the V.A.-V.L. complex, is the motor cortex, where the pyramidal tract begins.*

Cerebellum

In the foregoing paragraphs on the motor system the cerebellum has gone undescribed. Its omission would be inexcusable. Lesions of the cerebellum profoundly disable movement.

One way to essay an account of the cerebellum is to trace its inputs: its afferentation. We begin in the inner ear. There, in addition to Corti's organ, one finds five vestibular epithelia. In two of them, called the maculae, hair cells sense the tilt of the head. In the other three, the cristae, hair cells sense the angular acceleration. The five yield primary sensory data to fibers emitted by some 20,000 neurons in the nearby vestibular ganglion. The fibers, which form the vestibular nerve, attain the vestibular nuclei, a set of secondary sensory cell groups in the rhombencephalon. The vestibular nuclei project in turn to the cerebellum. There the projection distributes its fibers to part of the vermis (literally "the worm"), the midline district of the cerebellum, and also the flocculonodular lobe, the caudalmost part of the cerebellum, which con-

---

*The term extrapyramidal motor system was introduced in 1912 by the English neurologist S. A. K. Wilson. Over the years it has largely, but not entirely, replaced a much older term, basal ganglia, which initially referred to all the gray masses at the base of the cerebral hemisphere, including even the thalamus, but gradually became synonymous with the extrapyramidal triad: the corpus striatum, the subthalamic nucleus, and the substantia nigra.

sists of the caudalmost part of the vermis, called the nodulus, and a slender lateral wing that ends in a slight swelling called the flocculus. Remarkably, some of the fibers in the vestibular nerve bypass the vestibular nuclei: they go to the cerebellum directly. They, too, terminate in the vermis and in the flocculonodular lobe. No other instance is known in which the cerebellum gets primary sensory input. This suggests a close alliance between the cerebellum and the vestibular sense. Indeed, a survey of the vertebrates leads downward to the cyclostomes, the round-mouthed, jawless fishes, including lampreys and hagfishes, in which a flocculonodular lobe receiving vestibular input is all there is to the cerebellum. In more advanced animals, the cerebellum is greatly enlarged by the corpus cerebelli, a more rostral part of the organ. It includes a paramedian zone, which forms the greater part of the vermis, and a lateral expansion, most pronounced in mammals, the cerebellar hemisphere. Along with this augmentation come new and varied inputs. Somatic sensory information arrives from the spinal cord. It travels in spinocerebellar fibers. Information of obscure parentage arrives from the reticular formation. Most notably, information arrives from the entire expanse of the neocortex, by way of a projection interrupted in the pons. One may thus suppose that the cerebellum is a recipient of messages with parentage in all the senses (except, perhaps, olfaction). It is as if a number of structures in the brain and the spinal cord were corporations that had discovered the competition — the vestibular system — employs a valuable computer and had found a way to buy in.

What does the cerebellum do with its multitudinous input? To begin with, the cerebellum has a cortex. Figure 49 shows two representative cerebellar afferents (a spinocerebellar fiber and a pontocerebellar fiber) terminating there. Underneath it one finds a core of white matter — the cable basement of the cerebellar cortex — and embedded in the core are masses of gray matter called the deep cerebellar nuclei. The figure suggests only one; actually there are four on each side of the midline. The cortex projects to these four deeper masses. In turn, fibers that arise in the lateral three (the emboliform nucleus, the globose nucleus, and the dentate nucleus) make up the superior cerebellar peduncle, or brachium conjunctivum, the cerebellum's major outgoing channel, directed to the red nucleus in the midbrain and also the V.A.-V.L. complex of the thalamus. The red nucleus projects downward to the spinal cord; the V.A.-V.L. complex projects upward to the motor cortex. Fibers from the most medial of the deep cerebellar nuclei (the fastigial nucleus) also leave the cerebellum. They terminate largely in the vestibular nuclei and in the medial part of the rhombencephalic reticular formation. One concludes that signals generated in the cerebellar cortex must be processed for export by the deep cerebellar nuclei. There is, however, a notable exception: some of the fibers leaving the cortex of the flocculonodular lobe bypass the deep cerebellar nuclei and project to the vestibular nuclei. That again suggests the close alliance between the cerebellum and the vestibular sense.

A wealth of clinical evidence shows that lesions of the cerebellum characteristically entail a chronic disruption of the sequential order in bodily movement. Lesions of the cerebellar hemisphere, and especially lesions involving the emboliform, globose, and dentate nuclei (that is, the more lateral of the deep cerebellar nuclei), manifest themselves most strikingly in so-called extremity ataxia, which impairs movements of the ipsilateral limbs. When a patient with such an impairment is asked to extend his ipsilateral arm and then bring the index finger to the tip of his nose, he proves capable of obeying only with marked instability: his hand lurches from side to side, and the lurch grows worse as the finger nears its target. When he is asked to put the heel of the ipsilateral foot against the knee of the other leg and then bring the foot downward along that leg, he proves unable to do it with a normal smoothness of motion. In both cases, the essence of the deficit seems to be a temporal decomposition of the sequence by which the muscles of an extremity cooperate. Lesions of the vermis, the midline zone of the cerebellar cortex, and especially lesions involving the fastigial nucleus (the most medial of the deep cerebellar nuclei) often leave the extremities unimpaired. Instead they severely derange the movements of the trunk: they bring on trunk ataxia. Here the patient proves unable to balance his trunk over his legs. Attempting to walk, he staggers and tends to fall backward. Again the essence of the deficit is a temporal decomposition. It happens that several of the muscles employed for walking, notably the gluteus maximus and the iliopsoas (both of which span the hip joint), combine to move the leg or the trunk either backward or forward in the joint, depending on whether the leg or the trunk is kept fixed with respect to the joint. The muscles thus serve different functions at different times. In a patient with trunk ataxia the sequence for walking is disarrayed.

Cranial Motor Apparatuses

We close this discussion of the motor system with some notes on the local motor apparatuses intrinsic to the brain. In general they animate the head, and so they are responsible for actions such as chewing, swallowing, smiling, and grimacing. Most of the ones in the rhombencephalon are rather like the ones in the spinal cord. In both, the main source of afferents to the motor neurons is nearby interneurons. (In the rhombencephalon many interneurons occupy the lateral third of the reticular formation, a region of small neurons that have led to its designation as the parvicellular reticular formation.) In both, projections from the brainstem reticular formation (and elsewhere) converge on the interneuronal pools. In both, projections from the motor cortex do the same. And in both, some of the fibers arriving from the motor cortex bypass the interneuronal pools and affect the motor neurons directly. The last of these similarities encourages one to ask, Do the symptoms of a stroke include any not associated with the muscles governed by the spinal cord? Typically they do: the hemiplegia following a stroke tends to include a weakness of the facial musculature on the same side of the body as the limbs that are affected. The weakness is most pronounced around the mouth, and far less so in the upper half of the face. But much like the musculature of the trunk and of the neck, the weakened facial muscles eventually recover much of their strength.

One group of the local motor apparatuses intrinsic to the brain requires its own discussion. The group consists of three motor nuclei (groups of motor neurons and the associated interneurons) on each side of the midline. Two of them are in the mesencephalon; one is in the rhombencephalon. Together they animate six striated muscles on each side of the head. The muscles are the ones that turn each eyeball in its socket. It is easy to offer reasons why the group should be quite special. The eyes themselves are special. For one thing, they always move in synchrony. That makes them unique among all the paired parts of the body. Moreover, they turn like ball bearings. Hence the muscles that do the turning have no mechanical load; they act neither with gravity nor against it.

In any case, describing the vagaries of the oculomotor circuitry requires that we go well beyond the conduction lines of the generalized mammalian brain we have been displaying in these pages. (Figure 49 was its most recent iteration.) We shall briefly examine the cell groups called the gaze-control centers. In essence they are "function generators" serving different aspects of eye movement. One such center is in the dorsal midbrain, quite close to the superior colliculus; another is in the reticular formation at the level of the pons. The first one is known from clinical evidence to be involved in vertical gaze; in particular, lesions in the dorsal midbrain close to the superior colliculus compromise the ability of the eyes to turn upward. On evidence of a similar nature the second one is implicated in lateral gaze. From the second of the gaze-control centers, fibers project to the abducens nucleus, the most caudal among the three motor nuclei that control the eye-turning muscles (Figure 50). The fibers terminate within the nucleus itself. They also terminate in the surrounding tissue, which is gray matter consisting mostly of small cells. In turn, the motor neurons in each abducens nucleus animate the lateral rectus muscle on the same side of the head. The lateral rectus muscle rotates (abducts) the eye away from the nose. Plainly the abducens nucleus is an exit from the central nervous system. It is more than that, however. Intercalated among its motor neurons, and in the surrounding gray matter, are interneurons whose axons cross the midline, rise into the mesencephalon, and distribute themselves to the most rostral of the eye-moving nuclei, the oculomotor nucleus, on the opposite side of the brain. The oculomotor nucleus animates several eye-moving muscles. Among them is the medial rectus muscle, which rotates the eye toward the nose. The pattern of connections suggests a mechanism for activating the lateral rectus muscle of one eye in concert with the medial rectus muscle of the other. To put the matter another way, each lateral-gaze center appears to serve movements that direct the eyes in concert toward the half of the visual world on its own side of the midline.

The arrayal of this circuitry, and in particular the juxtaposition of the abducens nucleus with an interneuronal pool that coordinates lateral gaze, offers an irresistible opportunity to contrast two types of paralysis. A lesion involving the abducens nucleus and the surrounding gray matter means that the lateral rectus muscle serving the eye on that side of the head loses its governing motor neurons. The result is a nuclear paralysis. It is a flaccid paralysis: the muscle no longer has tonus, and it can no longer contract. Soon it will atrophy. In contrast, the medial rectus muscle serving the eye on the other side of the head loses none of its governing motor neurons. Instead its governing motor neurons lose some of the neural circuitry that would normally play on them. The result is a supranuclear paralysis. The muscle shows no loss of tonus. Indeed, a muscle affected by supranuclear paralysis can show

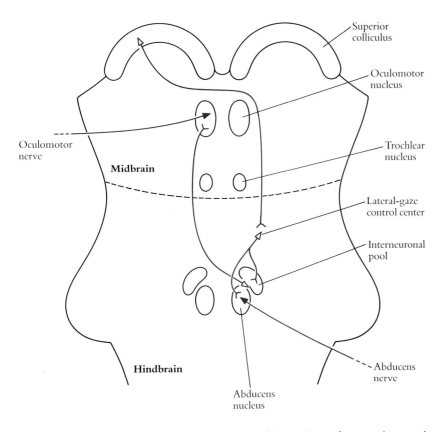

Figure 50: **Coordination of lateral gaze** is one of the tasks confronting the neural circuits that rotate the eyes. Here the coordination is shown in a diagram somewhat less schematic than the others employed in this part of the book. The coordination begins with a lateral-gaze control center high in the hindbrain reticular formation. The center projects to a local motor apparatus: the abducens nucleus and its surrounding interneurons. The nucleus rotates the ipsilateral eye (the eye on its side of the body) so that the axis of vision is directed away from the nose. In addition, the nucleus (and its surrounding interneurons) projects to the oculomotor nucleus on the other side of the brainstem. In this way the circuit rotates the contralateral eye toward the nose. In sum, the circuit turns the eyes in concert toward its side of the visual field. In all, three groups of motor neurons on each side of the brainstem join in rotating the eyes. They are the abducens nucleus, the oculomotor nucleus, and (between them) the trochlear nucleus.

increased tonus, and also more forceful reflexes. The paralysis itself is curious. Ask the patient to look toward the side of the lesion. The act requires that the ipsilateral eye rotate temporally while the contralateral eye rotates nasally. Not surprisingly, the ipsilateral eye (the one on the side of the lesion) proves to stop at midposition, with its gaze directed forward. Only the lateral rectus muscle could have turned it across the midline. Yet the contralateral eye also stops at midposition. Now ask the patient to focus on your finger as you move it from a distance toward the tip of his nose. Both his eyes rotate nasally, in a normal display of visual convergence. The medial rectus muscle that seemed to be paralyzed a moment ago now works perfectly well. Evidently the neural command to converge the visual axes reaches the motor neurons governing the medial rectus muscle by a pathway that does not include the interneurons in and around the abducens nucleus. The medial rectus muscle is paralyzed conditionally: that is, only in certain circumstances. This is the hallmark of a supranuclear lesion.

There is, however, a disturbing gap in the eye-moving circuitry. No projection from the neocortex has been found to terminate on the motor neurons of the abducens nucleus or the oculomotor nucleus. Moreover, no projection from the neocortex has been found to terminate on the interneurons in and around the abducens nucleus. Perhaps only the gaze-control centers project to this local motor apparatus.

What, then, projects to the gaze-control centers? Evidently both of them get fibers from the superior colliculus, which is reassuring, because it has long been known that electrical stimulation of each superior colliculus elicits conjugate movements of the eyes that turn them toward the opposite side of the world. What projects to the superior colliculus? Earlier in this chapter we suggested that it receives fibers from diverse parts of the neocortex. They include the visual cortex, and area 22, and, quite prominently, a field of the neocortex — area 8 — that is known as the frontal eye field. Area 8 is the strongest of the so-called contraversive eye fields: areas 19, 22, and 8. Electrical stimulation of any of the three elicits conjugate eye movements toward the contralateral side. Now area 19 and area 22 were mentioned at the outset of this chapter, when an analysis of their input suggested that they be classified (against the physiological evidence) as sensory. Are they motoric nonetheless? In particular, do areas 8, 19 and 22 constitute the neocortical level of motor control for the eyes, much as the motor cortex constitutes the neocortical level of motor control for the rest of the body? The notion is attractive. But it could be true only if some, at least, of the neurons in areas 8, 19 and 22 change their pattern of bioelectric activity just before eye movements, and quite to the contrary, most of the cells in area 8 are now known to change their pattern of activity not before eye movements, but after.

Where, in that case, is the neocortical level of control for the direction of the gaze? One demands that it exist, because one controls one's eyes quite as readily, and as willfully, as one controls a hand. Yet the surprising fact is that no part of the neocortex can be singled out as a "motor cortex" for the oculomotor system; the governance of eye movement is just too widely distributed. Perhaps the best corroboration is the clinical finding that essentially no amount of damage in the cerebral hemispheres can lastingly paralyze the conjugate movement of the eyes. Consider the survivor of a massive stroke who later suffers a massive stroke in the opposite cerebral hemisphere. In the wake of the second lesion comes a new and profound motor deficit. It is as if the lesion were in the spinal cord, where it destroyed motor neurons bilaterally, because the muscles of the extremities are paralyzed, not just weakened or ataxic. In the cranial musculature the deficit is similar. The patient can no longer chew, and so must be fed through a tube. His face is unmoving. It is as if the lesion were bilateral in the medulla oblongata. (The facial paralysis is thus called pseudobulbar palsy.) Yet even now his eyes will track you in unison as you move about his room.

Chapter Eight

Innervation of the Viscera

The motor system defies one's best attempts to call any behavior volitional. Suppose you are playing tennis. You make a splendid return, and for a moment you feel elated. Then you realize you simply made a freak shot; the racket just happened, somehow, to move the right way. The next time a tennis ball rushes at you on the same trajectory you will probably hit it badly. A moment ago you felt a wonderful sense of self-esteem: a sense of having desired movement and then of having controlled it. Now you decide you do not deserve any credit. Suppose you are walking in winter. You skid on an iced-over puddle. The skid elicits movements by which your body keeps itself from falling. Your arms flail about and release what they were holding; you stumble; but shortly you find you are still on your feet. You must admit the sequence was not at all volitional. Suppose you take this book from a shelf. Surely it is by volition that you initiate the act. But surely you have no control over the exact program of muscle contraction by which the act is accomplished. In particular, you cannot command any one muscle to contract, nor command others not to contract, yet all of your movements require a concert of muscle contractions. The act of picking up a book requires far more, in any case, than just the muscles of the arm and the hand, the muscles you may have been aware you were using at the time. Muscle groups in the trunk and the legs must also contract, as a matter of maintaining balance. If you try to pick up the book while you suffer from a sore back, you will know they have contracted.

Despite the essential mystery of the will to move, and despite the incompleteness of one's conscious control of one's body, the subjective experience of volition has given a name to the motor system that innervates striated musculature: it is the voluntary (or somatic) nervous system, as distinguished from the involuntary (or autonomic) nervous system, which innervates smooth musculature and glands: the active tissues of the viscera. A misunderstanding, however, is implicit in these terms. It concerns the word "autonomic," which literally means "self-governing." The autonomic nervous system is far less autonomic than the names of the system imply. Its functions are integrated with voluntary movements no less than with affects and motivations. In short, its roots are in the brain; one's experiences from moment to moment dictate not only contractions of striated muscles, but also, and in parallel — or even in anticipation — great functional shifts in the body's internal organs. The term autonomic has nonetheless won out.

The autonomic periphery is represented in our generalized mammal by an organ symbolizing, among other things, the intestinal tract, the urinary bladder, a bronchus, or an artery. In essence each is a tube whose width is modulated by the contraction of one or more coats of smooth-muscle tissue. The motor innervation of such a tube (or of a gland) employs chains (Figure 51) each consisting of two neurons. The first is in the central nervous system. It emits a rather thin axon (1.5 to four micrometers in diameter) that nonetheless is myelinated. The second is in the periphery. As a rule it is stationed in what is called an autonomic ganglion. It receives the axon the first cell emits, and in turn it sends its own axon, which is unmyelinated, to the organ or to the gland. This undermines a definition. In anatomical terminology a motor neuron dispatches its axon to innervate effector cells, namely striated-muscle fibers, smooth-muscle fibers, or gland cells. What, then, of the neuron whose axon leaves the central nervous system only to synapse with a neuron in an autonomic ganglion? Both are called motor neurons. Specifically, the central cell is called a preganglionic motor neuron and the peripheral cell is called a ganglionic or — illogically — a postganglionic motor neuron. (Obviously, only the axon emitted by the cell in the ganglion is "postganglionic.") The pattern contrasts with that of somatic motor innervation, in which a motor neuron in the central nervous system projects to effector cells directly.

The Sympathetic Periphery

Within the autonomic nervous system, two subsystems, the sympathetic and the parasympathetic, have long been distinguished by means of several criteria: anatomical, chemical, and functional. The sympathetic is the more extensive of the two. Its preganglionic motor neurons are in the spinal cord, where they occupy a district called the lateral horn of the spinal gray matter. Their longitudinal distribution extends through roughly the middle third of the spinal cord's length. In general, their axons are short, because the cells with which the axons synapse are in a ganglion at the side of the vertebral column (a paravertebral ganglion) or in front of the vertebral column (a prevertebral ganglion). In either case, the preganglionic fibers employ the neurotransmitter acetylcholine. In contrast, the postganglionic fibers often have a substantial distance to travel. As a rule, the postganglionic fibers employ the neurotransmitter norepinephrine.

The sympathetic division of the autonomic nervous system promotes the organism's ability to expend energy. Under its urging the bronchial trees widen, so as to facilitate respiration. The hairs of the skin stand on end. Sweating increases. Conversely, intestinal peristalsis is halted. At the same time, the glands connected to the gastrointestinal tract (the pancreas and the salivary glands, for example) decrease their activity. The smooth musculature in most hollow organs shows lessened activity, too. The sphincters of the anus and the bladder tighten, and the muscle essential for voiding urine — the detrusor muscle of the bladder — is inactivated. The walls of the bladder relax. The cardiovascular system undergoes a number of functional shifts. The heartbeat increases both in frequency and in intensity. The capsule and trabeculae of the spleen contract, so as to squeeze blood into the systemic circulation. (The spleen is built somewhat like a sponge.) The blood vessels supplying striated muscle, the lungs, and cardiac muscle grow wider. In those vessels, norepinephrine has a vasodilatory effect. Meanwhile, the vessels supplying the skin, the gastrointestinal tract, and organs such as the spleen are narrowed. In them the same transmitter has a vasoconstrictive effect. Thus the skin grows pale — an appearance typical of anger or fear. The overall pattern of vasodilation and vasoconstriction, in combination with the increased action of the heart and an increased volume of blood, serves to raise the systemic blood pressure. It also shunts blood toward those parts of the body that would be called on to support physical effort.

In and around the eye, the sympathetic has several effects. In the eye itself, the dilator muscle of the pupil contracts. Thus the pupil widens. Behind the eye, the orbital muscle contracts. Thus the eye stands forward in its socket. Above the eye, the tarsal muscle of the upper eyelid contracts. Thus the upper eyelid lifts. Both of these latter effects — the protrusion of the eyeball and the lifting of the eyelid — increase the size of the visual field. They also aid the caricaturist who wants to depict fright or anger. The caricaturist is sure to draw a face with bulging eyes and the whites of the sclera prominent around the iris.

Finally, the sympathetic governs an endocrine gland, the adrenal medulla, whose effects on the body augment the effects the sympathetic produces by means of its postganglionic ramifications. A number of circumstances combine to suggest that the adrenal medulla is a modified autonomic ganglion. First, the cells of the adrenal medulla and the cells of the autonomic ganglia arise (along with most primary sensory neurons) in the same part of the embryo, a part called the neural crest. Second, the chromaffin cells of the adrenal medulla (the type of cell most typical of the medulla) receive preganglionic fibers of the sympathetic nervous system and respond to the neurotransmitter acetylcholine. Third, the chromaffin cells of the adrenal medulla release a substance much like norepinephrine, the postganglionic transmitter of the sympathetic nervous system. Specifically, they release epinephrine (also called adrenalin), which differs from norepinephrine by the addition of a methyl group (CH_3). The epinephrine enters the systemic circulation. Thus it functions as a hormone, as opposed to a neurotransmitter. (In the brain itself it is implicated as a transmitter.) On arriving at visceral tissue, epinephrine is hundreds of times more potent than norepinephrine. In two ways, however, the effects of epinephrine differ from the effects of postganglionic sympathetic innervation. First, epinephrine injected into the systemic circulation of experimental animals promotes the production and release of glucose by the liver. Second, epinephrine does not promote sweating. The postganglionic fibers that innervate the sweat glands are atypical. They are emitted by the sympathetic ganglia, but their transmitter is acetylcholine, not norepinephrine.

The Parasympathetic Periphery

The sympathetic nervous system was well described by the Swiss physiologist W. R. Hess, who called it ergotropic, having coined the term from *ergos,* the

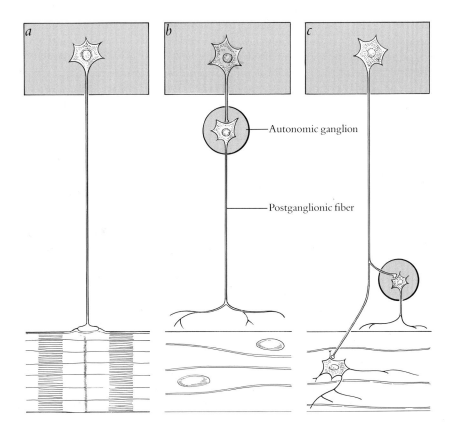

Figure 51: **Styles of motor innervation** are different for somatic innervation on the one hand and visceral, or autonomic, innervation on the other. In the somatic motor pattern a motor neuron in the spinal cord or the brainstem animates striated muscle directly (*a*). In the visceral motor pattern a two-neuron chain is required. The sympathetic nervous system stations a "preganglionic" visceral motor neuron in the spinal cord (*b*). It contacts a second visceral motor neuron, referred to—illogically—as postganglionic, in a ganglion just in front of the vertebral column (prevertebral) or just beside it (paravertebral). The second neuron completes the innervation. The parasympathetic nervous system also employs two-neuron pathways (*c*). The first neuron is situated in the brainstem or toward the bottom of the spinal cord, and the ganglion is close to the viscera (juxtamural) or even inside the viscera (intramural).

Labels in figure: Autonomic ganglion; Postganglionic fiber

Greek for "force," and *tropos*, meaning a "turning" or "switching toward." It is indeed a universal mobilizing mechanism, valuable in emergencies, with postganglionic ramifications throughout the visceral realm. In contrast Hess described the parasympathetic nervous system as trophotropic, having coined the term from *trophos*, meaning "growth." He intended his coinage to signify that the parasympathetic nervous system promotes the restitution of the organism. The parasympathetic is in fact the antagonist of the sympathetic. Yet the postganglionic ramifications of the parasympathetic are far less pervasive. No postganglionic parasympathetic fibers arrive, for example, at blood vessels in the limbs. Also, none arrive in the skin. Many of the functional shifts that countervail the actions of the sympathetic nervous system result, however, from the inhibition of the sympathetic. Thus the blood vessels nourishing the skin can be urged only to constrict, but when the urging is mitigated by inhibition of the sympathetic, the smooth-muscle layers in the wall of the vessels relax toward an innate tonus. Moreover, there are a limited number of what might be called positive parasympathetic effects — effects due to parasympathetic activation. In the cardiovascular system, the parasympathetic decelerates the heartbeat. In the eyes, it makes the pupil constrict. It also innervates the muscle of accommodation, the ciliary muscle, a contractile ring in which the lens of the eye is suspended. In a mammal the lens can move neither forward nor back, as it does in many reptiles. Instead it must accommodate by changing its curvature; the contraction of the ciliary muscle increases its convexity. Further still, the parasympathetic promotes the secretion of saliva from the salivary glands and tears from the lacrimal glands. In the gastrointestinal tract, the parasympathetic promotes peristalsis and the secretion of enzymes by the digestive glands. It also promotes peristalsis of the endgut and relaxation of the sphincter of the anus; it therefore facilitates the emptying of the bowels. Similarly, it relaxes the sphincter of the urinary bladder and activates the detrusor mechanism.

The preganglionic motor neurons of the parasympathetic nervous system are in the brainstem and in a short stretch of the spinal cord near the spinal cord's caudal tip. Like the preganglionic motor neurons of the sympathetic nervous system they employ acetylcholine as their transmitter. Their axons, however, are long, because the ganglia to which the axons project lie near the tissues of the viscera and sometimes even inside them. Cardiac muscle, for example, gets its parasympathetic innervation from a number of small ganglia on the walls of the atria. It gets its sympathetic innervation from the upper three paravertebral ganglia, in the neck. The stomach and intestinal tract get their parasympathetic innervation from the plexus of Auerbach and the plexus of Meissner, which consist of small, interconnected ganglia disseminated throughout the wall of the gut.* They get their sympathetic innerva-

---

*The plexus of Auerbach is disseminated throughout the interface between the outer and inner smooth-muscle layer of the gut; the plexus of Meissner is disseminated throughout the submucosal layer. Both defy traditional views of the autonomic ganglia, in that it now

tion from prevertebral ganglia. The eye gets its parasympathetic innervation from the ciliary ganglion, in the orbita a short distance behind the eyeball. It gets its sympathetic innervation from the superior cervical ganglion, the uppermost of the paravertebral ganglia, high in the neck. One final distinction between the sympathetic and the parasympathetic: the postganglionic transmitter of the parasympathetic is acetylcholine, not norepinephrine. Thus the postganglionic fibers innervating the sweat glands are anatomically part of the sympathetic nervous system; neurochemically, however, they are parasympathetic. As if in confirmation, the average secretion of sweat doubles during the hours of sleep, when the parasympathetic is maximally dominant over the body.

Hypothalamus

In the brain, neurons that affect the activity of the preganglionic motor neurons of the sympathetic and the parasympathetic nervous system appear to be concentrated in the ventral part of the diencephalon: that is, in the hypothalamus. The evidence is clear: when the hypothalamus of almost any animal, emphatically including man, is suddenly destroyed, the animal dies, with upheavals in what the French physiologist Claude Bernard called the internal milieu of the body, a term embracing tissue fluids and organ functions, as determined by blood pressure, heart rate, respiration rate, and so on. Neurosurgeons compelled to operate near the hypothalamus at the base of the forebrain are always concerned, therefore, lest the hypothalamus be so much as buffeted. Indeed, patients have died of hyperthermia (an acute rise in body temperature) after otherwise successful neurosurgery in which the surgeon's caution about injuring the hypothalamus seems to have been exemplary. This is not to say that the stability of the internal milieu is unyielding. The stability must be changeable if the organism is to adapt to changing circumstances. When the proverbial bull comes charging across the proverbial meadow, for example, one's heart rate and blood pressure had best be permitted a considerable increase to facilitate one's escape from a prospective goring. Perhaps homeostasis (the splendid term introduced by Walter B. Cannon of Harvard University) is best defined as the maintenance of certain limits of oscillation within which physiological functions can vary.

Nor is it to say that the hypothalamus has no forbearance whatever. Indeed, when a lesion of the hypothalamus develops slowly (in the form of a slow-growing tumor, for example), the damage may stay quite covert. This remarkable fact, well established by clinical experience, was demonstrated in a

seems they receive afferents from not only preganglionic motor neurons but also the wall of the intestine. They thus form a true intestinal nervous system, with the intrinsic capacity to integrate input and generate output. They are far more than mere stopovers on autonomic innervation paths from the central nervous system.

telling way by the German physiologist Rudolf Thauer, who tied a string around the rostral brainstem of a living rabbit just below the hypothalamus and passed the ends of the string through two small holes in the skull. Each day he tightened the string by about a millimeter. If a few weeks passed before the hypothalamus had been completely disconnected from the brainstem, the rabbit's vital functions were apparently undisturbed. Yet life in a laboratory cage is undemanding. A harsher environment would reveal that such a rabbit can no longer compensate effectively for marked changes in external temperature. In cold weather, the rabbit proves unable to shiver. Shivering, an automatism of striated musculature, is evidently under hypothalamic control. Moreover, the blood vessels supplying the skin of the rabbit fail to constrict, and the hairs on the skin do not erect. In hot weather, blood vessels in the ear of the rabbit fail to dilate. They evidently serve, under parasympathetic

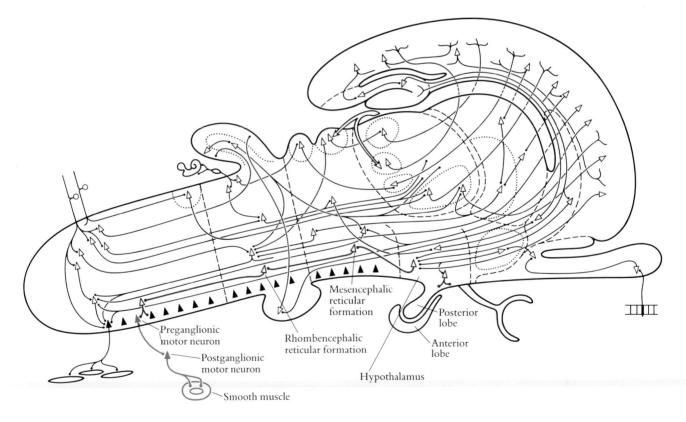

Mesencephalic
reticular
formation

Posterior
lobe

Preganglionic
motor neuron

Rhombencephalic
reticular formation

Anterior
lobe

Postganglionic
motor neuron

Hypothalamus

Smooth muscle

Figure 52: **Hypothalamus governs the viscera** in two ways. First, the hypothalamus emits axons that descend toward preganglionic visceral motor neurons, both sympathetic and parasympathetic. Although direct lines have been discovered, the more typical pattern (*dark color*) is a line interrupted in the midbrain, in the hindbrain, and in the spinal cord. A two-neuron innervation path characteristic of the autonomic nervous system (*light color*) leaves the spinal cord at the lower left. Second, the hypothalamus controls both lobes of the pituitary complex. Details of the control are schematized in the next two illustrations.

governance, to dissipate heat. Still, a remarkable amount of homeostatic control remains intact (or is regained) in the wake of a slowly made lesion. Thauer next began, in the same animals and using a similar technique, to interfere slowly with descending connections low in the mesencephalon. The deficits again were covert. It is as if there were a chain of command in the autonomic nervous system, or, as Bernard put it, an automatism of levels, so that when the hypothalamus is slowly incapacitated, regions of the brain below the hypothalamus can keep the internal milieu stable, albeit within abnormally narrow limits. Indeed, if the animal survives a sequence of slowly made lesions including a last one made in the spinal cord, a surprising proportion of visceral function persists.

The resilience of autonomic control accords well with what is known about the conduction lines descending from the hypothalamus. In particular, fibers passing directly from the hypothalamus to the lateral horn of the spinal cord's gray matter, where the preganglionic motor neurons of the sympathetic nervous system are situated, have recently been found. The fibers seem, however, to constitute a small minority of hypothalamic efferents; the hypothalamus has nothing like a pyramidal tract to carry its descending output. Instead it appears in large measure to project no farther than the midbrain, where neurons of the reticular formation take over. In fact, the pathways descending to autonomic motor neurons are interrupted at numerous levels (Figure 52). At each such interruption, further instructions can enter the descending lines. It is appropriate that this should be so. Life depends on the innervation of the viscera; in a way, all the rest is biological luxury. And vital systems ought to be organized on the principle that no single source of excitation should have hegemony over their workings. The convergence of information on motor neurons may be as prominent in the autonomic nervous system as it is in the somatic.

Paths to the Pituitary

The autonomic nervous system is not the only means by which the hypothalamus regulates the viscera. In addition the hypothalamus governs both the anterior and the posterior lobe of the pituitary complex. The earliest evidence of such governance derived from clinical cases in which internists made a tentative diagnosis of pathology of the pituitary. They suspected, for example, an adenoma: a tumor of the anterior lobe. After all, the symptoms included atrophy (or its opposite, hypertrophy) of the gonads or the adrenal cortex, which can be traced to a lack (or an overproduction) of certain hormones the anterior lobe releases into the systemic circulation. (All of the endocrine glands except the parathyroid gland, the adrenal medulla, and the beta cells of the islands of Langerhans in the pancreas are controlled — in fact they are kept from atrophy — by one or another of the hormones released by the pituitary complex.) Sometimes the symptoms were dramatic. A boy of five would appear in the clinic with fully developed genitals, hair on his abdomen and chest, a deep male voice, and a body markedly larger than one would expect of a child of that age. In brief, his puberty was precocious. The cause, one might assume, is oversecretion of somatotropin (growth hormone) on the part of the anterior lobe. Yet in some cases it later emerged that the pituitary gland was normal. The pathology lay instead in the hypothalamus.

The medical science of the time—say between the two World Wars—found this difficult to explain. For one thing, the anterior lobe is not a part of the brain. It is epithelial tissue that develops from the roof of the embryonic oral cavity. In addition, no hypothalamic fibers enter the anterior lobe. How, then, can the hypothalamus control it? A functional link between the two is established by blood vessels (Figure 53). Off from the circle of Willis, an arterial interchange at the base of the brain, come slender vessels known as the hypophysial arteries. In spite of their name they send many branches into the funnel-shaped, ventralmost part of the hypothalamus. There, in the region preceding the pituitary stalk (a region called the median eminence), the arterial branches produce a set of peculiar, looping capillaries. In turn, the capillaries collect to form blood-drainage channels. Morphologically, the drainage channels are veins, yet they enter the anterior lobe of the pituitary, where they ramify into a second bed of capillaries, much as if they were arteries. A vein that ramifies into capillaries is called a portal vein; the ones at issue are called the hypothalamopituitary portal system. They form the functional link. By now it is well established that certain neurons in the hypothalamus send their axons only as far as the first of the capillary beds (the one in the median eminence). There they release their neurotransmitters, or rather their chemical products. The products are known as releasing factors (R.F.'s) or releasing hormones (R.H.'s). One of them, thyrotropin releasing factor, is simply a tripeptide: a concatenation of three amino acids, in this case glutamate, histidine, and proline. Yet on its arrival in the anterior lobe (where the portal system takes it) each releasing factor proves capable of inducing certain cells in the lobe to release a hormone that the cells have synthesized and that they hold in reserve.*

A different functional link leads from the hypothalamus to the posterior lobe of the pituitary complex. This one is more direct, in that it is wholly

---

*The hormones released by the anterior lobe of the pituitary gland are called tropic hormones. Each is the second and final messenger in a sequence of chemical signals leading from the brain to a particular endocrine gland. Again consider a hypothalamic product: thyrotropin releasing factor. It induces certain cells in the anterior lobe to release thyrotropin, a tropic hormone. In turn, thyrotropin (which enters the systemic circulation) induces its target gland, the thyroid gland, to release its characteristic, biologically active secretion, namely the hormone thyroxin. By a similar cascade of directed chemical signals, corticotropin releasing factor induces certain cells in the anterior lobe to release adrenocorticotropic hormone (ACTH), which induces the adrenal cortex to release corticosteroid hormones. Several other cascades are known. All the tropic (literally "switch-on") hormones of the anterior lobe are at the same time trophic (growth-promotion or maintenance) hormones, in whose absence their target glands atrophy.

neural: it does not include a part of the circulatory system. It begins in two circumscribed, magnocellular nuclei: the supraoptic nucleus and the paraventricular nucleus. They are the first hypothalamic nuclei whose function has been identified with some precision. In the 1930's Ernst and Berta Scharrer, then in Germany and later successively at the University of Colorado and the Albert Einstein College of Medicine in New York, reported that cells of the supraoptic nucleus and the paraventricular nucleus contain inclusions, which the Scharrers described as colloid droplets. The Scharrers proposed that the cells secrete the stuff of the droplets, and thus that the cells, which undoubt-

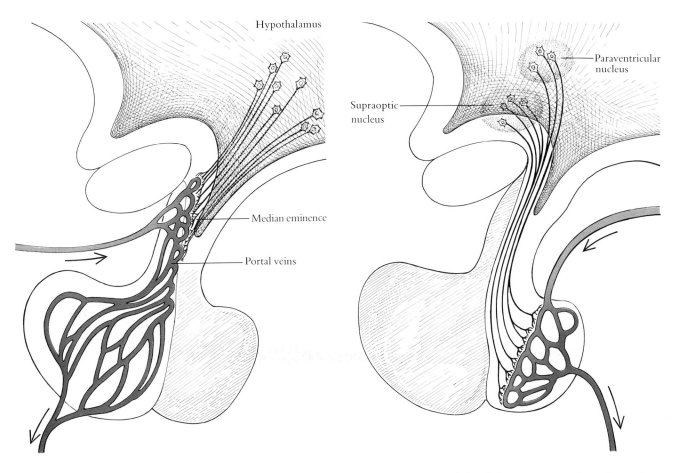

Figure 53: **Anterior lobe** of the pituitary complex makes several hormones and is induced to release them by chemical signals called releasing factors, which are secreted by hypothalamic neurons. The factors enter the hypothalamopituitary portal system, comprising first a capillary bed in the hypothalamus, then a venous drainage channel, and then, in the anterior lobe, a second capillary bed.

Figure 54: **Posterior lobe** of the pituitary complex makes no hormones; the two the lobe releases are supplied to it by axons. In particular, neurons in the hypothalamic cell groups called the supraoptic nucleus and the paraventricular nucleus make vasopressin and oxytocin. Their axons attain the posterior lobe and emit the hormones there.

edly are neurons, at the same time are glandular. It was an unpopular idea at the time the Scharrers proposed it. Later findings, however, confirmed it. In the late 1940's evidence showed that the droplet material is transported down the axons of the cells. Still later the electron microscope established that the droplets are aggregations of secretory granules. For their part, all (or nearly all) of the axons originating in the supraoptic nucleus, along with some 30 percent of the axons originating in the paraventricular nucleus,* pass through the pituitary stalk and so attain the posterior lobe of the pituitary (Figure 54). Unlike the anterior lobe, it is a part of the brain. Nevertheless it contains no neurons; hence the terminals of the supraoptic and paraventricular axons make no synaptic contacts. Instead they lie embedded in a tissue composed of the modified glial cells called pituicytes and a dense plexus of capillaries. There the glandular products of the supraoptic nucleus and the paraventricular nucleus are stored in the axon terminals until the neurons of those nuclei are called on to release them. And on release there seems nothing for the substances to accomplish in the posterior lobe except to enter the systemic circulation. The substances are the pair of chemically similar peptide hormones vasopressin and oxytocin.

Since they lie in the brain, a matrix of bioelectric communication, the neurons in the hypothalamus that secrete releasing factors and hormones may seem to be out of place. If so, three countering arguments can be offered. First, the neurons at issue are final common pathways. Numerous influences converge on them, just as numerous influences converge on motor neurons in the brainstem or the spinal cord, and they have only their axons by which to influence the periphery. Second, the neurons at issue are not the only instance of brain cells with endocrine function. Roger Guillemin of the Salk Institute has presented strong evidence, for example, that neurons disseminated throughout the brainstem secrete systemically active products: chemicals meant to mediate a biological effect in cells of the periphery. Among these chemicals is the peptide somatostatin, which is suspected to be both a neurotransmitter and a hormone. Somatostatin is implicated in the cessation of bodily growth. It acts in the anterior lobe of the pituitary, where it counters the secretion of somatotropin. Another hormone secreted by neurons turns out to inhibit the gonadotrophic influence of the pituitary. One need not give a catalog. The point is simply the growing intimations that the brain is secretly a gland.

The third argument is analogical. This book began with an account of recent opinion about the phylogenetic emergence of the nervous system, in which it was noted that secretory granules seem to be almost ubiquitous in the cells of simple invertebrate organisms. In brief, essentially all of the cells in

---

*The remaining 70 percent have several destinations, of which one is especially notable: the paraventricular nucleus is a substantial contributor to the pathway descending from the hypothalamus direct to the lateral horn of the spinal cord, which contains the spinal cord's preganglionic sympathetic motor neurons.

the simple invertebrate appear to be glandular. Now, most of the neurons in the human brain are not effector cells. In fact, none of them are effectors, in that none of them are contractile. Yet some of them, including the neurons of the supraoptic nucleus and the paraventricular nucleus, are committed to the production of a systemically active chemical. Perhaps they strictly adhere to the style of incipient neurons in primitive invertebrates. Others produce releasing factors. That is, they instigate a channeled chemical cascade that ultimately induces an endocrine gland to put its hormone in the systemic circulation. Still others—indeed all the rest of the billions—produce a chemical intended for the transmission of private messages to a specific set of postsynaptic loci. Such cells have nothing to say directly to the organism as a whole. In their specialized way, however, they, too, are secretory.

Chapter Nine

Affect and Motivation; The Limbic System

In the preceding chapter the hypothalamus emerged in two great functional realms: the regulation of the effector cells of the viscera and the regulation of endocrine glands. It will now emerge in a third, less tangible realm. Consider again the instances of precocious puberty initially attributed to the oversecretion of growth hormone by an adenoma of the anterior lobe of the pituitary complex but due in fact to an overgoading of the anterior lobe by a tumorous hypothalamus. If the tumor is inoperable and therefore continues its slow destruction of the hypothalamus, the child usually dies without having attained the size of an adult. (The immediate cause of death is often pneumonia.) Before then, he may have spells of extreme and spontaneous anger. Ultimately he shows apathy and dementia. Consider the electrical stimulation of certain parts of the hypothalamus in an experimental animal. Under such stimulation the animal — a cat, for example — may begin to pace back and forth. Its behavior suggests agitation. The cat may also be rendered liable to spit and lash out with its claws at anyone who attempts to stroke its fur or merely approaches its cage. Indeed, cats have been induced by the electrical stimulation of the hypothalamus to attack a laboratory rat with which they had hitherto shared their cage and their food. Consider, too, the reaction elicited by applying painful stimuli to a cat or a dog following the surgical excision of the animal's cerebral hemispheres and most of the diencephalon, leaving only the brainstem and the caudal half of the hypothalamus attached to the spinal cord. The reaction can be abolished by a further lesion that excises the caudal hypothalamus. As described by Philip Bard of Johns Hopkins University in the late 1920's, the reaction includes growling and spitting, dilation of the pupils, increased heart rate, and the erection of fur. The animal's teeth are bared, and so are its claws (in the case of the cat). In short, the animal presents a perfect picture of fury.

The first two pieces of evidence are straightforward. They suggest that the hypothalamus mediates emotional behavior. The third has been problematic, in part because the animals in Bard's experiments proved unable to direct their apparent anger toward any object in particular, and in part because the transection of the animals' brain eliminated the possibility that the cerebral cortex had brought on the anger. For both reasons the display observed by Bard was taken to represent only the outward appearance of emotion, and not the inner feeling. It was therefore called sham rage. Then, in 1953, James

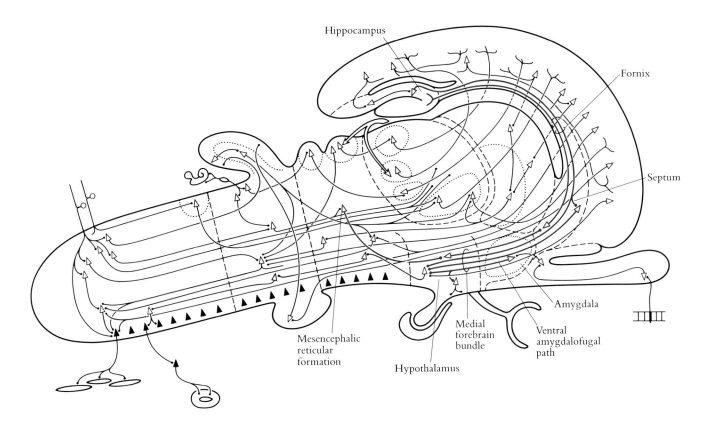

Figure 55: **Alliance with the hypothalamus** is the criterion distinguishing a continuum of brain tissue that reaches from the midbrain to the margin (or free edge) of the cerebral cortex. In this diagram the mesencephalic pole of the continuum is represented by an axon that ascends to the hypothalamus from a neuron in the mesencephalic reticular formation. The prosencephalic pole is more extensive. It includes the hippocampus and the septum, which are linked to the hypothalamus by a massive axon bundle, the fornix. Moreover, it includes the amygdala, which is linked to the hypothalamus by the ventral amygdalofugal path and the stria terminalis. (The latter does not appear in the illustration.) In the hypothalamus the links tend to coalesce into a heterogeneous tract, the medial forebrain bundle. The part of the continuum positioned in the forebrain is called the limbic system.

Olds and Peter Milner, at McGill University, reported that the weak electrical stimulation of sites for the most part in the hypothalamus or its rostral continuation, the septum, could elicit in experimental animals an internal state of pleasure, or in any case what psychologists describe as a state of reward. Olds and Milner had given laboratory rats the opportunity to press a lever in their cage and thereby close the circuit that delivered the stimulation. The rats had repeatedly done just that. Quite often, in fact, the rats had gone without eating and instead had persisted in their intracranial self-stimulation until they dropped from exhaustion. One might suspect the repeated pressing of the lever was a motor automatism, precipitated by a seizure that accompanied each instance of stimulation. It turned out, however, that the rats were willing to negotiate forbidding obstacles to get to the switch. Moreover, if the circuit was disconnected part way through the experiment, so that the pressing of the lever had no effect, the rats ran about in what an observer would surely describe as frustration. Further still, the weak electrical stimulation of sites that often lay no more than a millimeter away from a site at which stimulation had elicited a state of reward elicited either no state of reward or else the opposite of reward, namely aversion. After a single stimulation of such a site, the rat might retreat from the lever and show obvious reluctance to return.

The work of Olds and Milner gives a basis for the claim that the hypothalamus, and more generally a continuum of brain tissue in which the hypothalamus is central, involves itself not only in endocrine and visceral function (the measurable signs of emotion), but also in affect and motivation. The first term signifies the impact of the environment on an organism—the vital feelings, in other words, that are elicited in the organism by its internal and external milieu. Pleasure is an example. The second term signifies a state of need or desire: hunger is an example. The two are often related, because an affect can be the cause of a motivation. Still, an affect does not necessarily prompt the organism to take any particular action, whereas a motivation does so by definition.

Allies of the Hypothalamus

What composes the neural continuum in which the hypothalamus is central? For one thing, a part of the brainstem. Figure 55 shows a representative axon that ascends to the hypothalamus from a cell in the mesencephalic reticular formation—a cell that got its own input from a spinoreticular fiber. What the figure does not show (for lack of space) is a set of axons directed upward to the hypothalamus from the nucleus of the solitary tract, a cell group in the medulla oblongata. They are a fairly recent discovery. They are also quite revealing. The nucleus of the solitary tract is the only known instance of a circumscribed secondary sensory cell group whose primary sensory input is from the visceral domain. That is, its primary sensory afferents station their sensory endings in the wall of the respiratory tract, the wall of the digestive tract, and the walls of the heart and its vascular trunks. The endings fall into two classes. Some are positioned in the sliding planes between layers of smooth-muscle tissue. Such endings are baroreceptive, from the Greek *baros,* meaning weight: they report the stretching, or in some instances the relaxing, of the muscle. The other endings monitor some aspect of the chemistry of a fluid: the acidity of blood plasma, for example. Such endings are chemoreceptive. The point is plain: the conduction lines leading direct to the hypothalamus from the nucleus of the solitary tract amount to a visceral sensory lemniscus.

A second part of the continuum in which the hypothalamus is central lies rostral to the hypothalamus. It lies, then, in the cerebral hemisphere. A little more than a century ago, Pierre Paul Broca observed that an almost annular ring of tissue on the medial face of the cerebral hemisphere represents the free edge of the cerebral cortex. He called the ring *le grand lobe de l'ourlet:* the great lobe of the hem. It is a forceful expression of what he saw. In later years he was persuaded nevertheless to call the ring *le grand lobe limbique:* the great limbic lobe. The word *limbique* he took from the Latin *limbus,* meaning edge, border, or fringe. Still later, the ring came to be called the rhinencephalon—the nose-brain—as a result of the conviction that all of it serves the sense of smell. After all, the only sensory structure that clearly links itself to the ring is the olfactory tract, which attaches to the uncus, literally the hook, a place where the great limbic lobe turns back on itself at the base of the brain. In the 1930's, however, it became evident to James W. Papez of Cornell University that olfaction is not the principal source of rhinencephalic input. (The principal source, established three decades later, is association cortex.) Thus it became desirable to find a neutral term: a term in which olfaction is not dominant. Broca's term was resurrected; in English *le grand lobe limbique* is the limbic system, a name proposed in 1952 by Paul D. MacLean, who was then at Yale University. Its constituents vary, depending on who lists them; the limbic system's border is not sharp everywhere. In all accounts the list includes the hippocampus, a composite of two interrelated cortical gyri that occupies the medial wall of the cerebral hemisphere but is removed from sight on the medial face of the hemisphere by the infolding of the great limbic lobe. The list includes the ring-shaped gyrus fornicatus, the part of the great limbic lobe fully visible on the medial face of the hemisphere. (It can be seen in Figure 90.) It, too, is cortex, but cortex of various types. The list includes the amygdala, a large mass of gray matter, almost none of it cortex, that is hidden under the uncus.

Limbic Functions

What does the limbic system do? The evidence is varied. In fact, it is disconcertingly varied. On the one hand, it suggests that the hippocampus is a gatekeeper embodying the brain's ability to commit things to lasting memory. In that regard the single most telling piece of evidence emerged in the

1950's, when a neurosurgical procedure intended as a treatment of otherwise intractable forms of epilepsy served inadvertently to demonstrate that the removal of the hippocampus on both sides of the human brain entails a disorder now called hippocampal amnesia. The patient retains the memories he collected well before the surgery. But he cannot collect any new ones. As he reads toward the bottom of a printed page, he may already have lost all recollection of what he just read at the top. And as he speaks to a new acquaintance, he may interrupt the conversation to ask a second time for the name and the purpose of his visitor, whom he suddenly does not know. On the other hand, the evidence concerning the amygdala suggests a bewildering number of functions. In man the electrical stimulation of the amygdala is sometimes of diagnostic use to the neurosurgeon. The patient is conscious during the procedure. Often he reports undirected feelings of fear or anger. The feelings can be accompanied by abdominal or thoracic sensations — for example, the sensation that the stomach is churning. Urination can accompany the feeling of fear. In animals, the electrical stimulation of the amygdala elicits arousal. The animal stops what it was doing. If it was lying down, it gets up. It looks around as if it were searching. Often it exhibits snout automatisms: sniffing, licking, chewing, swallowing. In some instances the stimulation elicits behavior that investigators classify as fearlike, defenselike, or attacklike. In the African green monkey, or vervet, the excision of the amygdala on both sides of the brain yields still another finding. In the laboratory, the monkey is readily kept alive. Returned to nature, it cannot maintain itself, and soon dies. The reason is poignant: the monkey ostracizes itself from the group of monkeys of which it was part. Indeed, it exhausts itself evading its peers. It seems to be constantly anxious and depressed. According to Arthur Kling of Rutgers University, who made the investigation, the amygdalectomized monkey can no longer distinguish between friendly and unfriendly gestures on the part of other monkeys, and perceives all approaches as a threat.

It may seem surprising that structures as varied as the hippocampus, the gyrus fornicatus, and the amygdala are said to make up a system. Nevertheless, they share two attributes. First, they share a low threshold for epilepsy, the communal derangement of neuronal activity in which the cells produce synchronized action potentials. Epileptic seizures can thus remain confined to the great limbic lobe and not "spill over" to other parts of the brain. The signs of such seizures — which constitute temporal-lobe or psychomotor epilepsy — are several, but some of them are distinctive and seem to echo the evidence described in the preceding paragraph. To begin with, the seizure announces itself to the patient as hallucinatory sensations, which compose what is called the aura of the seizure. Common among the sensations is an olfactory or gustatory illusion: a peculiar, almost always disagreeable odor or taste that recurs with each new seizure. (Patients not on medication may have from one to five seizures per day.) Other initial sensations are of a more mental type. The patient may have a disturbing feeling of excessive familiarity with what is happening (*sentiment du déjà-vu*) or conversely a feeling of frightening strangeness (*sentiment de l'inconnu*). Further still, the patient may undergo a marked change in mood. Most typically, the patient's feelings modulate into anxiety or a pronounced sense of loneliness. In some cases the feeling is anger. After any of these beginnings the patient lapses into a dreamy state, becoming unresponsive to the environment and intensely preoccupied, it seems, with the internal self. In turn, this second phase of the seizure gives way to a final, motoric phase, which may vary from a grand mal seizure to minor automatisms such as aimless fumbling with articles of clothing. The motoric phase can take the remarkable form of perfectly coordinated serial actions: say, paying a waiter, putting on one's overcoat, and boarding the right bus home. The sequence draws faultlessly on stored memories; the sequence would otherwise be impossible. And yet it is characteristic of a pyschomotor seizure with a complex motoric phase that the patient, on "waking up" from the seizure, has no memory of what happened. Access to stored memories was unimpeded, but the recording of new ones stopped.

If one grants that the structures of the limbic system are prominent in creating déjà vu or a modulation in mood, among other signs of psychomotor epilepsy, one must conclude that the limbic system is a determinant of the organism's attitude toward its environment. Hippocampal amnesia can be analyzed in that context. Perhaps the brain assigns an affective value—a degree of meaningfulness—to passing events, and this assignment participates in making things memorable. The hippocampus, a limbic structure, would then assume a role in the brain much like that of the official in a government who is valued for his sagacity in affixing to certain documents the seals that will distinguish them in storage from what is deemed insignificant. The brain's storehouse for memory, however, remains unknown. Hippocampal amnesia, which does not obliterate memories already stored, suggests that the storehouse cannot be the hippocampus itself.

Limbic Circuitry

The second reason for grouping the hippocampus, the gyrus fornicatus, and the amygdala into a single system is that all of them participate in neural circuits linking them to the hypothalamus. The hippocampus projects to the hypothalamus by means of the fornix, literally the arch, a fiber bundle whose arcuate trajectory along the free edge of the cerebral cortex is suggested in Figure 55. The fornix is impressively massive: in the human brain it comprises a million fibers, which makes it the equal (in that respect) of the optic tract. About half of its fibers (in both the cat and the monkey) project directly from the hippocampus to the hypothalamus. The remaining half make their connections in the septum, from which new lines arise that extend to the hypothalamus. The amygdala projects to the hypothalamus by means of two distinct fiber systems. The one suggested in Figure 55 is the ventral amygdalofugal path. It is a loosely arranged group of fibers whose trajectory from the amygdala to the hypothalamus is short and direct. The other one, not shown in Figure 55, is the stria terminalis. A compact fiber bundle, it makes a bizarre and lengthy detour. In fact, it makes more than one complete spiraling turn around the diencephalon before it enters the hypothalamus.

Finally, the gyrus fornicatus is part of a far-ranging loop of projections extending from the hippocampus to the hypothalamus, then to the thalamus, then to the gyrus fornicatus, and finally back to the hippocampus. The first part of the loop is the fornix: it carries signals from the hippocampus to the mammillary body, a prominent, circumscribed cell mass at the caudal end of the hypothalamus. Then comes a projection (the mammillothalamic tract) directed from the mammillary body to the thalamic cell group designated the anterior nucleus, and after that a projection from the anterior nucleus to the cingulate gyrus, the dorsal limb of the gyrus fornicatus. Next the cingulate fasciculus, a fiber bundle intrinsic to the gyrus fornicatus, carries signals around the ring of the gyrus. It enters the ventral limb of the gyrus, called the hippocampal (or parahippocampal) gyrus. There a part of the parahippocampal gyrus called the entorhinal area proves to provide the hippocampus with its single most massive input; thus the loop is closed. It was the recognition of much of this loop of projections that led Papez to refute the notion that the hippocampus merely serves "in some obscure way the olfactory sector of functions." (The quote is from Papez.) Today the entire loop is called the Papez circuit.

Many of the connections we have named are reciprocated. Thus fibers project from the hypothalamus to the hippocampus, to the amygdala, and to the mesencephalic reticular formation. Figure 55 shows an instance of such reciprocity. The figure includes a fiber ascending toward the cerebral hemisphere along the trajectory of the fornix. The fiber gets no farther than the septum, where it synapses with a neuron whose axon attains the hippocampus. On its rise to the septum, however, the fiber is paralleled by a fiber going the opposite way, from septum to hypothalamus. In Figure 55 this two-way forebrain traffic represents the more complex reality of the medial forebrain bundle, a loose aggregation of fibers most apparent in the brain on their lengthwise course through the lateral hypothalamus. The fibers commingle with gray matter there, so that the lateral hypothalamus is an admixture of gray and white, much like the reticular formation of the midbrain and the hindbrain. The fibers that descend in the medial forebrain bundle have their most forward origins in places such as the amygdala and the septum. Some of them originate in the hypothalamus. They distribute themselves in the hypothalamus and beyond it, in the mesencephalic reticular formation. Conversely, the fibers that ascend in the medial forebrain bundle, roughly equal in number to the fibers that descend, originate largely in the mesencephalon. They ascend toward the cerebral hemisphere. Some of them contain a monoamine neurotransmitter, namely serotonin, norepinephrine, or dopamine. Indeed, the medial forebrain bundle has emerged in recent years as the great highway for monoaminergic fibers ascending from the hindbrain and midbrain into the forebrain. It is the only place in the brain where the main conduction lines for the three monoamines commingle. The lines employing serotonin are now suspected to be the ones that ramify most widely. Originating in the so-called raphe nuclei of the midbrain, they innervate essentially everything in the forebrain: the striatum, the limbic system, the neocortex. The lines employing norepinephrine originate mainly in the locus ceruleus, at the caudal border of the midbrain. They ramify almost as widely. In contrast to both, the lines employing dopamine are targeted preferentially on the striatum. (These are the lines from the substantia nigra implicated in Parkinson's disease.) In addition, they fastidiously choose some limbic targets: the amygdala, the septum, the entorhinal area. Most remarkable, perhaps, they choose in the neocortex only the frontal association fields. Still, all three monoaminergic projections ascending from the midbrain in the medial forebrain bundle attain the neocortex. Before the discovery of the monoaminergic projections, the fiber systems attaining the neocortex were thought to arise exclusively in the thalamus.

Limbic Inputs

To summarize: The caudal pole of the continuum in which the hypothalamus is central receives the downward discharge of the hippocampus and the amygdala by way of the fornix, the stria terminalis, the ventral amygdalofugal pathway, and the medial forebrain bundle. The rostral pole of the continuum receives the upward discharge of the mesencephalic reticular formation in part by way of the Papez circuit, which involves the anterior nucleus of the thalamus, and in part by way of a thalamic bypass including monoaminergic projections that ascend in the medial forebrain bundle. This does not mean the continuum is closed. We have already seen that lines extend from the hypothalamus, at the heart of the continuum, toward the visceral motor mechanisms of the autonomic nervous system and the endocrine mechanisms of the pituitary complex. Moreover, we have seen that sensory data—presumably visceral sensory data—enter the caudal pole of the continuum by way of ascending lines from the spinal cord and the brainstem.

The lines we now shall trace enter the rostral pole. That is, they enter the limbic system. As we shall see, they render it omnisensory. We start at the primary visual cortex: area 17 of Brodmann. It gets fibers bearing visual information from the lateral geniculate body of the thalamus, and it reciprocates the projection. In addition, it projects to thalamic gray matter that receives fibers from the superior colliculus and projects in turn to association cortex. For our present purpose we disregard these hails reverberating between neocortex and thalamus (and also the traffic passing from neocortex on one side of the brain to neocortex on the opposite side). Instead we examine the ipsilateral spread of visual information in the neocortical sheet (Figure 56). Area 17, the primary visual cortex, is at the posterior tip of the cerebral hemisphere. It projects to area 18, a band of surrounding neocortex. Area 18 projects to area 19, a second band surrounding the first; area 19 projects to the inferior parietal lobule, which lies on the side of the cerebral hemisphere; the

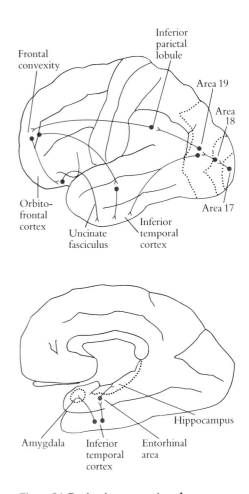

Figure 56: **Projections spanning the neocortex** carry cascading signals from primary sensory fields through a succession of association fields. The illustration shows the known visual sequence (*top drawing*). Basically, the primary visual cortex, at the posterior pole of the cerebral hemisphere, projects to a band of surrounding neocortex, which projects to a second band surrounding the first. From there paths extend toward two expanses of association cortex, one frontal, the other temporal, which communicate with each other. From the latter (*bottom drawing*) projections attain the amygdala and (with interruption) the hippocampus. Similar patterns emerge for the other senses represented in neocortex. A simplified pattern is part of the next illustration.

inferior parietal lobule projects to the side, or convexity, of the frontal lobe; and the frontal convexity projects to the underside, or orbital surface, of the frontal lobe. In addition, the frontal convexity projects to the superior and middle temporal gyri, which lie ventral to the inferior parietal lobule. They project to the inferior temporal gyrus, toward the underside of the brain. Area 19 projects to the inferior temporal gyrus directly.

The sequence is complex. Moreover, it lies in register with sequences of similar complexity that begin in the other primary sensory fields. Nevertheless, a pattern emerges. All of the senses represented in neocortex — vision, hearing, and the somatic sense — direct part of their traffic toward either or both of two cortical districts: the frontal association cortex and the inferior

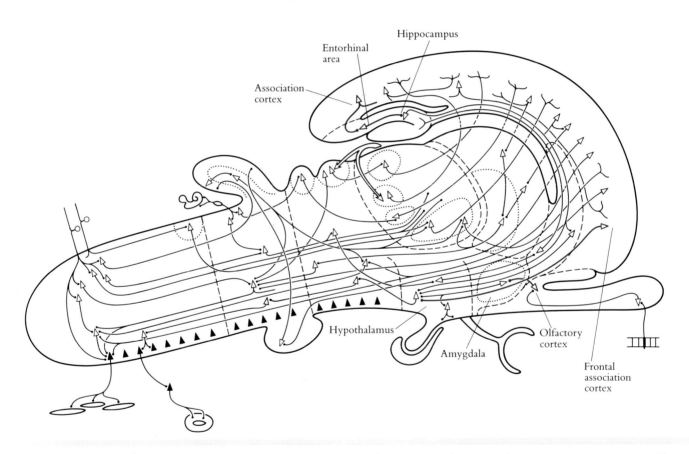

Figure 57: **Gateways to the limbic system** appear in color in this diagram, the last of 15 diagrams summarizing the neural circuitry of the mammalian brain and spinal cord. The principal gate is the entorhinal area, a cortical field near the edge of the cerebral cortex. The entorhinal area receives projections that cascade across the neocortical sheet; then it projects to the hippocampus. In this way it makes the limbic system a recipient of neocortical signals with ante-

cedents in vision, hearing, and somatic sensation. A comparable pathway running from neocortex to the amygdala does not appear in the illustration. Olfaction, too, has access to limbic structures. Its most straightforward access is shown by a projection from the primary olfactory cortex direct to the amygdala. One final projection subverts the notion that the limbic system is well delimited. The frontal association cortex projects to the hypothalamus.

temporal association cortex. The two are interconnected by a massive fiber bundle called the uncinate fasciculus. In turn, the inferior temporal cortex projects to the entorhinal area. The entorhinal area is the cortical gateway to the hippocampus (Figure 57). In addition, the inferior temporal cortex projects to the amygdala. In fact in primates it gives the amygdala its single most massive input. The projection is reciprocated. Indeed, the amygdala directs its cortical projections to the inferior temporal cortex and to the frontal cortex (specifically the orbital surface of the frontal cortex). It projects, therefore, to the parts of the neocortex in which the final stages in the cascade of sensory data toward the limbic system are embodied. Evidently the amygdala screens its neocortical input. Perhaps, then, it intervenes in ideation and cognition. Ordinarily, one thinks of brain function as working from sensory mechanisms inward—as being directed from sensory receptor organs over a sequence of synaptic way stations to sensory cortex, and from there (in what Papez called "the stream of thought") toward the limbic system. Here we encounter the opposite: a set of connections directed outward. It is as if the amygdala were participating in the brain's appreciation of the world.

The participation suggests a distinction between the interoceptive and exteroceptive data reaching the neural continuum in which the hypothalamus is central. The former, consisting of visceral sensory signals from the spinal cord and the brainstem, are probably unconditional stimuli pertinent to the maintenance of life itself. They may report, for instance, that blood pressure is dropping, and so they require that countermeasures (say an increase of sympathetic tonus and a concomitant inhibition of the parasympathetic) be activated unconditionally—that is, without regard to other aspects of the state of the organism. What enters the limbic system from the neocortex is fundamentally different. One might call it a repeatedly preprocessed, multisensory representation of the organism's environment. In this domain nothing is unconditional: the perception of the world is biased by physiological needs. One is reminded of a hungry child's visit to a restaurant. Entering, he sees what people have on their plates. Leaving, he sees that the diners also have faces.

What about olfaction? The relation between it and the limbic system, once thought to be a relation excluding the other senses, so that the limbic system was taken to be the nose-brain, really amounts to this: First, the primary olfactory cortex projects to the entorhinal area; the entorhinal area projects to the hippocampus. Thus we see reintroduced, after years of fervent affirmation followed by years of fervent denial, the idea that the hippocampus gets olfactory signals. In a way, the signals are privileged: the path from the olfactory epithelium to the hippocampus does not require a cascade of projections across the neocortical sheet. Hence the path from the olfactory epithelium is more direct than the path from sensory surfaces such as the skin. Second, the primary olfactory cortex projects to the amygdala, in large part to a particular cell group, the lateral nucleus of the amygdala. Again the paths are privileged in that they bypass the neocortex. It is reported that the olfactory bulb projects to the amygdala (specifically to the cortical nucleus of the amygdala), but one wonders whether this connection is present in man. It has been demonstrated in animals such as rodents, where it arises in the accessory olfactory bulb, a compartment of the bulb receiving input from a specialized area of the nasal mucosa called the vomeronasal organ. The two are thought to form an apparatus dedicated to the processing of sexually significant odors; in the fully formed human body neither one has been identified. Finally, the primary olfactory cortex projects to the hypothalamus.

One connection remains. The orbital part of the frontal cortex—alone in the neocortex—projects to the hypothalamus. Thus the limbic system founders as a circumscribed part of the brain, quite distinct from the neocortex. After all, the modern criterion for membership in the limbic system is a synaptic proximity to the hypothalamus, and the frontal cortex has that. In fact it has uninterrupted access to the visceral, endocrine, and affective mechanisms of the hypothalamic continuum. No other part of the neocortex has access so direct. What, then, is the frontal cortex? In the first place, the frontal cortex has long been notable for its lack of primary sensory fields. It is entirely association cortex. Indeed, as we have noted, the tracing of large-scale projections in the white matter underlying the cerebral cortex suggests that the frontal cortex is a neocortical end of the line: it is a destination for sequential projections that begin in the primary sensory fields. Second, the frontal cortex is a destination for signals with antecedents in the primary olfactory cortex. Like everything else about the olfactory circuitry, their pathway is idiosyncratic. It begins with fibers projecting from the olfactory cortex to the thalamus—belatedly, one might complain, because all other sensory conduction paths pass through the thalamus before they attain their field of primary sensory cortex. The scofflaw olfactory system makes its connections in the opposite order. The fibers end in a large thalamic cell group called the mediodorsal nucleus. Specifically, they end in the medial subdivision of the mediodorsal nucleus, a district of the nucleus in which the neurons are relatively large. The mediodorsal nucleus projects to the frontal association cortex; the medial subdivision contributes to that projection by directing its fibers to the frontal lobe's orbital surface. Third, the frontal cortex is a destination for signals representing the internal state of the organism. These arrive in part from the amygdala. They may also arrive from the mediodorsal nucleus. No massive, circumscribed fiber bundles afferent to the mediodorsal nucleus have ever been identified—nothing like an optic tract or a medial lemniscus. But the mediodorsal nucleus, and in particular its medial, magnocellular subdivision, is known to have numerous inputs from the continuum in which the hypothalamus is central. Some of these inputs are reported to arise in the septum, and others in the mesencephalic reticular formation. Still others arise in the amygdala.

The findings amount to this: The frontal cortex has access to all the sensory windows through which an organism apprehends the world. In addition, it has access to signals from the visceral domain. It projects to the hypothalamus. Might it be sending the hypothalamus a stream of neural code representing trains of ideation ongoing in the neocortex? And might the neural code sent back from the hypothalamus be a signal entering into ideation that a train of thought causes a feeling recognized interoceptively as pleasure or displeasure? The vernacular, at least, suggests such neural reentries. One says: "The thought of it makes me ill." Or: "I feel a little funny about that." One forms attachments, one chooses a livelihood, in part because a "gut feeling" augurs a more rewarding life. Perhaps it is little wonder that lesions of the human frontal cortex often lead to emotional flatness and a tendency toward insouciance and thoughtless acts. It is as if the victim of such lesions were placed in a state in which experiences and thought processes have lost their power to raise echoes from the interoceptive depths, and thus lost their power to guide.

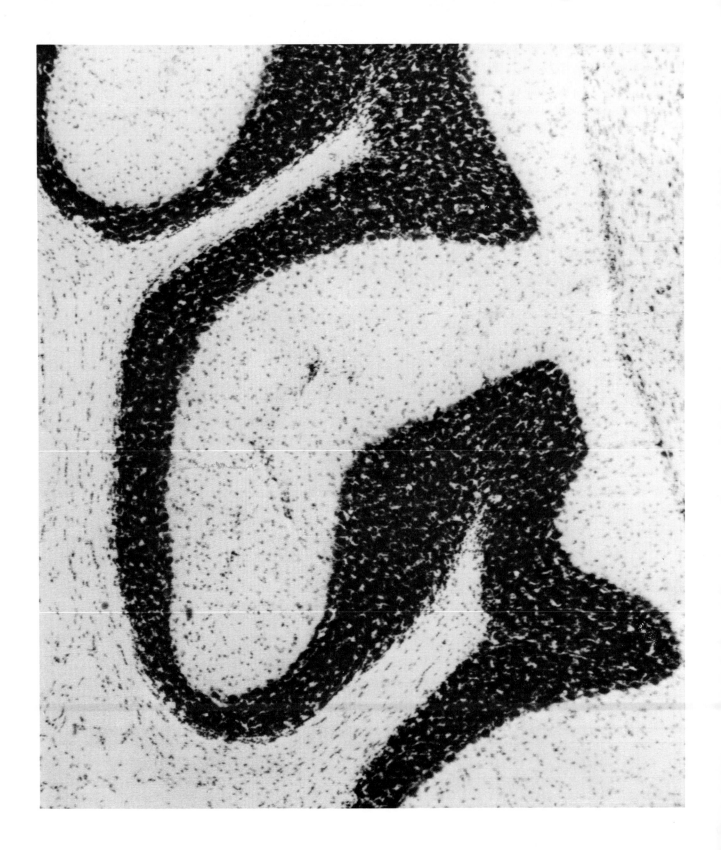

Part III

ANATOMY

Facing page: **Adjacent folia,** or convolutions of the cerebellar cortex, dominate this Nissl preparation of tissue from the brain of a rat. Each folium is three-layered. The dark-staining granular layer snakes through the field of view; it incorporates an extremely dense packing of the small neurons called granule cells. Superficial to the granular layer (or toward the right in this view) is the molecular layer, lightly stippled with the nuclei of glial cells. The third layer, positioned between the other two, is a file of the large, flask-shaped cerebellar neurons called Purkinje cells. The file is most easily discernible at the lower right, where it looks like a line of large black dots along the underside (actually the outer edge) of the granular layer. Each dot is a cell body some 30 to 35 micrometers in diameter. At the extreme right the cerebellar cortex abuts a mesencephalic structure, the inferior colliculus. The photograph was made by Peter Paskevich at the Mailman Research Laboratories of the McLean Hospital in Belmont, Massachusetts.

Chapter Ten

Ontogeny; Spinal Cord

The tracing of projections in the limbic system completes our survey of the connections in the mammalian brain and spinal cord. Its defects are several. In the first place, it did little justice to the true complexity of the connections. But then, if all the known systems of conduction were placed on a diagram of the mammalian brain and spinal cord, they would produce a hopeless tangle. The diagrams we did employ were quite complex enough, and at several unguarded moments our descriptions spilled well beyond them. Second, we seldom made distinctions between projections comprising millions of fibers and projections comprising only a fraction of that number. Recall, for example, that the spinothalamic fibers attaining the ventral nucleus of the thalamus may number no more than a few hundred in the primate, whereas the medial lemniscus has a million fibers, maybe more. Third, our survey largely neglected the bilateral symmetry of the central nervous system. In particular, we seldom described which projections cross to the opposite side of the central nervous system and which have destinations on the same side as their origin. The crossings (or their absence) are crucial in clinical diagnosis. For example, the symptom of alternating hemianalgesia (loss of pain sensation on one side of the face and the other side of the body) indicates a lesion in the lateral part of the rhombencephalon on the same side of the brain as the side of the facial sensory deficit. The conduction lines for pain from the body pass through the rhombencephalon after they have crossed; the lines for pain from the face pass through it before they cross. Most grievous of all, in addressing only the connectedness of the brain — that is to say, only the origins and destinations of the various fiber systems — we evoked no more than a rough

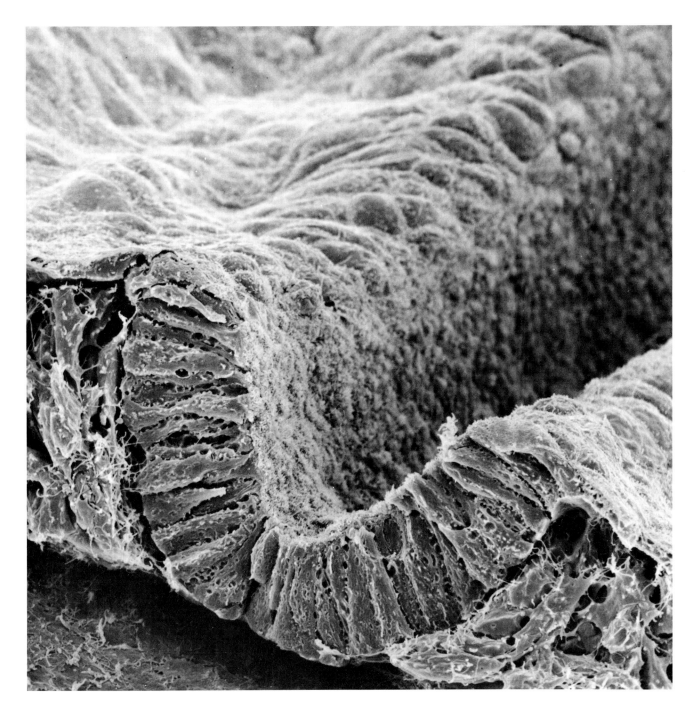

Figure 58: **Deepening of the neural groove** takes place early in the gestation of the central nervous system. In this scanning electron micrograph the groove is shown in the embryo of a hamster. It indents the ectoderm (the back of the embryo) at and around the midline; its walls are called neural folds. Fundamentally, the folds are epithelial: their cells pack closely together. (The looser cell ar-chitecture characteristic of connective tissue is apparent to the right and left of the folds.) Moreover, the epithelium is columnar: each fold consists of cells that span the thickness of the tissue. From the folds the full complexity of the brain and the spinal cord will develop. The micrograph was made by Robert E. Waterman of the University of New Mexico School of Medicine.

sketch of neuroanatomy: the three-dimensional architecture of the tissues stationed inside the cranium and down the core of the vertebral column. Our survey of the connections in the mammalian central nervous system is complete. Now we begin again, with the hope of remedying at least the last of these defects. The brain and the spinal cord are now to take shape before us. Our first concern is with certain events in ontogeny that dictate the broad-scale form of the nervous system.

Neuroembryology

The fundamentals of how the nervous system grows in the human embryo were known a century ago. By about the sixteenth day of gestation the neural plate is apparent. It is a thickening of the ectoderm, the outer layer of the embryo — a thickening that runs almost the length of the embryo at and about the dorsal midline. It is not a plate for long. Owing, perhaps, to the furious proliferation of its cells, it soon buckles inward. Thus, by about the twentieth day, the plate becomes divided into a left half and a right half by a groove that follows the embryo's dorsal midline. Each half thickens to form a neural fold (Figure 58). Meanwhile the groove grows deep and narrow. Then, by the twenty-second day, the lips of the folds begin to fuse, so that the neural tube takes shape. The tube separates from the rest of the ectoderm, which closes over it, and assumes a position just under the dorsal midline. At first the tube is only a single cell thick: each cell in the tube grips the limiting membranes that close off the tube at its inner and outer surface. Mitotic cell division is occurring, and at a high rate. One can see, however, that the mitosis is sequestered: the nucleus of each cell observed in the act of dividing lies near the inner limiting membrane. At such a time the cell becomes rounded in shape. In addition it loses its purchases on each of the limiting membranes. The cells engendered by the mitosis may reestablish both of their grips; each cell is therefore described as rounding off and then as elongating. At the times when the cell is not dividing, its nucleus and the surrounding cell body move away from the inner limiting membrane. It is now known that when the cell body reaches a position farthest from the inner limiting membrane, it synthesizes DNA, because only in that position does it take up thymidine, from which it synthesizes one of the four DNA bases. It also is known that the cycle of rounding off and elongating can be repeated many times, with a nucleus and its surrounding cell body shuttling toward and then away from the inner limiting membrane, making DNA and dividing. In the mouse the cycle takes eight hours; thus the number of cells increases exponentially at a rate of three doublings per day.

The district of the neural tube's cross section defined by the shuttlings of cell bodies is called the ventricular layer. It is the only district plain to see in the earliest neural tube. A second district soon appears: it is called the marginal layer (Figure 59). At first it contains only the processes with which the cells anchor themselves to the outer limiting membrane. Later it widens: it is swelled by the entrance of axons that sprout from the cell bodies. When the cells of the ventricular layer cease to divide, they leave the ventricular layer and settle at positions in the cross section intermediate between the ventricular layer and the marginal layer. Thus a third layer develops: the mantle layer. Its cells grip neither the inner nor the outer limiting membrane. They are cells, it seems, that never return to the ventricular layer and will never divide again. The mantle layer, like the marginal layer, augments as time goes on.

The development of neocortex permits us to examine neural ontogeny in greater detail. It also exemplifies some ontogenetic themes: That the brain is at bottom an epithelium, a tissue whose cells are separated from one another by a minimal amount of intercellular substance, somewhat like the bricks in a wall. That neurons arise far from their final locations and migrate to their homesteads. That neurons are postmitotic: they are recognizably neurons only when they have ceased to reproduce. That neurons arise in genetically programmed episodes and then interact with other cells, presumably in response to environmental cues. That neurons initially generate an overabundance of connections, which later pare themselves down.

Here, then, is how neocortex forms. Before the sixth week of human ontogeny the cerebral vesicle (the part of the neural tube that will become the cerebral hemisphere) has only a ventricular layer and a marginal layer. Then, in the sixth week, the mantle layer appears. Soon after that, some cells take up a position between the ventricular layer and the mantle layer. There they continue to divide. They compose what is called the subventricular zone. Next, in the seventh week, cells begin to accumulate high in the mantle layer. They compose what is called the cortical plate. By the eleventh week the plate is thick and compact; a wave of cell migration is ending. Thalamocortical axons arrive; some invade the plate. By the end of the thirteenth week the plate has two subdivisions, an inner district populated by large cells and an outer district populated by a denser packing of smaller cells. The inner, larger cells came first; the smaller ones passed through their ranks. In short, the cell migrations are building the cortex inside out. By the end of the fifteenth week the plate is uniform again; presumably the newer arrivals have enlarged. A

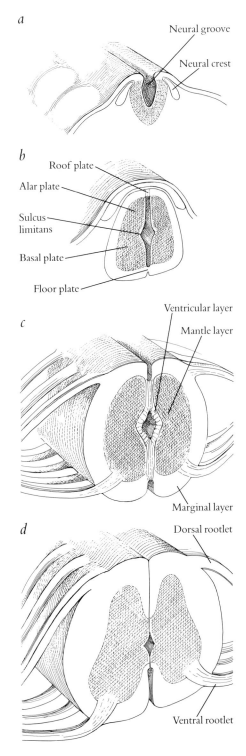

Figure 59: **Neural tube develops** when the lips of the neural folds join. Its districts have various fates in the fully formed central nervous system. The central canal of the tube becomes the ventricle system, a sequence of chambers filled with cerebrospinal fluid. The cells that line the canal become a ventricular lining. Two layers form most of the width of the tube. One is the mantle layer, which fills with neuronal cell bodies and thus becomes gray matter, or neuronal aggregations, in the central nervous system. The other, the marginal layer, fills with axons and thus becomes white matter, or axonal aggregations. The groove in each lateral wall of the central canal is the sulcus limitans. The part of the mantle layer dorsal to each sulcus is called the alar plate. Secondary sensory cell groups develop there, receiving sensory fibers from primary sensory neurons in ganglia flanking the central nervous system. The part of the mantle layer ventral to each sulcus is called the basal plate. Local motor apparatuses develop there, emitting motor fibers. In the spinal cord the motor fibers join with sensory fibers to form what are called the segmental nerves. In the brain the pattern is more complex.

further wave of migration is now occurring; it will populate the most superficial cortical cell-containing layers. How does each neuron migrate? A postmitotic neuron first entering the mantle layer is an elongated, bipolar cell no more than a few tens of micrometers long. It has a leading process, which adds, say, 70 micrometers to its length. It has ahead of it a journey of many thousands of micrometers. In the monkey the early arrivals accomplish their trip in a day or two. The ones arriving later, which traverse longer distances (and also seem to go slower), need two weeks or more. Pasko Rakic, who was then at Harvard University, has shown that a neuron migrating at a time when the ontogeny of the neocortex is well under way employs a safety line: it makes its journey apposed to the process of an immature glial cell — a radial glial cell, which spans the thickness of the wall of the cerebral vesicle (Figure 60). Evidently a number of neurons follow each radial line, thus becoming stacked in the cortex.* The later arrivals migrate past the early ones. Ultimately the radial glial cells disappear: many lose their long processes and turn into astrocytes.

In the fifth month of human ontogeny neurons are still arriving. (We here employ lunar months, which have the virtue of consisting of four weeks exactly.) Cell proliferation in the ventricular layer is over. It may, however, continue in the subventricular zone. Meanwhile, in the cortical plate, the cells are growing processes, and for the first time they are establishing synapses inside the plate. During the sixth month the deep cortical layers become distinguishable; the deep neurons are growing dendritic ramifications. The projection cells differentiate first, the local-circuit neurons later. In both cases, dendritic spines develop last: in even the deepest cortical layers they continue to show up after birth. By the seventh month the neocortex is six-layered, though layers 2 and 3 (the outermost cell-containing layers) are "immature." That is, they are not the adult layers; rearrangements continue well after birth. Association cortex matures last, long after the primary sensory fields and the motor cortex. Myelin sheaths develop. The myelination continues into old age. A word on projections. It seems they begin by being diffuse and overlapping, and later fine-tune themselves, gaining point-to-point topologic precision by the elimination of superfluous synapses, and even conduction lines. The visual system exhibits this dramatically. In the fully formed brain of a primate the optic nerve from each eye distributes its fibers to three of the six cell layers composing the lateral geniculate body of the thalamus. Thus each layer is innervated by the ipsilateral eye or the contralateral eye, but not by both. (The details will concern us later.) Initially in the embryo there is no such segregation: the geniculate projections from

---

*In other parts of the brain developing neurons may employ an alternative mode of migration. D. Kent Morest, then working at Harvard University with Valerie B. Domesick, found immature neurons in the superior colliculus growing a stout process to the site of their prospective location, then moving their nucleus inside the process. The final position of the nucleus dictated the final placement of the neuronal cell body.

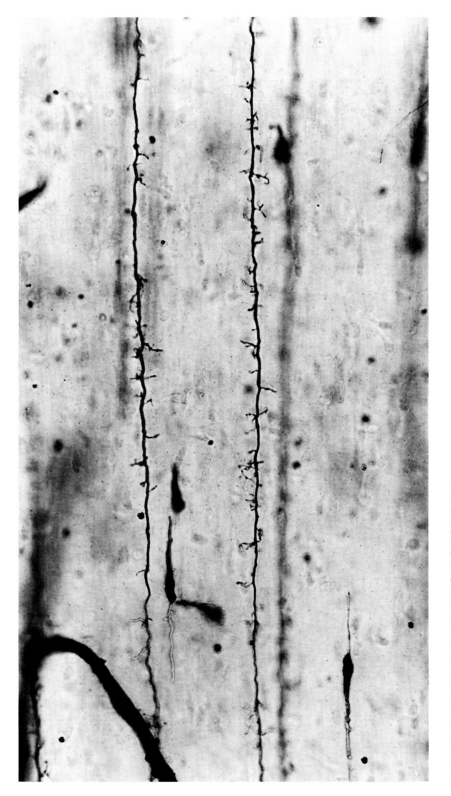

Figure 60: **Prospective neurons migrating** toward their final positions in the cerebral cortex are shown in Golgi-stained tissue from the part of the neural tube that becomes the cerebral hemisphere. The migrating neurons are spindle-shaped cells; one, in sharp focus, is toward the lower right. It emits a forward filament called the leading process and a rearward filament, the trailing process. Two long, black filaments, not part of any neuron, ascend through the field of view. In fact, they span the neural tube's width. They are processes emitted deep in the tube by cells called radial glia. The capricious Golgi stain marks only some neurons and only some of the radial-glial processes, but electron microscopy shows that each migrating neuron attains its destination by following one of the glial "safety lines." The thick black structures curving through the field of view are cerebral blood vessels. The micrograph was made by Pasko Rakic of the Yale University School of Medicine; the tissue is from the fetus of a rhesus monkey.

the two eyes intermingle in all six layers. In 1983, Rakic, working with Katherine P. Riley at Yale University, counted the number of optic-nerve axons along radial paths in cross sections of the optic nerve in monkeys and monkey fetuses, and from the counts they made some estimates of the total. In the adult monkey they found from 1.2 to 1.3 million axons. In a fetus killed at its sixty-ninth day of gestation they found 2.85 million. (The total gestation period is 165 days.) In older fetuses the number had progressively decreased. Meanwhile, in the lateral geniculate body the innervation of each cell layer had become more nearly monocular.

Patterns of Organization

Let us return to the fifth or sixth week of ontogeny. At that time the prospective brain is far smaller than the adult red nucleus will be. Nevertheless, the forward end of the neural tube shows the flexures, the ampulla-shaped swellings, and the budding side chambers — in a word, it shows the complexities — that portend the gross anatomy of the brain. Behind this forward end the greater part of the length of the tube remains straight and of even width. It will become the spinal cord. Its lack of flexures, ampullae, and side chambers ensures that the patterns governing its organization will remain relatively simple throughout its length. Consider, in that regard, the various districts of the neural tube. The lumen of the tube is called the central canal. As the spinal cord develops, the canal shrinks in diameter. Finally it becomes more or less occluded. (In the human spinal cord it is completely occluded.) In the developing brain, on the other hand, the central canal takes on a labyrinthine form as it becomes the ventricle system, a sequence of chambers filled with cerebrospinal fluid. The innermost zone of the neural tube itself is the ventricular layer. As the neural tube develops and cells irreversibly cast off their hold on the inner limiting membrane, the ventricular layer loses its cell population. Indeed, it is reduced to the ependyma, a remarkably regular epithelium consisting of a single rank of cuboidal cells. In a cross section of the fully formed spinal cord the ependyma is represented only by a small, irregular cluster of cells that mark the occluded central canal. In the brain, however, the ependymal cells form a lining of the ventricles. It is thought that the ependymal cells in the brain are the makers of cerebrospinal fluid. According to one hypothesis they filter it from the blood. The outer zones of the developing neural tube are the mantle layer, a homestead for postmitotic cell bodies, and the marginal layer, formed by the aggregation of their axons. The first becomes the gray matter of the fully formed central nervous system. The second becomes the white matter. Initially, therefore, white matter is superficial to gray matter throughout the length of the neural tube. In the developing spinal cord, this arrangement persists; nothing happens to change the relation between the two. In the developing brain, however, the initial relation can change. In the cerebral hemisphere, the final relation is just the reverse: gray matter — the cerebral cortex — comes to lie at the surface.

A further pattern of organization applies dorsoventrally. It, too, is readily seen when the development of the neural tube is not yet far advanced. When the tube first appears in the embryo, it is oval in cross section, and the central canal is a narrow slit with its long dimension oriented dorsoventrally. Soon, however, a groove called the sulcus limitans develops in each of the canal's lateral walls. The advent of the groove tends to widen the middle of the canal's cross section, so that it tapers both dorsally and ventrally. In sum, the cross section of the canal takes on the shape of an elongated diamond. Now if, at that time in development, one were to imagine a line passing through the two sulci limitantes, the line would divide the mantle layer into a dorsal district and a ventral district on each side of the neural tube's midline. The dorsal district is the alar plate — literally the wing plate. The ventral district is the basal plate. Two further names should also be given. The midline region that closes off the dorsal side of the central canal and separates the two alar plates is called the roof plate. The midline region that closes off the ventral side of the canal and separates the two basal plates is called the floor plate. Neither the roof plate nor the floor plate proliferates cells. Accordingly, neither develops a mantle layer as the brain and the spinal cord take form. In the end, the roof plate and the floor plate contribute only ependymal cells to the mature central nervous system.

Primary sensory neurons do not arise in the neural tube. Indeed, none of the neurons whose cell bodies occupy the periphery of the body seem to come from the neural tube. Such cells arise instead in the neural crest, a longitudinal ridge proliferating from the deep side of the ectoderm at the top of the neural fold on each side of the neural groove. At the time the folds fuse, producing the neural tube, the crest is largely detached from its ectodermal matrix; it is a continuous band atop the dorsum of the tube, markedly thicker at its lateral sides than it is along the midline. Soon — beginning in fact at the fourth week of gestation — the crest breaks into a sequence of epithelial nodes. At each side of the developing spinal cord there is a node for each of the segments that have formed in the embryonic body. Even before the nodes appear, cells are leaving the neural crest. Some will aggregate into a segmental sequence of interconnected sympathetic ganglia at each side of the vertebral column; these are the paravertebral ganglia, composing the sympathetic trunk. Others will travel farther and compose a large, unsegmented sympathetic ganglion ventral to the vertebral column. It is the prevertebral, or celiac, ganglion. A third group of cells will travel farther yet and become the chromaffin cells of the adrenal medulla. A fourth group will travel the farthest distance, to station themselves near peripheral organs or even inside them as the juxta-mural and intramural ganglia of the parasympathetic nervous system. The plexuses of Auerbach and Meissner, in the wall of the digestive tract, are in the intramural category.*

---

*The neural crest generates not only the neurons of the sensory and autonomic ganglia but also the glial cells in the periphery of the body. The latter comprise the so-called satellite

What remains of the neural crest at the close of these migrations is still a segmental sequence of nodes. From each of them a sensory ganglion develops; thus the nonmigratory neuroblasts engendered in the nodes become primary sensory neurons. They have a remarkable shape. Each primary sensory neuron begins by growing two processes, which emerge from opposite sides of the rounded cell body: the cell starts out bipolar. Then, however, the processes move progressively closer together. Ultimately they fuse, so that a single axonal stem process emerges from the cell body. The cell is now termed pseudounipolar. The stem retains its two branches. One of them travels outward to the periphery of the body, where it will terminate in a sensory ending, or several sensory endings. The other branch enters the developing spinal cord. A remarkable thing about the primary sensory neuron is that its cell body sprouts no dendrites. (The peripheral branch of the neuron's stem process conducts signals toward the cell body, but it cannot be viewed as a dendrite. For one thing, it usually has a myelin sheath.) Does the cell in fact have none? David Bodian of Johns Hopkins University has solved the long-standing riddle by finding that in the unique case of the primary sensory neuron the dendrites sprout from the peripheral end of the axon. Hence the somatic sensory endings in the periphery of the body are dendritic, not axonal. Like dendrites elsewhere they generate graded potentials that converge on an all-or-none site. Here, however, the all-or-none site is at the final node in the axon's myelination. Another remarkable thing about the primary sensory neuron is that the cell body receives virtually no synaptic contacts: it gets no input from other neurons. The earliest point at which incoming sensory data can be modified by other neurons is at the synaptic terminals of the centrally directed branch of the primary sensory axon — that is to say, in the spinal cord.

We are now in a position to specify the full dorsoventral pattern of organization. While primary sensory neurons and autonomic motor neurons are being generated and marshaled into ganglionic nests, cell proliferation and differentiation in the mantle layer of the neural tube is proceeding apace. In the alar plate, the dorsal zone of the neural tube, secondary sensory cell groups develop, in the company of other intermediate neurons and of glial cells. Correspondingly, the axon branches directed centrally from the primary sensory neurons in each sensory ganglion enter the spinal cord dorsolaterally, in a longitudinal row of fascicles called dorsal rootlets. Meanwhile, in the basal plate, the ventral zone of the neural tube, motor neurons develop, along with interneurons and glia. The basal events take a substantial lead. In fact, clusters of cells that are unmistakably neurons appear in the basal plate at a time when the alar plate shows utterly no differentiation. It seems that in the

---

cells, which populate ganglia, and the Schwann cells, which sheath axons in the periphery. Finally, the neural crest is thought to contribute cells to the pia and the arachnoid, the inner meninges.

developmental schedule of the central nervous system the motor side of the organization is given priority over the sensory side. In any case, the axons emitted by motor neurons leave the spinal cord ventrolaterally, in a longitudinal row of fascicles called ventral rootlets. The spinal cord's segregation of sensory and motor fibers into dorsal and ventral contingents became apparent in the early 19th century. In 1811 the Scottish surgeon and physiologist Charles Bell reported that the mechanical stimulation of ventral fascicles — but not dorsal ones — caused muscle contractions in experimental animals. Eleven years later the French physiologist François Magendie reported the complementary finding that the sectioning of dorsal fascicles rendered an animal's limb insensitive but failed to paralyze the limb.

Spinal Anatomy

The fully formed human spinal cord is in essence a long, slender column, nowhere much thicker than a finger. Figure 61 shows its dorsal aspect. Two rows of dorsal rootlets are visible, one on each side of the midline. Similar rows of ventral rootlets are hidden behind the cord. The dorsal and ventral rootlets collect into larger fascicles, the dorsal and ventral roots, and by this circumstance the segments of the spinal cord are distinguished: each segment is defined as that part of the length of the cord for which the dorsal rootlets converge into a single dorsal root on each side of the midline and the ventral rootlets converge into a single ventral root. By dividing the human spinal cord at levels between the fans of rootlets one finds from 33 to 35 segments. Beginning at the top and moving downward, there are eight cervical segments, followed by 12 thoracic, five lumbar, five sacral, and from three to five coccygeal. Still, the spinal cord itself shows no sign of segmentation. As each dorsal root extends away from the spinal cord, it enters a small lump of neural tissue wedged into an intervertebral foramen: an opening between successive vertebral arches. The lump is an intervertebral ganglion, also called a dorsal-root ganglion. In it are stationed the primary sensory neurons from which the fibers of the dorsal root arise. Next to each ganglion in the intervertebral foramen, or just proximal to the ganglion in the vertebral canal, the dorsal root fuses with the corresponding ventral root to form a segmental nerve.

A note on the meninges surrounding the spinal cord. The outermost of the three meningeal investments of the central nervous system is a tough sheet of fibrous connective tissue called the pachymeninx, Greek for "the thick membrane," or more often the dura mater, Latin for "the hard mother." (*Mater* was meant to evoke the image of a womb: a pouch in which the brain is enclosed.) The dura mater lines the vertebral canal, but only loosely so (Figure 62), with a space — the epidural space — intervening between it and the vertebrae. At the level of the spinal cord the epidural space is filled by fatty tissue and by a well-developed venous plexus. In contrast, the dura mater surrounding the brain is fused to the periosteum — the membranous sheath — of the bones of the skull. No venous plexus intervenes between the two.

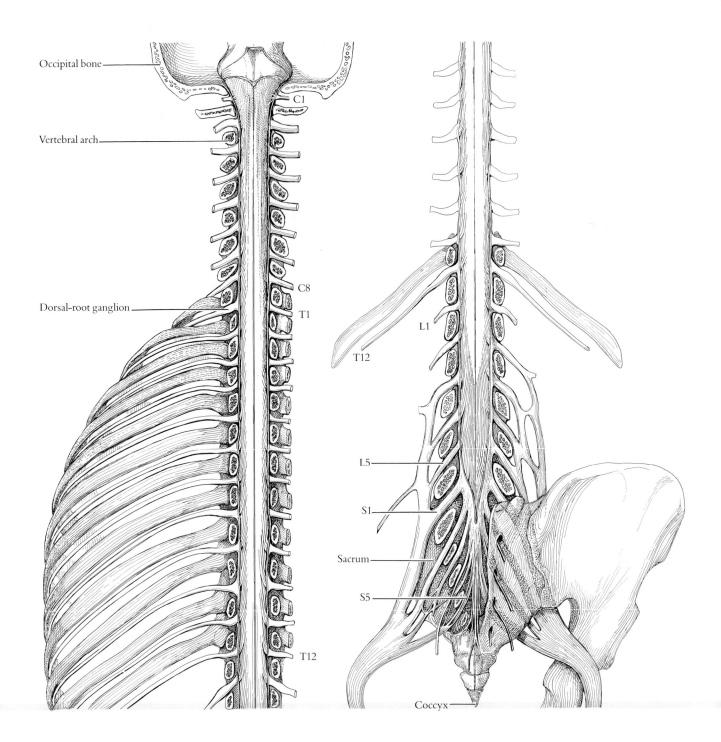

Occipital bone

Vertebral arch

Dorsal-root ganglion

C1

C8

T1

T12

T12

L1

L5

S1

Sacrum

S5

Coccyx

Figure 61: **Human spinal cord** is shown in a dorsal view; that is, a view from the back of the body. Fans of dorsal rootlets emerge at each side of the cord; they consist of primary sensory axons. Fans of ventral rootlets, consisting of motor axons, are hidden in this view. The rootlets coalesce into the dorsal and ventral roots, which co-alesce in turn to form the segmental nerves. On each side of the midline eight nerves are cervical, 12 are thoracic, five are lumbar, five are sacral, and from three to five are coccygeal. Each segment of the spinal cord is the part of the cord giving rise to one left-right pair of segmental nerves.

Around the brain, however, one finds great venous channels, the dural si-nuses, enclosed in the dura itself. Now, each dorsal-root ganglion lies in a funnel-shaped outpouching of the spinal cord's dura mater. The funnel en-closes a dorsal root and a ventral root. Just proximal to the ganglion, the lip of the funnel closes around these two roots to form a tight-fitting sheath that covers not only the ganglion but also the segmental nerve beyond it. In other words, no nerve truly pierces the dura mater.

The middle meningeal investment of the central nervous system is the arachnoid membrane. It is a delicate, semitransparent sheet of connective tissue. ("Arachnoid," from *arachne,* Greek for spider, indicates its resem-blance to a spider web.) Throughout its investment of the central nervous system the arachnoid adheres to the inner surface of the dura mater. Indeed, it adheres so closely that only a virtual space called the subdural space intervenes between the two. (The term virtual space refers to a joining of two tissues by no more than the surface tension of the intervening tissue fluid. The tissues can thus be readily separated, much like the pages of a wet newspaper.) The arachnoid faithfully follows the inner surface of the dura, even into the dural spouts. But just proximal to the place at which each spout closes around an intervertebral ganglion, the arachnoid leaves the inner surface of the dura and reflects onto each of the two roots enclosed by the spout. Then, back at the surface of the spinal cord, the arachnoid becomes continuous with the true capsule of the central nervous system — and the innermost of the meninges — the pia mater (Latin for "the soft mother"). Thus arachnoid and pia, which are really a single delicate tissue known as the leptomeninx (Greek for "the frail membrane"), line a space between the dura mater and the central nervous system. The space, called the subarachnoid space, is filled by cerebrospinal fluid and traversed by delicate fibers called subarachnoid trabeculae.

Figure 62 shows not only the meninges surrounding the spinal cord but also a cross section made through a high cervical segment. In this way we first encounter the spinal cord's internal structure. It is worth a detailed descrip-tion. For one thing, the spinal cord is a crucial part of the nervous system. It encompasses on the one hand the initial processing stations for most of the somatic sensory input to the brain, and on the other hand a substantial proportion of the lower motor system, through which brain function ex-presses itself in behavior. Then, too, the spinal cord demonstrates in most nearly explicit form the general plan by which the axial part of the central nervous system (the spinal cord and the brainstem, together called the neur-axis) is organized. Thus the brainstem, despite its complexity and longitu-dinal variation, and despite the presence of several structures without ana-logue in the spinal cord, is easier to comprehend if it is constantly compared with its spinal prototype.

Figures 63, 64, and 65 are a straightforward approach to the spinal cord's internal structure: they show pairs of spinal cross sections from different levels of the human spinal cord. Each pair consists of two closely spaced sections of a particular spinal cord segment. The pair in Figure 63 are from the seventh cervical (C7) segment, the pair in Figure 64 are from the fifth thoracic (Th5) segment, and the pair in Figure 65 are from the first sacral (S1) segment. In each case one section is Nissl stained, so as to emphasize gray matter, the main repository of neuronal cell bodies and dendrites. Since the Nissl technique leaves axons unstained, it tends to leave white matter white. The other section is stained the opposite way. The white matter is almost black; the gray matter is almost unstained. The German neuropathologist Carl Weigert developed the first such stain — that is, the first myelin stain — in the 1880's; he based it on hematoxylin, a common dyestuff purified from the wood of the logwood tree. The crucial step in the staining procedure is that the sectioned neural tissue is mordanted before the dyestuff is applied. Without that preliminary treatment hematoxylin stains both gray matter and white matter a fairly even purplish blue. The mordanting works a wholesale change in the tissue's chemical affinities. In particular, the mordant (potassium dichromate, ferric alum, or both) forms strong chemical bonds with myelin. It also binds to hematoxylin. In sum it forms a stable link between myelin and the dyestuff. The dyestuff's bonding to other tissue components is weaker. The Weigert stain and its subsequent modifications have found their greatest utility in surveys of neural tissue, both normal and diseased. The stain contrasts white matter with gray; in addition it marks off varying textures caused by comminglings of the two.

In all of the stained spinal sections white matter composes the perimeter of the cord; gray matter occupies the interior. Roughly speaking, the shape of the latter is constant: from one cross section to another it forms a figure often likened to the letter *H* or a butterfly. The top limbs of the *H*, or the butterfly's forward wings, are the dorsal horns: the end product of the alar plates' differentiation and the site of the spinal cord's secondary sensory cell groups. The bottom limbs of the *H*, or the butterfly's trailing wings, are the ventral horns: the end product of the basal plates' differentiation and the site of the spinal cord's somatic motor neurons. The cross rung of the *H*, or the butterfly's thorax, is a gray bridge connecting the left and right half of the spinal gray matter; at the midline the bridge encloses the obliterated central canal, which serves as a landmark dividing the bridge into a dorsal and a ventral gray commissure. A small prominence of gray matter protruding laterally between the dorsal horn and the ventral horn is the lateral (or intermediolateral) horn. It extends from C8 through L2 and thus appears only in Figure 64. It harbors the preganglionic motor neurons of the sympathetic nervous system; hence preganglionic sympathetic fibers leave the central nervous system exclusively in the ventral roots C8 through L2. The lateral horn is the most lateral part of a transverse zone of gray matter that also includes the gray commissures. Since the zone intervenes between the dorsal and ventral horn, it is often called the zona intermedia.

None of this is to say that the spinal gray matter is constant in detail. The cross sections in Figure 63 are from the middle of a sequence of five spinal cord segments (C5 through Th1) where the cord widens into a spindle-shaped enlargement, the cervical enlargement (or cervical intumescence), which accommodates sensory and motor circuitry serving the arm. The cross sections in Figure 65 are from the middle of the lumbosacral enlargement (or intumescence), a sequence of segments (L2 through the end of the cord) serving the leg. That leaves the cross sections in Figure 64. They come from the middle of a sequence of 12 segments (Th2 through L1) that lie between the two enlargements and have no extremity to serve. They serve only the trunk. Plainly the segments in the enlargements include more gray matter

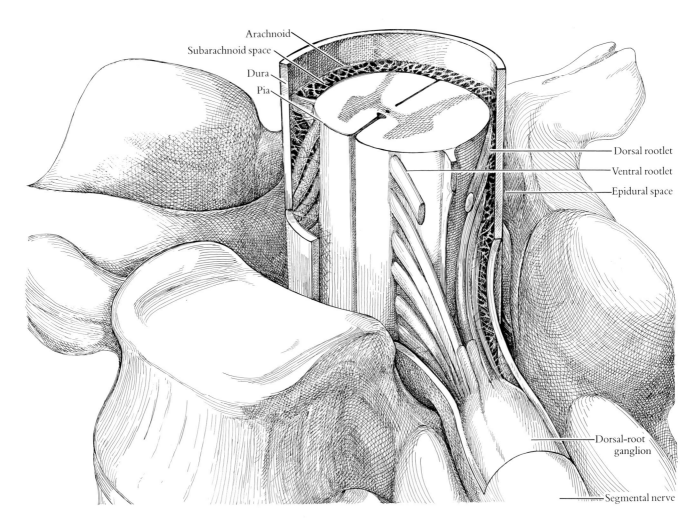

Figure 62: **Meninges,** three sheets of connective tissue surrounding the central nervous system, are shown surrounding the cervical spinal cord. The three are the dura mater, a tough sheet loosely lining the vertebral canal; the arachnoid membrane, which adheres to the dura's inner surface; and the pia mater, which is really the reflection of the arachnoid onto the surface of the central nervous system. The space between the vertebrae and the dura—the so-called epidural space—is filled with fatty tissue and veins; the space between the arachnoid and the pia—the subarachnoid space—is filled with cerebrospinal fluid and traversed by fibers called subarachnoid trabeculae. The dura mater forms sheaths around each pair of dorsal and ventral roots as they pass through an intervertebral foramen, becoming a segmental nerve. The ganglion containing the neurons giving rise to the dorsal-root fibers is often inside the foramen.

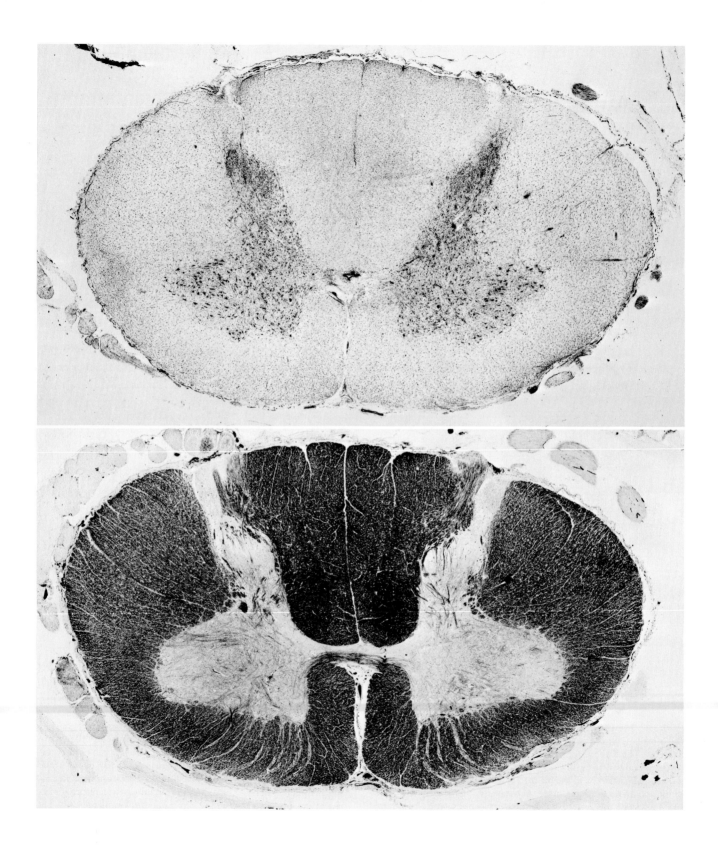

than the intervening, mostly thoracic, segments do. The difference is most striking in the ventral horn. Briefly, the ventral horn at thoracic levels lacks the large lateral expansion typical of intumescence segments. The explanation is straightforward; it derives from three facts. First, the spinal cord's motor neurons are arranged in longitudinal columns of varying length. A typical spinal cross section cuts through several such columns, so that they are seen in the ventral horn as clusters of motor neurons. Second, the columns are arranged in a functional sequence: the ones innervating limb (or distal) mus-

originates - dorsal root

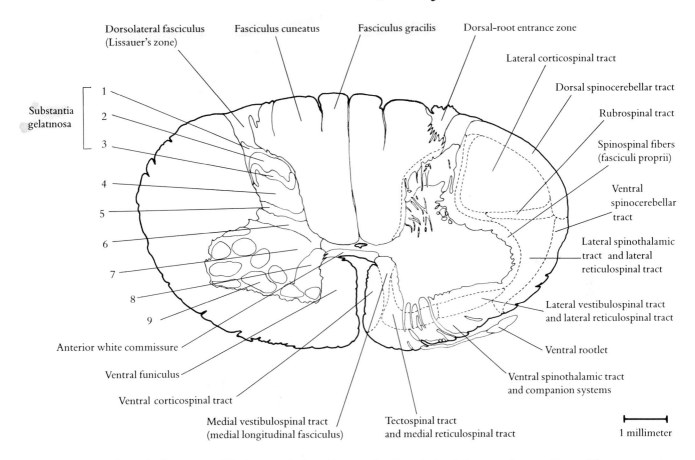

Figure 63: **Seventh cervical segment** of the human spinal cord is part of the cervical enlargement, a widening of the cord where the spinal gray matter accommodates sensory and motor circuitry serving not only the axial part of the body but also the arm. Two cross sections are displayed. The top one is Nissl stained; thus cell bodies are stipples, and gray matter, which forms the core of the spinal cord, is emphasized. The gray matter has the overall shape of a butterfly. The upper wings, which differentiate from the alar plates of the neural tube, are the dorsal horns; the lower wings, which differen-tiate from the basal plates, are the ventral horns. The accompanying map shows the nine laminae distinguished in the spinal gray matter by the Swedish anatomist Bror Rexed. The bottom section is Weigert stained. The method, developed by the German neuropathologist Carl Weigert, marks myelin; thus white matter is rendered black. On each side of the midline the white matter forms three districts: the dorsal, the lateral, and the ventral funiculus. The accompanying map locates some of the spinal cord's ascending and descending fiber contingents.

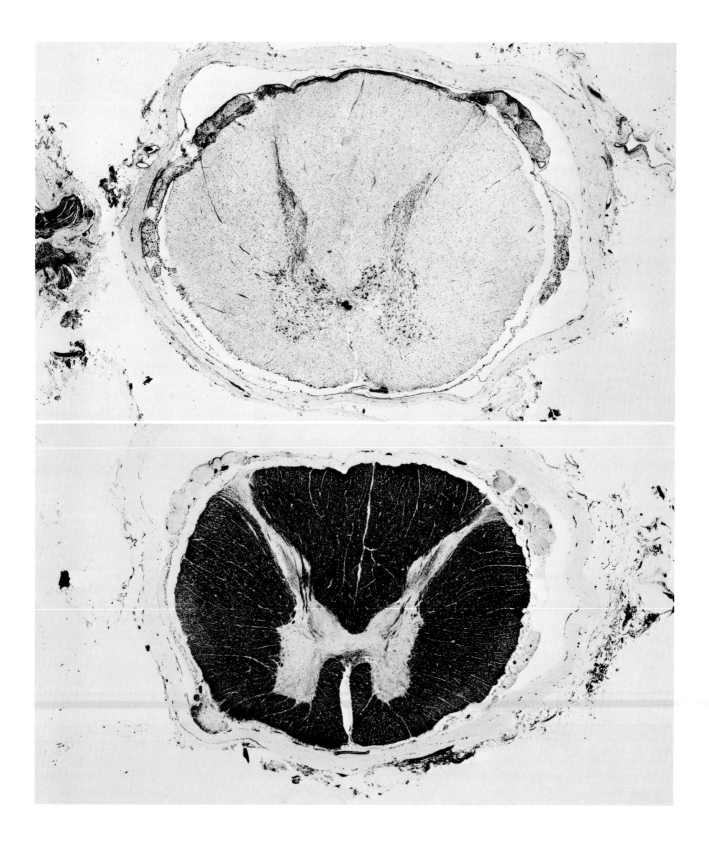

cles are lateral to the ones innervating trunk (or axial) muscles — the muscles of the neck, the back, and the abdominal wall. Third, all spinal cord segments have axial muscles to govern. The erector trunci muscle, for instance, extends from the base of the skull to the sacrum. In addition, the intumescence segments animate distal muscles. Hence a survey of the motor-neuronal columns in a thoracic spinal cord segment encounters only columns innervating trunk muscles. In contrast, a survey of the columns in an intumescence segment, proceeding laterally along the circumference of the ventral horn, encounters columns innervating trunk muscles such as the erector trunci; trunk-to-girdle muscles such as the rhomboidales and the serratus anterior; girdle-to-limb muscles such as the deltoid; proximal limb muscles such as the brachialis and the triceps; and distal limb muscles such as the long finger flexors. Finally, at extreme positions lateral and dorsal in the horn, one finds columns innervating the small muscles of the hand or the foot, including the interossei and the muscles of the thenar (the ball of the thumb). The small

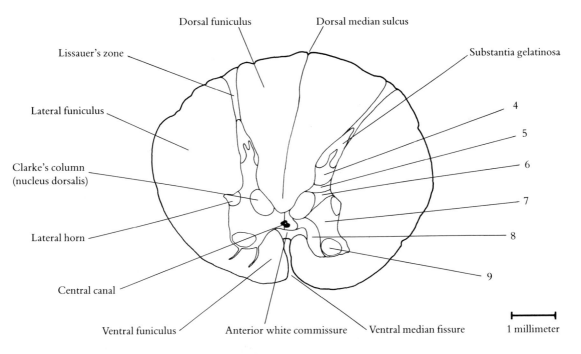

Figure 64: **Fifth thoracic segment** of the human spinal cord is in a stretch of the cord serving only the axial part of the body. It does, however, include two specialized structures. A lateral bulge of the gray matter in Rexed's lamina 7, between the dorsal horn and the ventral horn, is the lateral horn. Extending only from the eighth cervical (C8) segment to the second lumbar (L2) segment, it contains the preganglionic motor neurons of the sympathetic nervous system. A rounded, medial bulge of the gray matter in Rexed's laminae 5 and 6, at the base of the dorsal horn, is the dorsal column of Clarke. Extending, like the lateral horn, from C8 through L2, it contains secondary sensory neurons that project to the cerebellum. Specifically, Clarke's column emits the dorsal spinocerebellar tract.

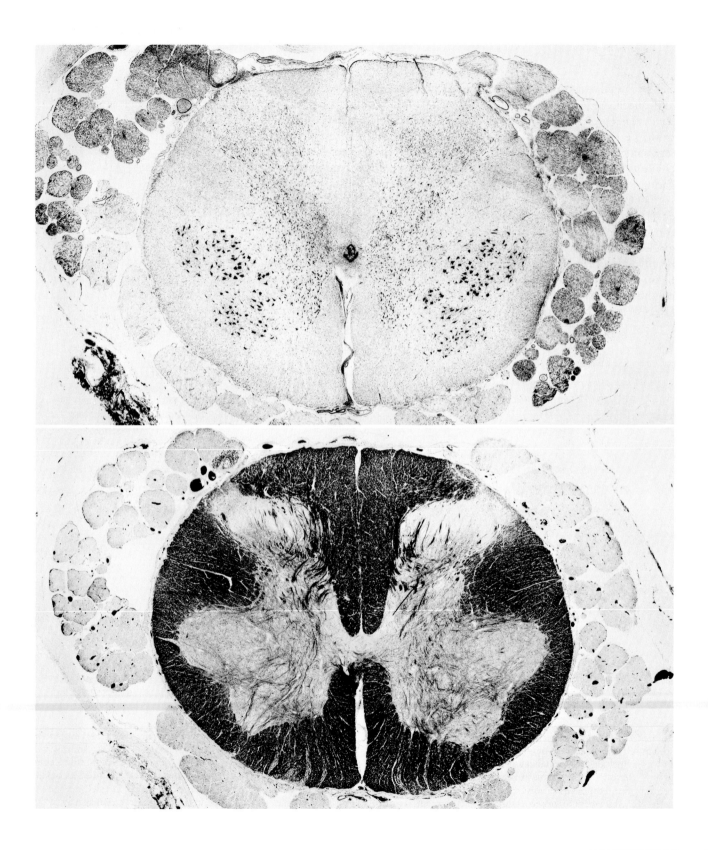

muscles of the hand are crucial for manual skills requiring discrete finger movements. They are also the muscles most severely impaired by a lesion of the pyramidal tract. But then, pyramidal-tract fibers terminating within clusters of motor neurons (instead of among the interneurons between the clusters of motor neurons) are commonest by far in the clusters positioned dorsally and laterally in the ventral horn. Such fibers are all but absent from the most medial clusters.

The dorsal horn shows variations, too. In the classical nomenclature it has three chief divisions, each accounting for about a third of the horn's cross section. The cap-shaped, apical third of the horn consists mostly of small, closely spaced neurons seven to 12 micrometers in diameter. This is the substantia gelatinosa of Rolando. It is notably poor in myelin; in the Weigert preparations of Figures 63, 64, and 65 it is the lightest spot on the section. Its involvement in nociception will concern us shortly. Next is the middle third of the dorsal horn. Here the cells are more widely spaced and for the most part

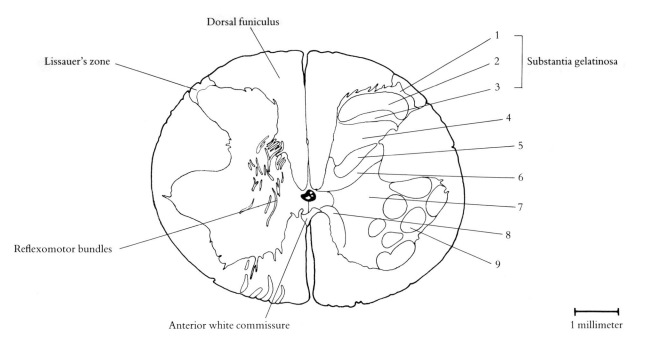

Figure 65: **First sacral segment** of the human spinal cord is part of the lumbosacral enlargement, a widening of the cord where the spinal gray matter accommodates sensory and motor circuitry serving not only the axial part of the body but also the leg. Here the spinal gray butterfly is squatter than elsewhere. Still, the overall pattern is similar. For example, the ventral horn contributes more markedly to the enlargement than the dorsal horn does. Clusters of motor neurons in the ventral horn are collectively lamina 9 of Rexed. Yet some of the largest stipples in the Nissl-stained ventral horn are interneurons, not motor neurons. The cross sections are surrounded by dorsal roots and ventral roots descending in pairs to intervertebral foramina at lower levels of the vertebral column.

of medium size, from 15 to 20 micrometers across. A few are as large as 30 micrometers. The region includes a dense plexus of myelinated fibers; thus in Weigert preparations it is the darkest part of the dorsal horn. It has traditionally been viewed as the principal part of the horn and so was long known as the nucleus proprius cornu dorsalis, meaning, in rough translation, the dorsal horn's real nucleus. The name is not entirely unfit: the nucleus proprius harbors most of the neurons emitting the fibers of the spinothalamic tract. Last is the ventral third of the dorsal horn. In general it is a district of large and medium neurons. It has, however, a notable feature: the dorsal column (or dorsal nucleus) of Clarke, an almost perfectly cylindrical volume of large, rotund neurons that produce a medial bulge at the base of the dorsal horn. (Clarke was the 19th-century English anatomist Jacob A. L. Clarke.) The column of Clarke occupies spinal cord segments C8 through L2. That makes the column coextensive with the lateral horn. It also means the column appears only in Figure 64. The column emits the dorsal spinocerebellar tract, one of two spinal paths to the cerebellum.

In 1954 the Swedish anatomist Bror Rexed proposed a new system of subdivision for all the spinal gray matter, dorsal and ventral. He had observed a lamination—a layered pattern—in cross sections of the spinal cord's gray matter. In his scheme, which now is widely employed, the substantia gelatinosa consists of three zones: laminae 1, 2, and 3 of Rexed. Lamina 1 is a file of widely spaced, strikingly elongated neurons of medium size arrayed atop the dorsal horn like seals on a rock. The neurons are called the marginal cells of Waldeyer, after Heinrich Waldeyer, the German anatomist who described them some six decades before Rexed published his study. Lamina 2 is the bulk of the substantia gelatinosa; it contains the smallest neurons in the spinal cord. Lamina 3 is composed of somewhat larger cells. The nucleus proprius corresponds more or less to a single layer, lamina 4; the basal third of the dorsal horn corresponds to laminae 5 and 6. (The dorsal column of Clarke occupies the medial part of laminae 5 and 6.) The zona intermedia and the polymorphous cell population at the core of the ventral horn together form lamina 7; a narrow medial strip of lamina 7, enclosing the ventral horn's most medial motor neurons, is lamina 8. The columns of motor neurons are collectively lamina 9.

The white matter of the spinal cord has an uncomplicated description. Fundamentally, the dorsal and ventral horn divide it into three districts on either side of the midline. Each district is called a funiculus, the diminutive of the Latin *funis,* or rope. Some anatomical landmarks make the parcellation precise. At the dorsal midline, a shallow groove, the dorsal median sulcus, indents the spinal cord's surface. A second groove, the dorsolateral sulcus, marks the line at which the dorsal rootlets arrive. The sector of white matter, triangular in cross section, between the two indentations is the dorsal funiculus, also called the dorsal or posterior column. Nearly all the fibers of the dorsal rootlets enter the spinal cord there. In particular they enter at the dorsolateral corner of the funiculus, which is known as the dorsal-root entrance zone. Having entered, most if not all of them bifurcate: each one divides into an ascending and a descending branch. In carnivores and primates, including man, such branches compose nearly all of the dorsal funiculus. It follows that in these species the dorsal funiculus is essentially a bundle —in primates the largest bundle—of primary sensory fibers. As yet there have been no synaptic interruptions in the ascending conduction paths; the code of the messages arriving from the sensory periphery cannot yet have been transformed.

Two funiculi remain. One of them, the lateral funiculus (or lateral column), is circumscribed by the dorsal rootlets, which enter along the dorsolateral sulcus, and the ventral rootlets, which emerge along a similar groove, the ventrolateral sulcus. The other one, the smallest of the three, is the ventral funiculus (or ventral column). It lies between the ventrolateral sulcus and a very deep cleft at the spinal cord's ventral midline that is called the ventral median fissure. The lateral funiculus and the ventral funiculus contain no primary sensory fibers. They are composed exclusively of higher-order fibers —fibers that arise in the central nervous system and not in dorsal-root ganglia. Some of these fibers ascend from the spinal cord into the brain; they compose the spinocerebellar and the lemniscal channels. Others descend; from all levels of the brain—hindbrain, midbrain, and forebrain—fibers course into the spinal cord. Doubtless the ultimate targets for many of the messages they convey are the spinal cord's motor neurons. Nevertheless, few of them synapse with motor neurons directly. Still others among the higher-order fibers are given several names: they are called spinospinal fibers, or intersegmental fibers, or propriospinal fibers, or spinal association fibers. Some of them ascend, some descend. Some cross the midline to reach the opposite side of the spinal cord, some remain ipsilateral. Some are short, some span the length of the cord. What they all have in common is that they originate and terminate in the spinal gray matter: they serve to interconnect different levels of the cord. As a rule, spinospinal fibers stay in the spinal gray matter if they have dealings only in their segment of origin. If, however, they travel beyond that segment, they ascend or descend just outside the gray matter, then turn back into the gray. Accordingly, the zone of spinal white matter immediately surrounding the gray matter in all three funiculi is a zone in which spinospinal fibers are numerous. One particular spinospinal system is rather distinct in the spinal white matter. It is the dorsolateral fasciculus (or marginal zone, or simply zone) of Lissauer, named after the 19th-century German neurologist Heinrich Lissauer. The dorsolateral fasciculus caps the apex of the dorsal horn, thus completing the partition of the dorsal and lateral funiculi. In thoracic cross sections it is narrow and elongated; in intumescence cross sections it is wider and flatter. At all spinal levels, however, it consists mainly of thin, sparsely myelinated fibers that originate in the substantia gelatinosa, ascend or descend a short distance, and return to the substantia gelatinosa. In addition it contains thin dorsal-root fibers that make their synaptic connections in the substantia gelatinosa. Moreover, from about C4 on up, it contains an increasing number of primary sensory fibers that enter the brain but end in the spinal cord. They are the longest constituents of the descending (or spinal) tract of the trigeminal nerve, a bundle with which Lissauer's zone imperceptibly blends as it crosses the spinorhombencephalic border.

The First Central Connections

How do the primary sensory fibers composing the dorsal roots link up with the circuitry of the spinal cord? Much of the understanding of the somatic sense depends on the answer to that question. It is therefore unfortunate that the answer is incomplete — incomplete even at this first synaptic step into the central nervous system. To be sure, the overall spread of a given dorsal root's centrally directed fibers can be determined. The distribution of each class of somatic sensory data — touch, proprioception, nociception, and so on — is far more problematic. The fundamental difficulty is that many dorsal-root fibers ascend long distances in the dorsal funiculus while repeatedly sending collaterals into the spinal gray matter. As a result it is unclear whether the primary sensory data led into the three basic secondary sensory channels — local reflex, cerebellar, and lemniscal — are separate and specific for each channel. We have already seen that the rootlets of each dorsal root enter the dorsal funiculus at its dorsolateral corner and that within the funiculus the rootlet fibers divide into ascending and descending branches. The further course of the branches is best described in three parts.

First: Great numbers of fibers invade the spinal gray matter at and near their level of entry into the spinal cord, very largely in the form of collaterals issued by the ascending and descending branches of the primary sensory fibers. This local distribution of the dorsal root is most massive in the segment of entrance but also involves, in decreasing volume, the three segments above the segment of entrance and the two segments below it. Thus the local distribution of a dorsal root includes no fewer than six spinal cord segments. By the same token, each spinal cord segment receives primary sensory data from no fewer than six dorsal roots. Within each segment the collaterals synapse mostly in the dorsal horn. Many, however, pass into the zona intermedia and even into the ventral horn, where they synapse with interneurons of Rexed's laminae 7 and 8 or with motor neurons directly. The latter connection is the monosynaptic reflex arc. The dorsal-root collaterals invading the ventral horn tend to group themselves in fascicles resembling horse tails; Cajal named them reflexomotor bundles. In the Weigert preparations of Figures 63, 64, and 65 several such bundles are visible. It seems to be an unbroken rule that no primary sensory fibers cross the midline. Accordingly, any communication of sensory data to the contralateral side of the spinal cord must come through interrupted paths: the crossing fibers must be emitted by neurons of the spinal gray matter.

Second: Many dorsal-root fibers (or their collaterals) attain their secondary sensory cell group by ascending the dorsal funiculus for a distance exceeding the local range of "three segments up." The column of Clarke, for example, gets proprioceptive input from the lower half of the body, in particular the leg; thus some of its afferents enter the cord at sacral levels. Yet the column's caudal limit is at spinal segment L2. The fibers must climb to get there. Strangely, fibers conveying proprioception from the arm, which enter the spinal cord at segments as high as C5, do not descend to Clarke's column. Instead fibers bearing such data ascend. Their destination is the lateral cuneate nucleus, a cell group at the top of the spinal cord and well into the hindbrain whose cells look much like those of Clarke's column. For its part Clarke's column emits the dorsal spinocerebellar tract, which occupies the dorsal half of the lateral funiculus near the surface of the spinal cord. The tract delivers data to the ipsilateral side of the cerebellum. That is, the tract is uncrossed: it makes no decussation on its way to the brain. That makes it unusual, though not unique, among ascending secondary sensory bundles. The lateral cuneate nucleus emits the cuneocerebellar tract. It, too, is uncrossed.

The ventral spinocerebellar tract forms something of a contrast. For one thing, it is crossed. Its fibers decussate in the ventral white commissure, a thin plate of white matter separating the spinal gray matter from the ventral median fissure. Then, having crossed the midline, the fibers assemble in the ventral half of the lateral funiculus (the so-called ventrolateral quadrant of the cord) to begin their ascent to the brain. In addition, the ventral spinocerebellar tract originates throughout the length of the spinal cord. Finally, the ventral spinocerebellar tract originates from a wide part of the cross section of the spinal cord's gray matter, including not only the dorsal horn — in particular laminae 4, 5, and 6 of Rexed — but also the ventral horn — lamina 7. The different origins of the two spinocerebellar tracts are mirrored in the nature of the data they transmit to the cerebellum. The column of Clarke gets most of its input from primary sensory neurons whose peripheral endings are stationed in muscles and tendons; many are stationed in muscle spindles. Accordingly, the dorsal spinocerebellar tract carries mostly proprioceptive data. Rexed's laminae 4 through 7 get input from a wider range of somatic sensory endings, including ones responsive to touch and pressure at the body surface. Accordingly, the ventral spinocerebellar tract carries a greater proportion of exteroceptive data. It should be said that the signals conveyed by the spinocerebellar tracts, important as they must be to the cerebellum, seem to play little if any role in conscious perception. Massive destruction of the cerebellum in the human brain impairs neither the patient's position sense — the awareness of the body's arrayal — nor the perception of touch and pressure. The conscious sensations arising from dorsal-root input seem to require the spinal lemnisci.

Third: The most notable instance of primary sensory fibers attaining their secondary sensory cell group by ascending the dorsal funiculus for a distance exceeding "three segments up" occurs because all dorsal roots deliver data to the dorsal-column nuclei — that is to say, the source of the medial lemniscus, at the top of the spinal cord. Some of the dorsal-root fibers that enter the caudalmost spinal cord segments must therefore climb the full height of the dorsal funiculus. Throughout the ascent they are joined on their lateral side by the fibers of successively higher dorsal roots. As a result, the dorsal funiculus at cervical levels is somatotopically divisible into a medial part representing the leg and trunk and a lateral part representing the arm. At about C6 and higher the division is expressed by a shallow groove, the intermediolateral sulcus, which delineates the fasciculus gracilis on its medial side from a larger lateral district, the fasciculus cuneatus. The two are visible in Figure 63. Each fasciculus ends synaptically in the eponymous dorsal-column nucleus. A lesion of the dorsal-column nuclei or of their input system, the dorsal funiculus, or of their output system, the medial lemniscus, entails no loss in nociception. Losses do emerge, however, in exteroception and proprioception. The exteroceptive loss can be found both in two-point discrimination and in the sensing of vibration. Normally it is easy for a person to tell whether a tuning fork applied to the skin covering a bony prominence is vibrating or at rest. But spinal cord lesions interrupting the dorsal funiculus eliminate the capacity to make that distinction on the ipsilateral side of the body. The proprioceptive loss affects position sense. Stand behind the patient and ask him to close his eyes. Then place one of his arms in a half-outstretched position. Ask him to bring the other arm to the mirroring position. The patient cannot do it.

The spinal cord's other lemniscus, the spinothalamic tract, does not require that primary sensory data climb farther than "three segments up." The fibers composing the tract originate throughout the length of the spinal cord, mostly from cells in Rexed's laminae 1, 3, and 4. Within their segment of origin the fibers cross to the opposite side of the cord, employing the ventral white commissure as their bridge across the midline. Their decussation complete, they assemble in the ventrolateral quadrant: the ventral half of the lateral funiculus. There they turn rostrally. They will maintain a ventrolateral position throughout their spinal and rhombencephalic trajectory. Ascending with them are a variety of companions, including not only the ventral spinocerebellar tract but also spinoreticular fibers, directed to the brainstem reticular formation; spino-olivary fibers, directed to the inferior olivary nucleus, in the medulla oblongata; spinosolitary fibers, directed to the nucleus of the solitary tract, also in the medulla; spinoannular fibers, directed to the central gray substance of the midbrain; and spinotectal fibers, directed to the superior colliculus. Some of these companions are part of the spinothalamic tract, in that they share its origin. Others are more nearly independent; perhaps they are best seen as spinal association fibers transcending the spinal cord's upper limit, so that they associate the spinal cord with the brainstem. In any case, only a modest fraction of the fibers composing the bundle called spinothalamic actually attain the thalamus.

Clinical evidence clearly implicates the spinothalamic tract as the principal conveyor of nociceptive and thermoreceptive information to the brain. Specifically, lesions or compressions of the spinal cord's ventrolateral quadrant result in the loss of pain and temperature sensation below the level of the lesion on the opposite side of the body. (Tactile sensation is also compromised, especially if the ventral part of the ventrolateral quadrant is affected by the lesion; thus a "ventral spinothalamic tract," allotted chiefly to tactile sensation, is distinguished from a predominantly nociceptive and thermore-ceptive "lateral spinothalamic tract.") Even so, the details of how the spinothalamic tract comes to be nociceptive remain in dispute. The few points of agreement are worth noting. In the first place, the primary nociceptive afferents to the spinal cord are among the thinnest fibers found in peripheral nerves.* They tend to enter Lissauer's zone. Physiologically, they are charac-

*Neurophysiologists classify the sensory axons in peripheral nerves into an *A* category of myelinated fibers and a *C* category of unmyelinated ones. In turn the *A* category embraces three subcategories: *A*-alpha fibers, which range from 12 to 22 micrometers in diameter

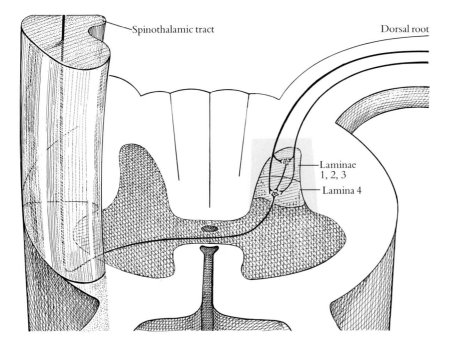
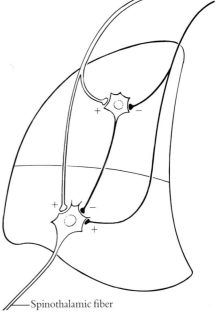

Figure 66: **Wall-Melzack theory** of nociception, or pain sensation, proposes that signals reporting tissue-threatening stimuli are transmitted to the brain by what amount to party lines. In this illustration of the theory a neuron in lamina 4 of Rexed emits a spinothalamic axon, which ascends in the lateral funiculus on the opposite side of the spinal cord. The cell gets two classes of primary sensory data. Tactile input comes from a thick dorsal-root fiber, nociceptive input comes from a thin one. A small neuron somewhere in lamina 1, 2, or 3 (the spinal cord's so-called substantia gelatinosa) gets the same two sensory inputs. The tactile input excites the small neuron, so that it inhibits the large one, putting a brake on the latter's spinothalamic output. In contrast, the nociceptive input inhibits the small neuron, so that the small neuron releases its inhibitory hold on the large one. The resulting volley of spinothalamic traffic conveys nociception on a transmission line that otherwise serves tactile sensation.

terized by a high excitation threshold: they are activated only by stimuli strong enough to threaten—or cause—tissue damage. Like many other primary sensory fibers, they distribute their central ramifications mostly to the dorsal horn in the local six-segment range. Some of the ramifications terminate in lamina 4 of Rexed, others in the substantia gelatinosa: laminae 1, 2, and 3. Some lead into reflex channels, notably the nociceptive, or withdrawal, reflex, which recruits mainly flexor muscles in an often massive mobilization designed to remove the jeopardized part of the body from harm.† Other ramifications (perhaps collaterals of the reflex connections) must connect, somehow, with the spinothalamic tract.

The fundamental controversy surrounding the neurology of pain sensation is expressed by a question: Is pain a specific submodality of the somatic sense, with unique conduction lines in not only peripheral nerves but also the central nervous system? Or is pain sensation mediated by intense signal strength impinging on central conduction lines that otherwise mediate only touch and pressure sensation? Both notions have their defenders. Edward Perl, working at the University of Utah, has found neurons in lamina 1 of Rexed—the layer of the marginal cells of Waldeyer—that respond only to peripheral stimuli intense enough to threaten the integrity of the body's soft tissues. Perl holds that these selectively nociceptive neurons, with their secondary sensory axons, compose a specific spinothalamic channel for central pain conduction. On the other hand, Patrick D. Wall and Ronald Melzack, who were then at the Massachusetts Institute of Technology, have proposed a more complex arrangement (Figure 66). In their scheme a spinothalamic neuron, say in lamina 4 of Rexed, receives tactile input by way of a thick dorsal-root fiber and nociceptive input by way of a thinner fiber. Both inputs excite the neuron. In addition, both inputs affect a small neuron of the substantia gelatinosa—a so-called gate neuron, which inhibits the spinothal-

---

and correspond to proprioceptive endings; *A*-beta fibers, from five to 12 micrometers in diameter, which correspond to touch-, pressure-, and vibration-sensitive endings; and *A*-delta fibers, from two to five micrometers in diameter, which correspond to nociceptive and temperature-sensitive endings. The *C* category, ranging from .1 to 1.5 micrometers in diameter, consists exclusively of fibers with nociceptive endings.

†The nociceptive reflex marks an extreme among the spinal cord's reflexes. It is notably multisegmental. Indeed, it is potentially pansegmental: the nociceptive input conveyed to the spinal cord by a minimal number of dorsal roots (the overlap among dermatomes, or dorsal-root innervation fields on the skin, suggests that the minimum is two) can recruit motor neurons throughout much, even all, of the spinal cord's length. Thus the circuits serving the nociceptive reflex include great numbers of spinospinal fibers. In brief, the reflex is notably polysynaptic. The stretch reflex is different on both counts. Elicited, as we have seen, by the passive stretching of a muscle, it tends to limit its recruitments to the motor neurons that innervate the muscle. Thus it keeps its signals within a small number of spinal cord segments. In addition its circuits are largely monosynaptic. That, too, serves to limit the spread of the signals.

amic neuron. The crux of the scheme is that the tactile and nociceptive inputs affect the gate neuron in opposite ways. The tactile input excites the gate neuron, and so promotes the inhibition of the spinothalamic neuron. The nociceptive input inhibits the gate neuron, and so disinhibits the spinothalamic neuron. The resulting increase in the latter's rate of discharge conveys nociception to the brain. The Wall-Melzack scheme is appealing, not least because it accounts for a prosaic but suggestive phenomenon. When you bark your shin, you find that rubbing it ameliorates the pain. Perhaps the rubbing overwhelms the gate neurons with a torrent of tactile input, a torrent that drowns the nociceptive traffic. And yet one cannot deny the well-documented observations of selectively nociceptive neurons atop the dorsal horn. Perhaps the competing ideas will ultimately coalesce into a more encompassing understanding.

Chapter Eleven

Hindbrain

We come now to the first of the events that give the brain its shape. During the third week of human gestation two flexures become apparent at the cranial end of the neural tube (Figure 67). The more caudal of the two appears just behind the swell of the primary rhombencephalon and renders the tube convex in the dorsal direction; it is called the cervical flexure. The more rostral of the two appears at the level of the primary mesencephalon; it is called the mesencephalic, or simply the cephalic, flexure. It, too, is dorsally convex, but more sharply than the other. Indeed, it bends the neural tube at nearly a right angle. Between them a third bend, the pontine flexure, develops. It alone is dorsally concave. Perhaps that explains why the ventricle of the rhombencephalon, which is called the fourth ventricle, has a rhomboid shape. If a bean pod with a dorsal seam running its length has its ends squeezed together so that a flexure develops with the seam along the concavity of the bending, the seam will split so as to open a rhomb-shaped cleft. We conclude — though the logic is shaky — that the roof plate of the neural tube (the analogue of the bean pod's seam) must be weaker than the floor plate. For when the neural tube bends in one direction, that of the cervical and the cephalic flexure, the floor plate does not give. But when the neural tube bends in the opposite direction, that of the pontine flexure, the roof plate does give.

Unlike a bean pod, however, the roof plate does not split. Instead it stretches, and as the central nervous system develops, the stretched part of the plate becomes the inner, ependymal layer of a double-layered tissue called choroid membrane. The outer layer is formed by vasculated pia mater. As the embryo grows further, the membrane throws itself into folds. At first the folds are gentle. Then side folds develop, and the membrane grows serpentine. In this way a choroid membrane becomes a choroid plexus; the brain of a mammal has three (one for each of its ventricles). Because of its infolding, the surface area of each plexus is considerable. At the eighth or ninth week of ontogeny the plexuses begin their life's work: the production of cerebrospinal fluid. The fluid fills the ventricle system. Soon the roof plate in the caudal part of the fourth ventricle grows thin at the midline. Indeed, like a worn spot in an automobile tire, it begins to bulge outward: it forms an ependymal diverticulum that protrudes into the meningeal tissue that is in place around the brainstem. Eventually the roof plate bursts at the site of the bulge. The result is the median aperture of the fourth ventricle, also called the foramen of Magendie. It is a hole through which the cerebrospinal fluid finds free passage from the fourth ventricle into the subarachnoid space that surrounds the central nervous system. Two similar holes develop in the roof of the fourth ventricle, one at the tip of each lateral recess, the spoutlike lateral expansion of the ventricle. These openings are called the lateral apertures of the fourth ventricle, or the foramina of Luschka, after Hubert Luschka, a 19th-century German anatomist.

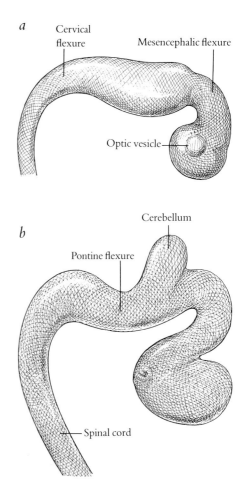

Surface Structure

Figure 68 shows the fully formed human brainstem. The view is from the ventral side. In this perspective the rightness of distinguishing two major subdivisions of the hindbrain is clear. The caudal subdivision is the myelencephalon, or medulla oblongata. Its ventral surface exhibits a characteristic relief. The midline is marked by a deep groove that continues the spinal cord's ventral median fissure. The groove is flanked on each side by the pyramid, a bandlike prominence. The pyramid seems at first to be a rostral extension of the spinal cord's ventral funiculus. Actually it corresponds to the pyramidal tract, which emerges from deep in the brainstem. At the surface of the hindbrain the tract courses caudalward for a distance of about three centimeters. Then it undergoes an almost total decussation. Only a tenth of the fibers in the tract continue their descent uncrossed as constituents of the ventral funiculus. The remaining nine-tenths cross the midline in the form of fascicles that interdigitate with those of the tract of the opposite side. The crossing fibers will disappear from the surface to continue their downward course in the lateral funiculus. As a consequence of the decussation the ventral median fissure is more or less obliterated over a distance of about a centimeter. The level of the obliteration is considered by convention the border between the spinal cord and the medulla oblongata.

The upper boundary of the medulla oblongata is a sharp incisure called the pontomedullary groove. Then comes the metencephalon, the rostral subdivision of the hindbrain. It includes the pons, the cerebellum, and the brachia pontis: two huge bundles of fibers that course around the brainstem from the pons to the cerebellum. (The pons, the cerebellum, and the brachia pontis

Figure 67: **Flexures in the neural tube** begin to develop in the third week of human gestation. They are three in number. The cervical flexure and the mesencephalic flexure bend the tube so that it is dorsally convex (*a*). Between them the pontine flexure bends the tube in the opposite direction (*b*). The pontine flexure develops after the other two have appeared.

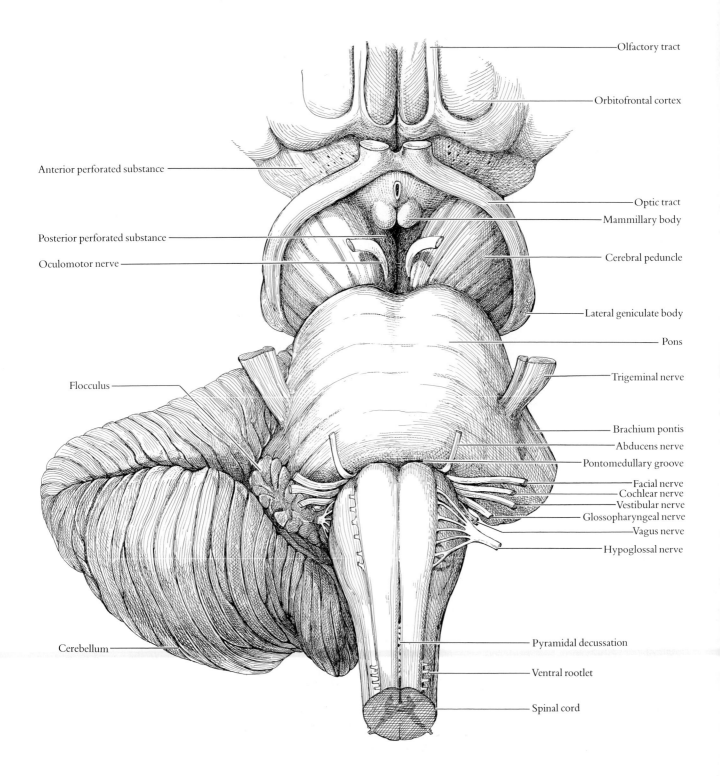

Olfactory tract

Orbitofrontal cortex

Anterior perforated substance

Optic tract

Mammillary body

Posterior perforated substance

Cerebral peduncle

Oculomotor nerve

Lateral geniculate body

Pons

Flocculus

Trigeminal nerve

Brachium pontis

Abducens nerve

Pontomedullary groove

Facial nerve

Cochlear nerve

Vestibular nerve

Glossopharyngeal nerve

Vagus nerve

Hypoglossal nerve

Pyramidal decussation

Cerebellum

Ventral rootlet

Spinal cord

form a ring that encircles the core of the brainstem.) The rostral border of the pons is the rostral border of the hindbrain. Above it is the midbrain. In this ventral view, however, the midbrain is hard to see. For one thing, the mesencephalic flexure gives the rostral part of the brainstem a strong curve that makes its dorsal, convex surface more extensive than its ventral, concave surface. Then, too, the ventral side of the midbrain is mostly hidden behind the largest fiber bundle in the brainstem. The bundle is the cerebral peduncle; it is a corticofugal fiber system that includes the pyramidal tract.

Figure 69 is a dorsal view of the human brainstem. It is partially dissected. On one side of the drawing a cut has been made through the pedestal of white matter connecting the cerebellum to the rest of the brainstem. The pedestal consists of the millions of fibers entering or leaving the cerebellum as components of three cerebellar peduncles. The brachium pontis, or middle cerebellar peduncle, is the largest of the three; it occupies the heart of the mass. Above it is the brachium conjunctivum, or superior cerebellar peduncle; below it is the restiform body, or inferior cerebellar peduncle. The cerebellum itself has been half removed; it would have hidden the hindbrain. The roof of the fourth ventricle has also been half removed. The caudal part of the roof is choroid membrane. In contrast, the rostral part, where the fourth ventricle narrows to become an estuary of the cerebral aqueduct (a narrow channel through the midbrain to the ventricles of the diencephalon and the cerebral hemispheres), is a whitish plate called the anterior medullary velum. Fused to the velum is the most anterior part of the cerebellum, a part called the lingula because of its tonguelike shape. The dissection in Figure 69 ensures that the floor of the fourth ventricle — the so-called rhomboid fossa — is almost completely exposed. A groove called the median sulcus marks the midline. Lateral to it runs a second groove that is less pronounced but nonetheless visible. This second groove is the sulcus limitans, which demarcated the alar plate from the basal plate in the embryo's neural tube. The apparent caudalmost tip of the ventricle is called the obex. The real tip is slightly lower: the ventricle extends a few millimeters farther caudalward as a pocket that ends blind at the occluded central canal of the spinal cord. Caudal to the obex at the surface of the brainstem is the dorsal median sulcus. Here, as in the spinal cord, it identifies the midline. Lateral to the sulcus is a pair of whitish

Figure 68: **Ventral surface of the human brainstem** best shows the two divisions of the hindbrain. The caudal division, the myelencephalon, or medulla oblongata, includes a deep groove, the ventral median fissure, flanked on each side by the pyramidal tract, which raises the bulge called the medullary pyramid. The rostral division, the metencephalon, includes the pons. Above the pons is the midbrain, largely hidden behind the cerebral peduncles. All but one of the cranial nerves emerge from the brainstem's ventral surface. The vagus and the glossopharyngeal emerge ventrolaterally from the medulla oblongata; the hypoglossal emerges there, too, in a more medial position. The cochlear, the vestibular, the facial, and the abducens emerge from the pontomedullary groove. The trigeminal emerges at the surface of the pons. The oculomotor emerges between the cerebral peduncles.

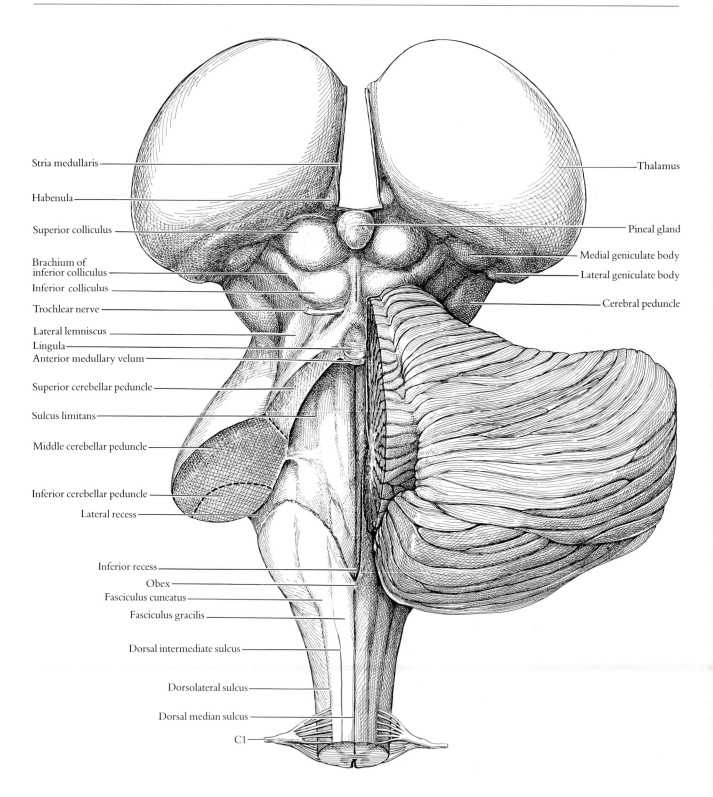

Stria medullaris

Habenula

Superior colliculus

Brachium of
inferior colliculus

Inferior colliculus

Trochlear nerve

Lateral lemniscus

Lingula

Anterior medullary velum

Superior cerebellar peduncle

Sulcus limitans

Middle cerebellar peduncle

Inferior cerebellar peduncle

Lateral recess

Inferior recess

Obex

Fasciculus cuneatus

Fasciculus gracilis

Dorsal intermediate sulcus

Dorsolateral sulcus

Dorsal median sulcus

C1

Thalamus

Pineal gland

Medial geniculate body

Lateral geniculate body

Cerebral peduncle

prominences, separated from each other by a groove called the dorsal intermediate sulcus. The prominences veer laterally and become markedly swollen near the level of the obex. They are the fasciculi cuneatus and gracilis, which compose the rostral end of the dorsal column, and they grow swollen in the caudal rhombencephalon due to the advent of the dorsal-column nuclei: the nucleus gracilis and the nucleus cuneatus. At the top of Figure 69 are the superior and the inferior colliculi. Together they form the four-hilled roof of the midbrain, called the tectum mesencephali, the corpora quadrigemina, or the lamina quadrigemina. Overhanging and even flanking it is the diencephalon: in particular, the thalamus, which is so large in the human brain that it overflows, so to speak, its pocket in the forebrain.

Motor and Sensory Columns

The rhombencephalon and the mesencephalon are sometimes regarded as composing a part of the brain utterly different from the spinal cord. A growing familiarity with the brain brings with it a different opinion. Certainly a survey of the similarities and differences between the brainstem and the spinal cord is a useful beginning to the study of the brainstem's internal structure.

In the first place, it is comforting, as one studies the spinal cord, to find a sharp and ever present boundary between gray matter and white matter. A cross section at any level of the cord displays at its center the characteristic spinal gray butterfly, defined on a field of white. In the hindbrain this boundary is progressively effaced. Only certain fiber systems remain circumscribed: the pyramidal tract, for instance, and the dorsal spinocerebellar tract. Most of the rest are commingled with gray. In the second place, it is comforting, as one studies the spinal cord, to find secondary sensory cells and motor neurons in familiar positions. Every cross section shows both. The former are in the dorsal horn and the latter are in the ventral horn. In the hindbrain things seem to be different. Secondary sensory cells lie lateral, not dorsal, to the sulcus limitans. Motor neurons lie medial, not necessarily ventral. But this is simply a consequence of the stress put on the brainstem as the pontine flexure develops. In effect the flexure opens the neural tube, so that the alar plate on each side of the midline ends up in a position lateral, not dorsal, to the basal plate. In both the spinal cord and the hindbrain the position of motor neurons

Figure 69: **Dorsal surface of the human brainstem** is fully visible when the cerebellum is ablated. On one side of the midline the cerebellar pedestal has been transected. It includes three divisions, or cerebellar peduncles: the inferior peduncle, or restiform body; the middle peduncle, or brachium pontis; and the superior peduncle, or brachium conjunctivum. Of the cerebellum on that side, only the lingula remains. Above it is the midbrain, whose dorsal surface exhibits four bulges, the inferior and superior colliculi. Just under them a cranial nerve, the trochlear, emerges. The dissection exposes half of the floor of the ventricle of the hindbrain: the fourth ventricle. The floor is flanked, on each side of the midline, by a pair of elevations raised by the dorsal-column nuclei.

and secondary sensory cells is dictated in a straightforward way by the embryonic position of the basal and alar plates.

Beyond that, there are complications. Consider first the arrayal of motor neurons. In the spinal cord one finds two great classes of motor neurons. Somatic motor neurons are in the ventral horn; visceral motor neurons are in the lateral horn. It is convenient to regard the somatic motor neurons as composing a single "column"—a somatic motor column exhibiting local variations but extending nonetheless through the length of the spinal cord. Similarly, it is convenient to regard the visceral motor neurons as composing a visceral motor column. True, the visceral motor neurons do not occupy the full length of the spinal cord. The preganglionic motor neurons of the sympathetic nervous system lie only in spinal cord segments cervical 8 through lumbar 2 and those of the parasympathetic nervous system lie only in sacral segments 2, 3, and 4. One is content to say they compose a column because they all are motor neurons: indeed, all of them are preganglionic and autonomic. Moreover, they all appear at the same position on the spinal cord's cross section.

In the brainstem one finds again a somatic motor column and a visceral motor column (Figure 70). Both, however, are interrupted. In particular, the somatic motor column on each side of the brainstem consists of four cell groups near the midline just under the floor of the fourth ventricle or, farther rostrally, the cerebral aqueduct. The most caudal of the four is the hypoglossal nucleus, in the caudal hindbrain. It innervates all the muscles of the tongue. Next comes a gap in the column, and then the abducens nucleus, in the rostral hindbrain. It is the most caudal of the three somatic motor nuclei on each side of the brainstem that innervate muscles attached to the eyeball and thus turn the eye in its socket. The other two are the trochlear nucleus and the oculomotor nucleus, which lie low and high respectively in the midbrain. The visceral motor column on each side of the brainstem consists of three cell groups. Each is preganglionic and parasympathetic, and each is lateral to the

Figure 70: **Motor and sensory cell groups** in the brainstem occupy six interrupted columns on each side of the midline. Motor columns are schematized on the left. The somatic motor column comprises four motor nuclei, or communities of motor neurons and interneurons. They are the hypoglossal nucleus, the abducens nucleus, the trochlear nucleus, and the oculomotor nucleus. The visceral motor column comprises three motor nuclei. They are the dorsal motor nucleus of the vagus nerve, the salivatory nucleus, and the nucleus of Edinger-Westphal. The branchial motor column comprises three motor nuclei. They are the nucleus ambiguus, the facial motor nucleus, and the motor nucleus of the trigeminal nerve. Sensory columns are schematized on the right. The special somatic sensory column comprises six secondary sensory nuclei; two are cochlear (that is, auditory) and four are vestibular. They cluster in the hindbrain. The visceral sensory column is a single nucleus: the nucleus of the solitary tract. Its meeting with its contralateral counterpart in the medulla oblongata is called the commissural nucleus. The general somatic sensory column is also a single nucleus: the sensory nucleus of the trigeminal nerve. Its rounded head, however, is known as the main sensory nucleus of the nerve; its long tail is the descending nucleus of the nerve.

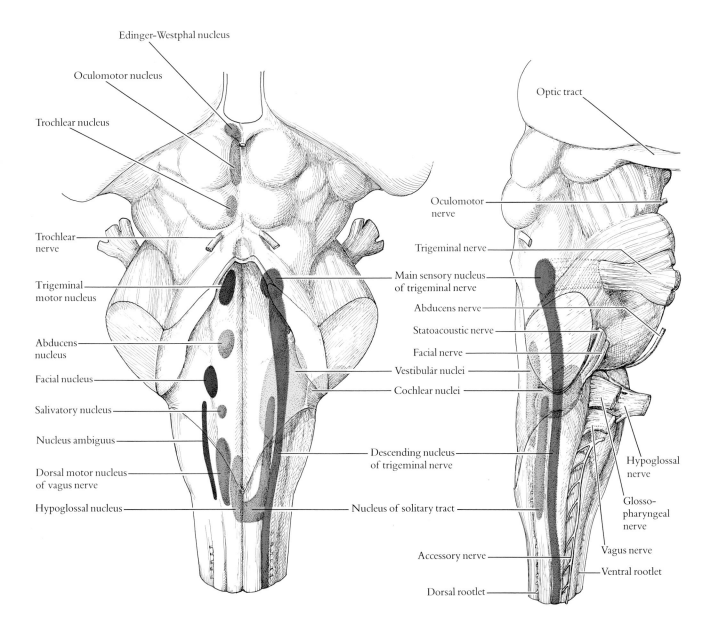

Edinger-Westphal nucleus

Oculomotor nucleus

Trochlear nucleus

Trochlear nerve

Trigeminal motor nucleus

Abducens nucleus

Facial nucleus

Salivatory nucleus

Nucleus ambiguus

Dorsal motor nucleus of vagus nerve

Hypoglossal nucleus

Optic tract

Oculomotor nerve

Trigeminal nerve

Main sensory nucleus of trigeminal nerve

Abducens nerve

Statoacoustic nerve

Facial nerve

Vestibular nuclei

Cochlear nuclei

Descending nucleus of trigeminal nerve

Nucleus of solitary tract

Accessory nerve

Dorsal rootlet

Hypoglossal nerve

Glosso-pharyngeal nerve

Vagus nerve

Ventral rootlet

Motor nuclei

 Somatic motor column

Visceral motor column

Branchial motor column

Sensory nuclei

General somatic sensory column

Special somatic sensory column

Visceral sensory column

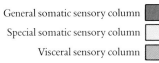

somatic motor column just under the ventricle system. The most caudal of the three, the dorsal motor nucleus of the vagus nerve, lies at much the same level as the hypoglossal nucleus. By way of postganglionic motor neurons in or near its target organs it supplies parasympathetic governance to the heart and the smooth muscle and gland cells of the intestinal tract and the respiratory tract. The middle representative of the three, the salivatory nucleus, is better known to physiologists than it is to neuroanatomists. By way of ganglia near its target organs it innervates the three salivary glands, and also the lacrimal gland, in the orbita of the eye. The uppermost of the three, the nucleus of Edinger-Westphal (named after the German anatomist Ludwig Edinger and the German neurologist Karl F. O. Westphal), occupies the rostral pole of the oculomotor nucleus. By way of the ciliary ganglion, within the orbita, it innervates two smooth muscles in the eye: the ciliary muscle and the constrictor pupillae muscle.

Close to the somatic motor column and the visceral motor column but in a more ventral position on a cross section of the brainstem one finds a third motor column. It, too, is interrupted: it consists of three separate cell groups, all in the hindbrain. In ascending order they are the nucleus ambiguus, which governs the muscles of the pharynx and the larynx, the muscles of swallowing and vocalization; then the facial motor nucleus, which governs the muscles of facial expression; and then the motor nucleus of the trigeminal nerve, which governs the muscles of mastication. In the embryo of a mammal all these muscles arise from a set of four incomplete rings of tissue that encircle the developing foregut. The rings are called branchial arches, from *branchion,* the Greek word meaning gill. Hence the column is called the branchial motor column. The muscles, incidentally, are striated.*

The secondary sensory cell groups of the brainstem are also said to form columns. But one such column, the special somatic sensory column, consists of cell groups clustering at and about the level of the lateral recess of the fourth ventricle, at the middle of the length of the hindbrain. There they receive primary sensory information from the sensory epithelia of the inner ear. They are the cochlear nuclei and the vestibular nuclei. A second sensory

---

*In the spinal cord we encountered no branchial motor nucleus. We would have found one, though, if we had paid closer attention to the upper four cervical segments. There a group of motor neurons centrally placed in the ventral horn composes what is called the spinal nucleus of the accessory nerve. It might well be considered a spinal extension of the nucleus ambiguus. Its efferent axons emerge from the spinal cord in a segmental series of rootlets along the lateral — not the ventral — side of the cord. The rootlets combine to form a slender longitudinal fascicle, the spinal accessory nerve itself. The nerve is unique: instead of directing itself through an intervertebral foramen it ascends alongside the cervical spinal cord, entering the cranial cavity through the foramen magnum. Within the cranium it is joined by fibers from the nucleus ambiguus. The augmented bundle then leaves the cranial cavity through the jugular foramen, immediately behind the vagus nerve. Back in the neck, its contingent of spinal efferents innervates the sternocleidomastoid muscle and the upper part of the trapezoid muscle. Both are thought to develop from branchial arches 5 and 6, which are rudimentary in a mammalian embryo.

column consists of a single cell group confined mostly to the medulla oblongata. It is the visceral sensory column, which is to say, the nucleus of the solitary tract. It receives primary sensory information from baroreceptive and chemoreceptive sensory endings in the viscera.* (Its rostral third, sometimes called the gustatory nucleus, receives information from the taste buds.) Only the third and last of the sensory columns found in the brainstem really impresses one as being a column. It is the general somatic sensory column. It, too, consists of a single cell group, the sensory nucleus of the trigeminus. In its case, however, the cell group extends without interruption through the length of the hindbrain. In fact, the cell group becomes continuous at the caudal boundary of the brain with the dorsal horn of the spinal cord. The cell group is thus the cranial part of a column of gray matter that continues upward without interruption from the lower end of the spinal cord to the upper end of the rhombencephalon. The general somatic sensory column receives all its primary sensory input from a single cranial nerve: the most massive one, the trigeminus. It thereby gets proprioceptive, tactile, and nociceptive information from the face, the mucosa of the nasal and oral cavities, the dentition, and the nonoptic tunics of the eye: the sclera, the cornea, and the chorioidea. The dorsal horn gets the same great classes of information from the trunk and the limbs. In sum, then, the general somatic sensory column is both anatomically and functionally a cranial extension of the dorsal horn, and the dorsal horn is the general somatic sensory column, so to speak, of the spinal cord. It should be added that the rostral end of the general somatic sensory column, which lies near the rostral limit of the hindbrain, is a rounded mass of gray matter called the main (or principal) sensory nucleus of the trigeminal nerve. The long taper of the column merging into the dorsal horn is called the descending (or spinal) nucleus of the trigeminus.

The sensory and motor columns of the brainstem, each three in number, are schematized in Figure 71. So are the cranial nerves. None of them fully mimics the spinal pattern; that is, none of them arises, like a spinal nerve, from the fusion of a dorsal, sensory contingent and a ventral, motor contingent. Still, in one of the cranial nerves the spinal model reappears in lessened form. The trigeminal nerve emerges from the brain as a large sensory root, the portio major, and just medial to it a much smaller motor root, the portio minor.

Of the remaining cranial nerves four are purely motor. They are the hypoglossal nerve, the abducens nerve, the trochlear nerve, and the oculomotor nerve. They are much like ventral roots. For one thing, all but one of them consist exclusively of axons directed from the somatic motor column to

---

*In the spinal cord we encountered no circumscribed visceral sensory nucleus. In fact none is known. It is a remarkable lack, especially when one considers that numerous sensory axons follow the peripheral ramifications of the sympathetic nervous system and enter the spinal cord by way of dorsal roots. Perhaps the secondary sensory neurons receiving these visceral afferents are diffusely distributed in the dorsal horn and so have escaped detection.

striated muscle tissue of the tongue or the extraocular muscles. The exception is the oculomotor nerve, which includes a visceral motor contingent: the preganglionic parasympathetic fibers arising in the nucleus of Edinger-Westphal. Moreover, all but one of them leave the brainstem near the ventral midline. The exception is the trochlear nerve, which breaks with all convention by exiting the brainstem near the dorsal midline. (It leaves just caudal to the inferior colliculus.) In the course of its exit it commits a further aberration: it decussates. Three cranial nerves are almost purely sensory. They are the acoustic or cochlear nerve, the vestibular nerve, and the trigeminal nerve, or at least its massive portio major. They are much like dorsal roots. For one thing, they consist almost exclusively of primary sensory fibers directed from a sensory ganglion to either the general somatic sensory column or the special

Figure 71: **Arrangement of brainstem columns** is dictated by ontogenetic modifications in the positions of the alar and basal plates; thus the brainstem elaborates the simpler pattern found in the spinal cord. These schematized cross sections offer some particulars. In the spinal cord (*top drawing*) secondary sensory neurons in the dorsal horn form what amounts to a general somatic sensory column. Somatic motor neurons in the ventral horn form a somatic motor column. Preganglionic sympathetic motor neurons in the lateral horn form a visceral motor column. (In sacral spinal cord segments the latter has a further installment consisting of preganglionic parasympathetic motor neurons.) The hindbrain (*bottom drawing*) looks quite different: the somatic and visceral motor neurons are medial, not ventral, to the somatic sensory column. But that is simply because the pontine flexure opens the part of the neural tube that develops into the hindbrain, so that the basal plate is medial, not ventral, to the alar plate. On the other hand, the special somatic sensory column and the visceral sensory column have no spinal cord analogues, and the branchial motor column has only a covert analogue, in the form of cervical motor neurons innervating two neck muscles. Three cranial nerves—the cochlear, the vestibular, and the trigeminal—are somewhat like dorsal roots. (The trigeminal, however, includes a motor contingent.) Four cranial nerves—the hypoglossal, the abducens, the trochlear, and the oculomotor—are much like ventral roots. Three cranial nerves—the facial, the glossopharyngeal, and the vagus—are mixed: they are visceral sensory, visceral motor, and branchial motor.

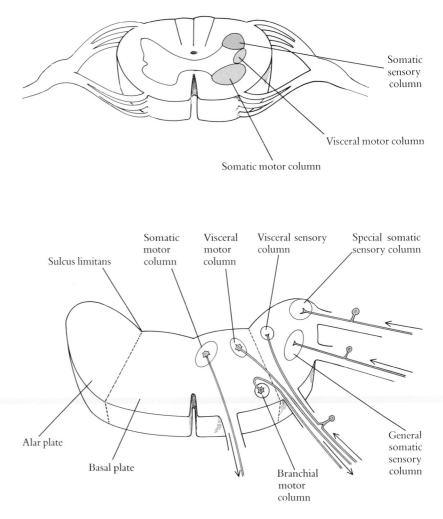

somatic sensory column. (The acoustic nerve includes some axons efferent to the brainstem that synapse on some of the hair cells of Corti's organ and are thought to adjust the response threshold of those auditory signal transducers.) Moreover, the nerves in question enter the brainstem laterally. (One must remember that the pontine flexure unfolds the developing rhombencephalon and shifts the brainstem's dorsal-root entrance line to a lateral position on the cross section.) Finally, three cranial nerves are mixed — that is, both sensory and motor. They are mixed in a curious way: each of them carries fibers from a branchial motor nucleus and from a visceral motor nucleus, plus visceral sensory fibers directed to the nucleus of the solitary tract. They are the vagus nerve, the glossopharyngeal nerve, and the facial nerve. They emerge at intermediate positions on the ventral surface of the hindbrain; closer, however, to the line of the purely sensory cranial nerves (the brainstem's "dorsal roots") than to the line of the purely motor nerves (the brainstem's "ventral roots"). The vagus emerges as a longitudinal series of rootlets, the glosso-pharyngeus as a single trunk. The facial nerve often emerges as two fascicles, a large medial one and a smaller lateral one. The former is branchial motor; it innervates the facial musculature. The latter, called the nervus intermedius of Wrisberg, is visceral motor and visceral sensory (in particular gustatory).

Internal Structure: The Spinomedullary Transition

We turn to a series of Weigert-stained cross sections of the human rhomben-cephalon. We cannot be exhaustive; our intent is to suggest the complexity of the rhombencephalon's internal structure — a complexity poorly acknowl-edged by the exercise of stringing motor nuclei and secondary sensory cell groups into columns. Figure 72 shows the approximate positions of the sections we have chosen; then Figure 73 shows the two most caudal sections. Both transect the neuraxis at the spinomedullary transition: the level at which some 90 percent of the fibers in each pyramidal tract cross the midline to begin their descent as the lateral corticospinal tract in the lateral funiculus of the contralateral half of the spinal cord. Here the progressive effacement of the spinal cord pattern begins. The section at the top of the figure (the more caudal of the pair) could pass as a spinal cord segment, were it not for some notable changes. In the first place, the section, labeled *a*, does indeed show the sweep of the medullary pyramids across the midline and into the dorsal half of the opposite lateral funiculus. At the midline itself, the pyramids consist of fascicles intertwining like the fingers of two clasped hands. After emerging from the decussation, the fascicles cut a wide, straight swath obliquely across the gray matter, severing the ventral horn from the rest of the gray. About 10 percent of the fibers in each medullary pyramid stay clear of the decussation: they keep their ventral, uncrossed position and become the ventral cortico-spinal tract, which flanks the spinal cord's ventral median fissure. The aggre-gation of crossed pyramidal fibers in the dorsal half of each lateral funiculus narrows the basal part of the dorsal horn and displaces it dorsalward, together

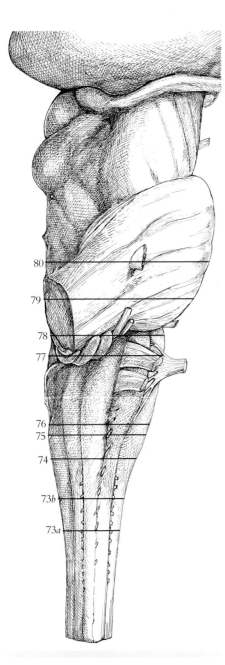

with the gray bridge that connects the two halves of the spinal gray matter: the ventral and dorsal gray commissures. As a result the dorsal horn in Figure 73a has an almost horizontal orientation.

Note the apical (here the most lateral) part of the dorsal horn. It seems markedly increased in size; still, the cross section shows it as a large, rounded mass of gray matter comprising a wide, sickle-shaped outer zone with little myelination (quite plainly this is the substantia gelatinosa, or laminae 1, 2, and 3 of Rexed) and a core region richer in myelin (plainly the rostral extension of the nucleus cornu proprius, or lamina 4 of Rexed). Separating the substantia gelatinosa from the pial surface of the section is a layer of thin, weakly myelinated fibers that invites the designation Lissauer's zone. At this level, however, the zone consists chiefly of primary sensory fibers of the trigeminus (the longest of which extend as far caudally as the third or fourth cervical segment). From here on rostralward, the zone of Lissauer becomes, therefore, the descending, or spinal, trigeminal tract. By the same token, Rexed's laminae 1 through 4 become the so-called subnucleus caudalis of the descending, or spinal, trigeminal nucleus. The subnucleus caudalis is the only division of the nucleus with a substantia gelatinosa; this being so, it is notable that the subnucleus processes the nociceptive input from the sensory realm of the nerve. At the most medial part of the dorsal horn, a narrow column of gray matter invades the fasciculus gracilis of the overlying dorsal funiculus. It is the caudal end of the nucleus gracilis, the most medial of the dorsal-column nuclei. In section b of Figure 73 the nucleus is more conspicuous. Moreover, it is joined on its lateral side by a similar invasion, the nucleus cuneatus, a broadly triangular region. The dorsum of the section thus includes the alignment of three somatic sensory nuclei. The nucleus gracilis, most medial of the three, represents the leg; the nucleus cuneatus, in the middle of the three, represents the arm and the hand; the spinal trigeminal nucleus, most lateral of the three, represents the head. The alignment illustrates the tendency of the somatic sense to conserve the topology of the body.

The ventral horn, like the dorsal, shows modifications that signal its arrival in the brain. In a, the more caudal of the cross sections in Figure 73, the ventral horn has been severed from the rest of the section's gray matter by the sweep of the lateral corticospinal tract. Even so, it contains motor neurons. Along its medial border lie small motor-neuronal clusters: the so-called supraspinal nucleus, which constitutes the rostral extreme of the spinal cord's most medial motor-neuronal "column." Like the latter, it innervates axial muscles—in particular, the "strap muscles" under the hyoid bone in the neck. (The sternohyoid and omohyoid muscles are examples.) At a slightly higher level the column will end. Then, somewhat more rostrally, the column will reappear, in the form of a somatic motor nucleus that innervates axial muscles above the hyoid bone. It will reappear, that is, as the hypoglossal nucleus, innervating the musculature of the tongue. More lateral in the ventral-horn remnant are the most rostral motor neurons of the spinal accessory nerve. They, too, are at the end of a column that will reappear farther rostrally, in the form of a branchial motor cell group, the nucleus ambiguus.

Figure 72: **Nine hindbrain cross sections** are displayed in Weigert preparations in the next eight illustrations; here their levels are shown on a lateral view of the human brainstem. Five of the nine are in the medulla oblongata, or myelencephalon; the remaining four are in the metencephalon.

In *b,* the more rostral of the sections in Figure 73, a remarkable change is occurring. What appears to be ventral horn is no longer really the equivalent of the ventral horn of the spinal cord. For one thing, the "ventral horn" in Figure 73*b* contains no notable assemblies of motor neurons. Then, too, it is traversed by longitudinal fiber bundles. Most telling, perhaps, its border with the spinothalamic tract and other components of the lateral funiculus has become rather indistinct. It is as if the region were making a lateral diffusion. The region is in reality the caudal end of the brainstem reticular formation.

One more point concerning Figure 73*b.* Immediately ventral to the nucleus cuneatus is an assemblage of delicate, ventrally oriented fascicles. They are the most caudal representatives of a system of fibers sweeping from the nuclei gracilis and cuneatus in arciform trajectories across the medulla oblongata; they are in fact called internal arcuate fibers. The fascicles cross the midline dorsal to the medullary pyramids (the ones in Figure 73*b* find their path blocked by the pyramidal decussation and deflect rostrally before crossing). Immediately across the midline they turn upward to form the medial lemniscus.

Internal Structure: Myelencephalon

The next several cross sections lie well rostral to the spinomedullary transition. All of them exhibit the configuration of gray and white matter typical of the myelencephalon, or medulla oblongata. In spite of the changes that take place over the sequence—some are gradual, others are more abrupt—our description can be, at least to some extent, collective of some or all of the sequence.

The sections appearing in Figure 74 and Figure 75 are well worth describing together. Both represent a long jump upward from the level of Figure 73*b.* The more caudal section (Figure 74) is at the level of the obex: the central canal has not yet opened to become the fourth ventricle. The more rostral section (Figure 75) is several millimeters higher and involves the caudal part (the inferior recess) of the ventricle. Neither section exhibits anything immediately reminiscent of the spinal cord. Yet one knows there must be secondary sensory cell groups comparable to those in the spinal cord's dorsal horn, positioned dorsally in Figure 74 and farther laterally in Figure 75, where the unfolding of the neural tube has produced the fourth ventricle. One also knows there must be three columns of motor nuclei, representing a ventral-horn analogue, in ventral and medial positions. The main obstacle to a prompt recognition of these spinal cord counterparts in the medulla oblongata is twofold. First, the ventral horn's assemblies of intermediate neurons (chiefly in laminae 7 and 8 of Rexed) have now "exploded" into a large, poorly delineated, central field of gray and white matter, the brainstem reticular formation. Second, a serpentine sheet of gray matter, forming a large, ovoid structure called the inferior olivary nucleus, or simply the inferior olive, has now appeared lateral and dorsal to the pyramidal tract. The

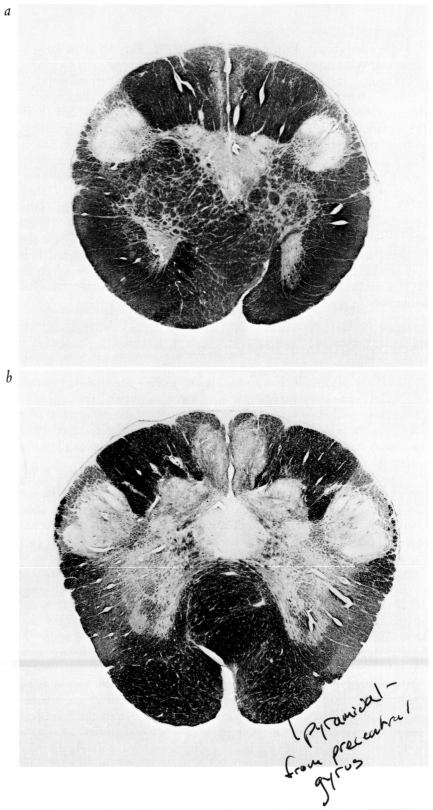

a

b

Figure 73: **Progressive effacement** of the spinal cord's pattern characterizes the caudal rhombencephalon, shown here in a pair of Weigert-stained cross sections from a human brain. In the more caudal section (*a*) the decussation of the pyramidal tract severs the ventral horn while giving the dorsal horn an almost horizontal orientation. The ventral horn includes the rostralmost spinal cord motor neurons, which innervate neck muscles. The dorsal horn now includes the descending nucleus of the trigeminus. In the more rostral section (*b*) the dorsal-column nuclei are visible: the nuclei gracilis and cuneatus. With the descending trigeminal nucleus they complete a somatic sensory map of the body. The "ventral horn" in the section is really the caudal end of the brainstem reticular formation.

pyramidal – from precentral gyrus

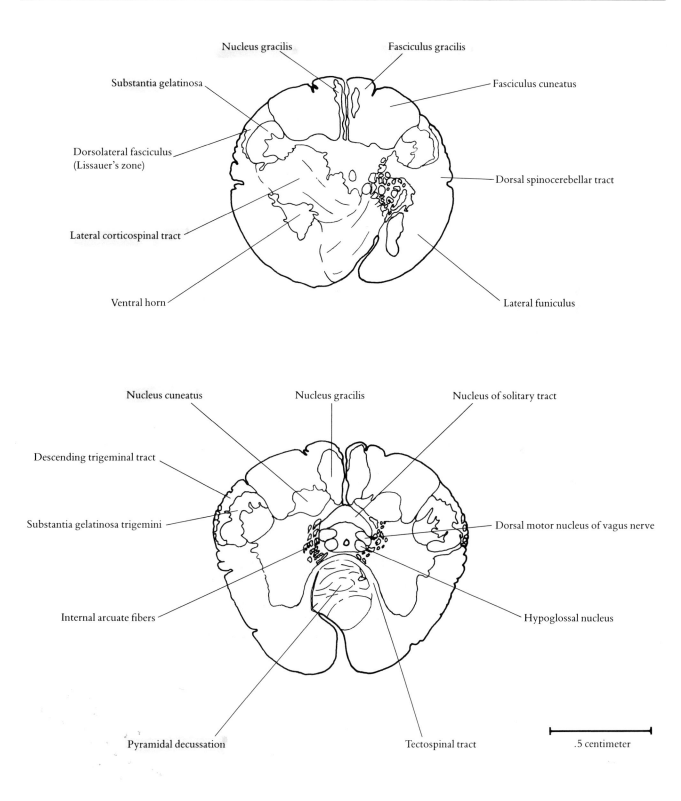

Nucleus gracilis

Fasciculus gracilis

Substantia gelatinosa

Fasciculus cuneatus

Dorsolateral fasciculus
(Lissauer's zone)

Dorsal spinocerebellar tract

Lateral corticospinal tract

Ventral horn

Lateral funiculus

Nucleus cuneatus

Nucleus gracilis

Nucleus of solitary tract

Descending trigeminal tract

Substantia gelatinosa trigemini

Dorsal motor nucleus of vagus nerve

Internal arcuate fibers

Hypoglossal nucleus

Pyramidal decussation

Tectospinal tract

.5 centimeter

inferior olive has no spinal cord analogue; it is one of two formations of uniquely rhombencephalic gray matter that project massively to the contralateral half of the cerebellum. The other one, the pons, will appear in subsequent sections. Both occupy a ventral position on the cross section, in spite of their derivation from the alar plate.

Our survey of Figure 74 and Figure 75 begins with an identification of the three motor columns. The most conspicuous of the three is the somatic motor column, represented in both of the sections by a round, lightly myelinated area: the caudalmost constituent of the column, the hypoglossal nucleus. In

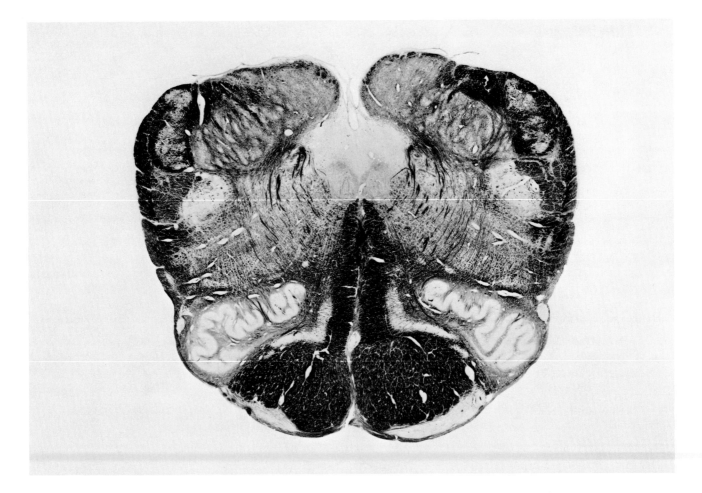

Figure 74: **Level of the obex** in the caudal rhombencephalon marks the uppermost limit of the spinal cord's occluded central canal. Dorsal to the canal, and spanning the width of the section, are the nucleus gracilis, the nucleus cuneatus, and the external cuneate nucleus, an array of secondary sensory cell groups receiving input from dorsal-column fibers. The nuclei gracilis and cuneatus emit internal arcuate fibers, which sweep through the section, decussate, and join the medial lemniscus. The oval of gray matter ventral to the nucleus cuneatus is the descending trigeminal nucleus, which now lacks a substantia gelatinosa. A further district of gray matter, this one ven-

Figure 74 the nucleus lies just ventral to the obliterated central canal; in Figure 75 it lies just under the floor of the fourth ventricle. Its central root fibers (a term denoting motor axons before they emerge at the surface of the brain) follow a nearly ventralward course to leave the brainstem in a longitudinal row of rootlets between the medullary pyramid and the olivary prominence. (One such rootlet is visible on the right side of Figure 75.) Lateral to the hypoglossal nucleus and slightly dorsal to it, the caudalmost constituent of the visceral motor column, the dorsal motor nucleus of the vagus, appears as a strikingly pale-staining (that is, poorly myelinated) region. In Figure 75 it

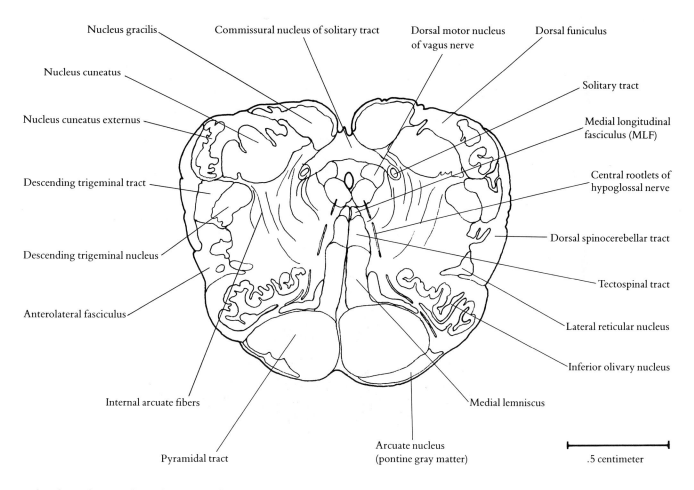

Nucleus gracilis

Nucleus cuneatus

Nucleus cuneatus externus

Descending trigeminal tract

Descending trigeminal nucleus

Anterolateral fasciculus

Internal arcuate fibers

Pyramidal tract

Commissural nucleus of solitary tract

Dorsal motor nucleus of vagus nerve

Dorsal funiculus

Solitary tract

Medial longitudinal fasciculus (MLF)

Central rootlets of hypoglossal nerve

Dorsal spinocerebellar tract

Tectospinal tract

Lateral reticular nucleus

Inferior olivary nucleus

Medial lemniscus

Arcuate nucleus (pontine gray matter)

.5 centimeter

tral to the nucleus gracilis, is the nucleus of the solitary tract, which meets its contralateral counterpart as the commissural nucleus. Ventral to the occluded central canal is the hypoglossal nucleus. The strikingly pale-staining region dorsal and lateral to it is the dorsal motor nucleus of the vagus. A third motor nucleus, the nucleus ambiguus, is virtually impossible to find: it lies deep in the reticular formation. Ventral to the reticular formation is the inferior olivary nucleus, a convoluted sheet of gray matter folded into an oval shape. Its neurons project to the cerebellum. Ventral to the olive is the pyramidal tract.

lies beneath the ventricular floor. The third motor column—the branchial motor—is represented at the levels of Figure 74 and Figure 75 by the nucleus ambiguus. Unfortunately the nucleus is nearly impossible to find in a Weigert preparation. The nucleus is shaped like a needle; no more than six of its motor neurons are likely to appear on any one cross section. Still, its location can be approximated. Imagine a line extending from the center of the hypoglossal nucleus to the lateral margin of the olivary prominence. The nucleus

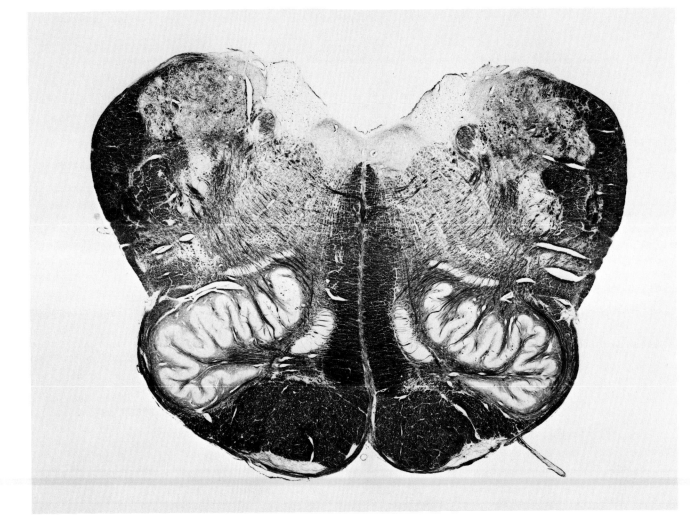

Figure 75: **Fourth ventricle's caudalmost district,** the inferior recess, is transected in a section several millimeters higher than the section in Figure 74. The hypoglossal nucleus is now in the floor of the ventricle; its efferents leave the ventral face of the section between the inferior olive and the medullary pyramid. The dorsal motor nucleus of the vagus is subventricular, too. Sensory cell groups, including the nucleus of the solitary tract, are in more lateral positions. Again the gray oval ventral to the nucleus cuneatus is the descending nu-

is in the midst of the medullary reticular formation, about two-thirds of the way to the lateral end of the line. The motor fibers leaving the nucleus describe a dorsally directed arch to join the central root fibers of the vagus and glossopharyngeus.

We turn next to an identification of the secondary sensory cell groups in Figure 74 and Figure 75. In the former they occupy much of the dorsal fourth of the section. Three large ones are side by side; they are the nucleus gracilis,

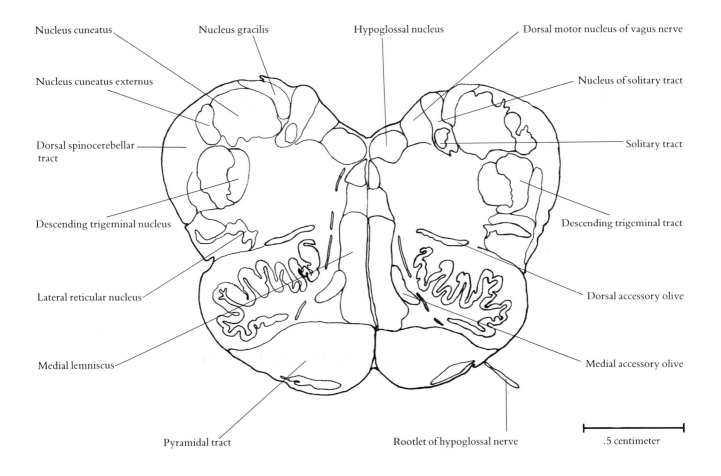

cleus of the trigeminus, accompanied on its lateral side by the descending trigeminal tract. Here, as in Figure 74, three longitudinal fiber systems, the medial lemniscus, the tectospinal tract, and the medial longitudinal fasciculus, form a band abutting the midline. Another three systems, the spinothalamic tract, the ventral spinocerebellar tract, and (going the opposite direction) the rubrospinal tract, compose a more lateral group. A further system, the olivocerebellar projection, emerges from the hilus of each inferior olive.

the nucleus cuneatus, and the nucleus cuneatus lateralis, or external cuneate nucleus. All three are dorsal-column nuclei: they get their primary sensory input from the spinal cord's dorsal-root fibers, by way of the dorsal column. Along their ventral borders, the nuclei gracilis and cuneatus can be seen issuing numerous slender fascicles of internal arcuate fibers, which sweep through the reticular formation to join the contralateral medial lemniscus. The external cuneate nucleus issues no such fibers. Instead its efferents join the dorsal spinocerebellar tract, which runs dorsally over the lateral face of the nucleus on a trajectory toward the inferior cerebellar peduncle. (Recall that the external cuneate nucleus is the medullary equivalent of the spinal cord's column of Clarke, which projects to the cerebellum.) In Figure 75 the nucleus gracilis is already nearing its rostral limit; in Figure 76 its two companions will also be gone, replaced by two of the four vestibular nuclei. A short distance ventral to the nucleus cuneatus in Figure 74 and again in Figure 75 a circumscribed oval of gray matter appears, accompanied on its lateral side by the comma-shaped cross section of an equally circumscribed fiber bundle. The gray matter is the descending, or spinal, nucleus of the trigeminus, which no longer includes a substantia gelatinosa: the obex is well rostral to the subnucleus caudalis. The bundle is the descending trigeminal tract, the conveyor of its primary sensory input.

The descending trigeminal nucleus is the sole rhombencephalic representative of the general somatic sensory column. (The dorsal-column nuclei, being innervated by the spinal cord's dorsal roots, fit no scheme of rhombencephalic sensory columns.) The special somatic sensory column has not yet made its appearance. That leaves the visceral sensory column — which is to say, the nucleus of the solitary tract. Figure 74 shows its most caudal part, immediately ventral to the nucleus gracilis. There the nucleus of the solitary tract expands medially to fuse at the midline with its contralateral partner, thus forming the commissural nucleus, a broad arch of extremely pale-staining gray matter. The arch composes the dorsal half of a ring of gray matter that surrounds the occluded central canal; farther rostrally, in Figure 75, the ring has opened, producing a bowl-shaped mass of subventricular gray matter. From there on upward, the nucleus of the solitary tract on each side of the rhombencephalon is a lateral subdivision of the subventricular gray, accompanied on its ventral and lateral sides by the solitary tract: the slender, circumscribed fiber bundle from which the nucleus gets its primary sensory input.

The tract (to take that first) consists of primary sensory fibers from three of the cranial nerves: the vagus, the glossopharyngeus, and the facial. The vagus and glossopharyngeus contribute fibers from mechanoreceptive endings and chemoreceptive transducer cells in the wall of the heart and its great trunk vessels, in the respiratory tract, and in the wall of the digestive tract. In addition, the vagus and glossopharyngeus innervate a special class of chemoreceptive transducer cells: the gustatory receptor cells of the taste buds on the posterior third of the tongue. The facial nerve contributes fibers from the taste buds on the anterior two-thirds of the tongue. The fibers all make synaptic connections in the nucleus of the tract. The rostral third of the nucleus receives the gustatory fibers. It is therefore no surprise that a lemniscal channel, the gustatory lemniscus, has been traced from the rostral third of the nucleus to a thalamic cell group: the semilunar nucleus, a distinct, crescent-shaped, ventromedial subdivision of the ventrobasal nucleus. In turn, the semilunar nucleus projects to a district of neocortex on the ventral, hidden face of the postcentral gyrus. As described by Ralph Norgren and Christiana Leonard, who traced it in the rat in a study done at the Rockefeller University, the gustatory lemniscus is peculiar in three respects. First, it is rather diffuse. Second, it is largely uncrossed. All other known lemnisci are at least half crossed. Third, it is synaptically interrupted low in the mesencephalon, in a region of gray matter called the parabrachial nuclei. (In this third respect the gustatory lemniscus resembles the auditory, or lateral, lemniscus, which also is interrupted by a caudal-mesencephalic way station: the inferior colliculus.) The caudal two-thirds of the nucleus of the solitary tract, including the commissural nucleus, is the brainstem's true visceral sensory cell group: it receives the primary visceral sensory fibers that the vagus and glossopharyngeus bring to the brain. In turn, it directs a widespread reflex channel at rhombencephalic mechanisms controlling cardiovascular, respiratory, and gastrointestinal function. Such mechanisms include the dorsal motor nucleus of the vagus and the reticular formation of the medulla oblongata. In addition, the caudal two-thirds of the nucleus of the solitary tract issues a long ascending tract that parallels the gustatory lemniscus. It, too, is interrupted (but only in part) in the parabrachial nuclei. Its destination, however, is not the thalamus, but the hypothalamus. Presumably this visceral sensory analogue of a lemniscus enables the nucleus of the solitary tract to involve the hypothalamus in the mechanisms serving autonomic homeostasis.

The final aspect of our survey of Figure 74 and Figure 75 is the identification of some of the principal fiber systems appearing on the sections. A group of three longitudinal fiber systems compose a prominent dark-staining band abutting the midline of each section. The most ventral part of the band, positioned immediately dorsal to the pyramidal tract, is the medial lemniscus. Then comes the tectospinal tract, a direct, crossed pathway from the superior colliculus to the cervical motor mechanisms controlling the neck muscles. The dorsalmost tip of the band, just under the ventricular floor, is the medial longitudinal fasciculus, a bundle that spans the length of the brainstem and the cervical spinal cord. At the levels of Figure 74 and Figure 75 it consists largely of crossed and uncrossed fibers descending from the vestibular nuclei to the cervical motor mechanisms. Both the tectospinal tract and the medial longitudinal fasciculus follow the spinal cord's ventral funiculus to their cervical destinations; they course alongside the ventral corticospinal tract.

A further group of fiber systems follow a lateral trajectory, passing longitudinally through the region bordered ventrally by the inferior olive, dorsally by the descending trigeminal tract, and laterally by the pial surface of the medulla. The group, sometimes called the superficial anterolateral fasciculus, comprises at least two ascending systems, the spinothalamic tract and the ventral spinocerebellar tract, and at least one crossed, descending system, the rubrospinal tract, from the red nucleus, in the midbrain. No borders can be drawn between the three. Moreover, the fasciculus as a whole grades imperceptibly, on its medial side, into the longitudinal fascicles of the reticular formation. Still, the fasciculus plainly represents a rostral continuation of the ventrolateral quadrant of the spinal cord's white matter. In our series of brainstem cross sections it maintains the same relative position until the level

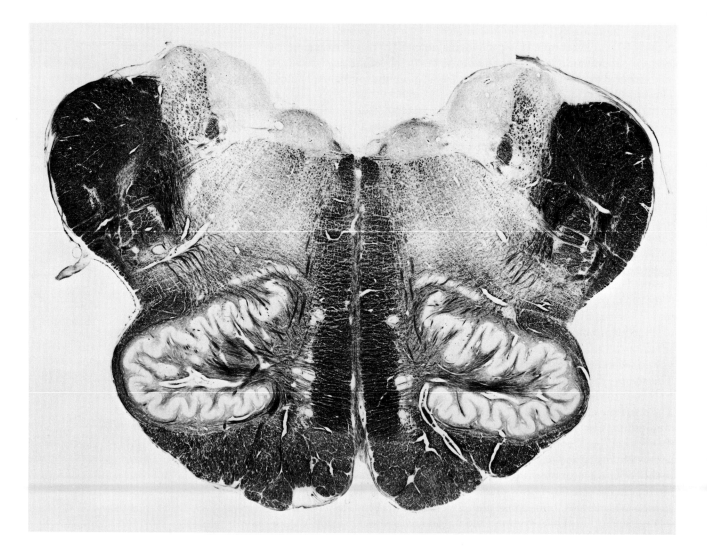

Figure 76: **Reticulated fabric** formed by the more or less even commingling of gray and white matter at the core of this cross section, high in the medulla oblongata, marks the brainstem reticular formation. Broadly speaking, the formation participates in the maintenance of three postures: that of behavioral alertness, that of the stance of the body (for example, the balancing of the trunk over

of Figure 77. Beyond that, in the metencephalon, it becomes separated from the surface of the brainstem by the brachium pontis, or middle cerebellar peduncle.

One principal fiber system in Figure 74 and again in Figure 75 is transverse, not longitudinal. Also, it is unique to the medulla oblongata. The olivocerebellar projection originates from all parts of the inferior olivary nucleus and is distributed to all parts of the cerebellum. Its fibers emerge through the hilus,

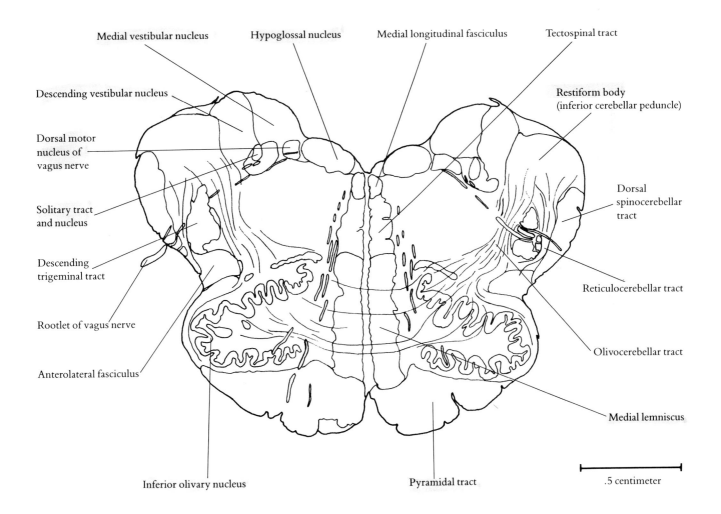

Medial vestibular nucleus

Hypoglossal nucleus

Medial longitudinal fasciculus

Tectospinal tract

Descending vestibular nucleus

Dorsal motor nucleus of vagus nerve

Solitary tract and nucleus

Descending trigeminal tract

Rootlet of vagus nerve

Anterolateral fasciculus

Restiform body (inferior cerebellar peduncle)

Dorsal spinocerebellar tract

Reticulocerebellar tract

Olivocerebellar tract

Medial lemniscus

.5 centimeter

Inferior olivary nucleus

Pyramidal tract

the limbs), and that of homeostasis: the visceral posture. Within the reticular formation, on each side of the section, a massive aggregation of olivocerebellar fibers virtually occludes the descending tri-

geminal nucleus. Dorsal to the reticular formation, again on each side of the section, the dorsal-column nuclei are gone, replaced by two vestibular nuclei, the descending and the medial.

or mouth, of each olive, traverse the medial lemnisci in widely dispersed fascicles, and then pass sequentially through the dorsal lamella of the contralateral olive, the medullary reticular formation, and the descending trigeminal nucleus and tract to join the restiform body, or inferior cerebellar peduncle. An impression of the volume of the projection is conveyed by Figure 76, which shows on both sides of the midline a massive aggregation of olivocerebellar fibers obscuring almost the entire cross section of the descending trigeminal nucleus. Note, too, the rapidly increasing size of the restiform body as it ascends from the level of Figure 74, where it comprises only the dorsal spinocerebellar tract and the cuneocerebellar tract, to the level of Figure 77, where it includes in addition the olivocerebellar fibers. The increase, to be fair, is not entirely the result of the olivocerebellar projection. The restiform body also is joined by uncrossed reticulocerebellar fibers sweeping dorsalward at the lateral side of the descending trigeminal tract from the lateral reticular nucleus, a small, circumscribed part of the reticular formation visible in Figure 74 and Figure 75 just dorsal to the inferior olive. The nucleus is known to get input from the motor cortex.

What can one say about the reticular formation? In the foregoing paragraphs we have mentioned it several times, but then, it is prominent throughout the length of the brainstem: at the core of each brainstem cross section it is a more or less even commingling of gray matter and fascicles of ascending and descending fibers that give the formation a netlike weave, or indeed, in Weigert preparations, the appearance of a homespun tweed fabric. Early observers aptly (and prudently) called it the *formatio reticularis alba et grisea:* the white and gray reticulated formation, a purely descriptive term.

Let us try to define the formation. Suppose that in an effort to master the anatomy of the brainstem you draw the outline of a cross section through the medulla oblongata. You place in it the motor nuclei and the secondary sensory cell groups stationed in the medulla. (As it happens, most of them are fairly well delineated.) Then you add the outline of the inferior olive and the outlines of the circumscribed fiber bundles passing longitudinally through the medulla: the pyramidal tract and the medial lemniscus, among others. A large, central part of the cross section remains alarmingly blank. It includes a wealth of neurons, but they resist all classifications as simple as "motor" or "sensory." More than 40 years ago, W. F. Allen of the University of Washington called them the "leftover cells"—a description that met with little favor. Yet Allen's phrase is apposite: the reticular formation, extending through the length of the brainstem, is the realm of the neurons that remain when all motor neurons and secondary sensory neurons have been accounted for. What they do is most impressive. For one thing, they appear to generate, in part as their response to the sensory, cerebellar, cortical, striatal, and limbic inputs converging on the reticular formation, a baseline state, or "posture," of activity that they broadcast, by a widespread system of efferent connections, to neurons in all the main divisions of the brain and spinal cord. In the forebrain the broadcasts are essential for the maintenance of what amounts to perceptual and behavioral alertness. Indeed, the impulses serving alertness appear to arise especially in the reticular formation of the mesencephalon and the rostral rhombencephalon. The evidence is well known to clinicians. In cases of irreversible coma following severe head injury, either or both of two parts of the brain are usually found to be extensively damaged. One is the cerebral cortex. The other is the midbrain. Second, the reticular formation contributes to posture in the conventional sense of the word. That is, it contributes to the stance of the body, acting, in this respect, through somatic motor neurons in the brainstem and spinal cord. H. G. J. M. Kuypers, who was then at the Erasmus University in the Netherlands, has found that bilateral lesions in the medial, magnocellular reticular formation of the rhombencephalon render animals unable to balance their trunk over their limbs. Thus the magnocellular reticular formation seems to find its somatic motor expression, at least in part, in the stabilization of the joints. Third, many neurons of the reticular formation participate in maintaining homeostasis, the postural stability of the internal milieu (that is, the visceral domain). In the lateral part of the medullary reticular formation, for example, close to the medial border of the descending trigeminal nucleus, a group of cells discharge in synchrony with the rhythm of respiration. Presumably they function as the pacemaker for that rhythm. No other neurons in the brain have been found to do the same. Farther rostrally, at the transition from rhombencephalon to mesencephalon, a reticular region concerns itself with another aspect of respiration, the turnover from inspiration to expiration. The region is referred to as the pneumotaxic center. Neurosurgeons have long known that the inadvertent compression of the region can lead to respiratory arrest in deep inspiration.

The reticular formation does look chaotic. Its inputs are heterogeneous and dismayingly convergent. Its output fibers compose few circumscribed bundles: they tend to be widespread, and organized only diffusely. Yet many of the effector mechanisms embodied in the reticular formation are highly specific and precise. The heterogeneity of the inputs to the reticular formation may thus reflect no more — and no less — than the need for life functions such as respiration to adapt to circumstances as diverse as the acidity of the blood plasma, the oxygen content of the air one inhales, and the amount of physical exertion one undertakes — or anticipates undertaking — from moment to moment.

Internal Structure: Metencephalon

Our survey of rhombencephalic cross sections resumes with Figure 77, which transects the lateral recess of the fourth ventricle. It is a section made at the transition from the medulla oblongata to the metencephalon: the pontine region of the hindbrain. In confirmation of the transition, the base of the section grazes the caudal part of the pons, which in Figure 77 has the shape of an inverted arch of gray matter under the ventral margin of each pyramidal tract. The surface of the pons (that is, its basal and lateral margins) is a layer of

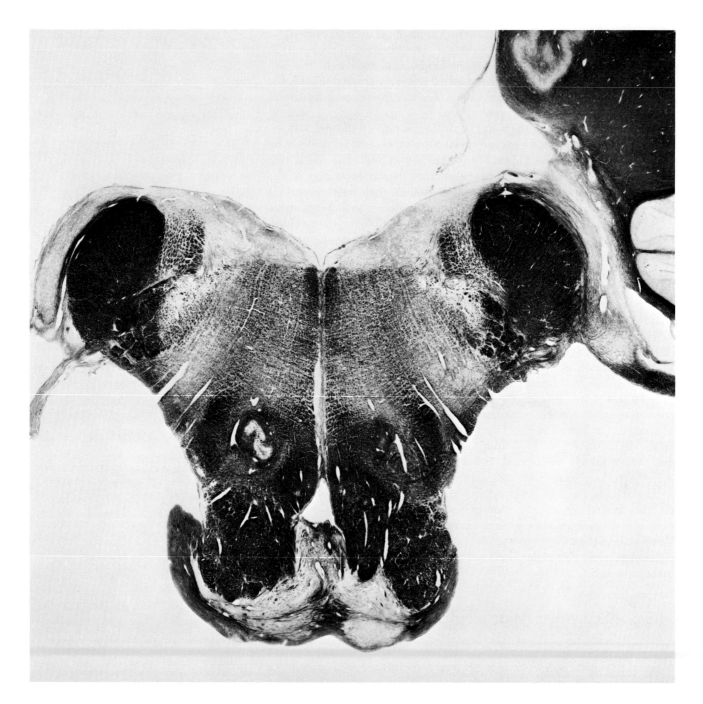

Figure 77: **Advent of the pons** indicates the transition from one hindbrain subdivision, the medulla oblongata, or myelencephalon, to the other division, the metencephalon. The caudalmost tip of the pons is at the base of the section. Its surface is a layer of decussating fibers that are joining the brachium pontis, or middle cerebellar peduncle. A second mass of cerebellar afferents, the restiform body, or inferior cerebellar peduncle, is at the opposite, dorsal side of the figure. It includes the dorsal spinocerebellar tract, the cuneocerebel-

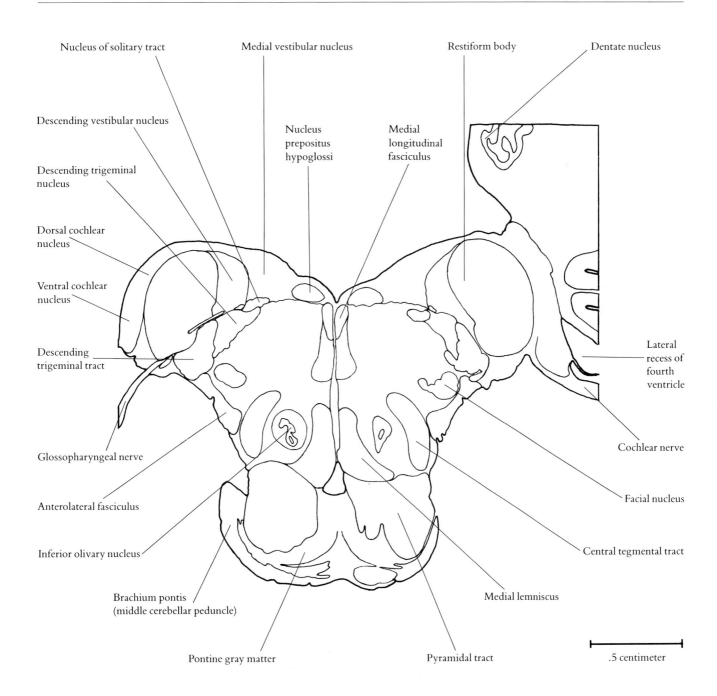

Nucleus of solitary tract

Medial vestibular nucleus

Restiform body

Dentate nucleus

Descending vestibular nucleus

Nucleus prepositus hypoglossi

Medial longitudinal fasciculus

Descending trigeminal nucleus

Dorsal cochlear nucleus

Ventral cochlear nucleus

Descending trigeminal tract

Lateral recess of fourth ventricle

Glossopharyngeal nerve

Cochlear nerve

Anterolateral fasciculus

Facial nucleus

Inferior olivary nucleus

Central tegmental tract

Brachium pontis (middle cerebellar peduncle)

Medial lemniscus

Pontine gray matter

Pyramidal tract

.5 centimeter

lar tract, the olivocerebellar projection, and reticulocerebellar fibers. Almost surrounding the restiform body is the special somatic sensory column. Medial to the restiform body, two vestibular nuclei (again the medial and the descending) compose the vestibular triangle.

Dorsal and lateral to the restiform body, the cochlear nuclei appear; in the right half of the section the cochlear nerve enters them from the ventral side. Elsewhere in the section the inferior olive is flanked by its principal afferents, which compose the central tegmental tract.

transverse fibers: pontine efferents that are crossing the midline to join the contralateral brachium pontis, or middle cerebellar peduncle. They constitute the main input to the great lateral expanse of cerebellar cortex called the cerebellar hemisphere. A smaller bundle, the restiform body, or inferior cerebellar peduncle, conveys inputs from a greater variety of sources to a more medial zone of the cerebellar cortex including the paramedian district called the vermis but extending laterally beyond it. The part of the cross section dorsal to the pons looks much like the medulla oblongata. Still, some changes have taken place. The inferior olive has reached its rostral limit: only its uppermost tip can be seen. With its disappearance, the cross section of the medial lemniscus has begun to change in profile from vertical (that is, dorsoventral) to horizontal (mediolateral). The change will be complete in Figure 79. The fiber bundle lateral to the rostral pole of the olive is the central tegmental tract, a remarkably compact bundle, considering its widespread origin from the mesencephalic reticular formation. The tract is thought to be the chief system of afferents to the olive. We failed to notice it earlier: at more caudal levels its axons are part of the fiber capsule surrounding the olive.

Figure 77 is notably lacking in motor nuclei. The somatic motor column is missing: the hypoglossal nucleus reached its rostral limit a few millimeters lower. Its position on the cross section is occupied by the nucleus prepositus hypoglossi, a longitudinal mass of subventricular gray matter that is known to contain interneurons serving the abducens, the trochlear, and the oculomotor nuclei. The visceral motor column also is missing, or rather the column is indistinct. The dorsal motor nucleus of the vagus is no longer apparent, yet scattered at this level of the hindbrain, in the subventricular gray matter and the adjoining reticular formation, are the preganglionic parasympathetic motor neurons composing the salivatory nucleus. Their axons join two cranial nerves, the glossopharyngeus and the facial. The branchial motor column is somewhat plainer. The nucleus ambiguus is gone. In its place, on the right side of the section though not yet on the left, the next more rostral constituent of the column, the facial motor nucleus, shows its caudal pole.

Finally, some changes are apparent in the dorsolateral, alar-plate, or "dorsal-horn" district of Figure 77. A convenient landmark is afforded by the large, comma-shaped cross section of the restiform body, which now has almost attained its definitive size. (Some olivocerebellar and reticulocerebellar fascicles are still joining it from the ventral side.) The restiform body is tunneling under the lateral recess; farther rostrally it will initiate a steep dorsal curve into the core of the cerebellum. Medial to the restiform body lie two constellations of secondary sensory cell groups. In the more ventral one the general somatic sensory column is represented by the descending trigeminal nucleus; the descending trigeminal tract is at its lateral margin. On the left side of Figure 77 the visceral sensory column—that is, the nucleus of the solitary tract—makes a final appearance, in the form of a small gray structure fusing into the dorsal margin of the descending trigeminal nucleus. (Its companion on the right side has already lost its identity.) Extending laterally from the nucleus is a slender central root fascicle of the glossopharyngeus. (A peripheral root of the nerve emerges just under the restiform body, in the lateral position typical of the mixed cranial nerves: the ones both sensory and motor.) The more dorsal constellation of secondary sensory cell groups, abutting the floor of the fourth ventricle, is the vestibular triangle, which forms the medial part of the special somatic sensory column. In Figure 77, as in Figure 76, the triangle consists of the dark-staining, heavily myelinated inferior, or spinal, vestibular nucleus and the larger, pale-staining medial vestibular nucleus. Farther rostrally, at the level of Figure 79, the inferior nucleus will be replaced by two further vestibular nuclei, the lateral and the superior. Adjoining the vestibular triangle in Figure 77 is the lateral part of the special somatic sensory column, which has the protuberant shape of a layer of gray matter slung over the dorsal and lateral sides of the restiform body. The gray matter comprises the cochlear nuclei: the dorsal and the ventral. Together they form the floor of the lateral recess; their arc matches the strong, almost right-angled downward curve of the lateral recess itself.

The key to the aggregate of the special somatic sensory cell groups is the cranial nerve that serves them: the statoacoustic nerve, also called the vestibulocochlear. The nerve is really two almost separate bundles, which enter the brainstem in the far lateral, quasi-dorsal-root position characteristic of the purely sensory cranial nerves. The vestibular nerve carries signals from mechanoreceptive hair cells in the sensory epithelia of the vestibular part of the membranous labyrinth: the maculae of the utriculus and the sacculus and the cristae of the semicircular canals. The cochlear nerve, also called the acoustic or auditory nerve, arrives slightly more caudally. It carries signals from further mechanoreceptive hair cells, these stationed in Corti's organ, in the wall of the cochlear duct of the membranous labyrinth. The two nerves diverge when they enter the brainstem. The vestibular nerve, visible in Figure 78, directs its fibers in a straight line past the medial side of the restiform body, thus attaining the vestibular triangle at its lateral corner. The fibers terminate chiefly in the four vestibular nuclei, but some pass to the cerebellum, providing that organ with its only known instance of primary sensory input. Meanwhile, the cochlear nerve, visible on the right side of Figure 77 and the left of Figure 78, directs its fibers along the lateral side of the restiform body. It distributes the fibers in such a way that each cochlear nucleus receives a complete tonotopic map of Corti's organ.

In turn the cochlear nuclei begin the central auditory connections. In particular the dorsal and ventral cochlear nuclei on each side of the midline emit fibers that sweep medially to form a plate called the trapezoid body, just dorsal to the pons in Figure 78 and again in Figure 79. It is a hemidecussation: roughly half of the fibers from each side of the brainstem participate in the crossing. At the lateral margin of the trapezoid body they join the uncrossed fibers to begin their ascent as the lateral lemniscus. At first they climb with two other fiber systems, the spinothalamic tract and the ventral spinocerebellar tract, from which they are hard to distinguish. Later, however, at the caudal border of the midbrain (Figure 82), the lateral lemniscus extricates itself from its companions and curves steeply dorsalward as a circumscribed

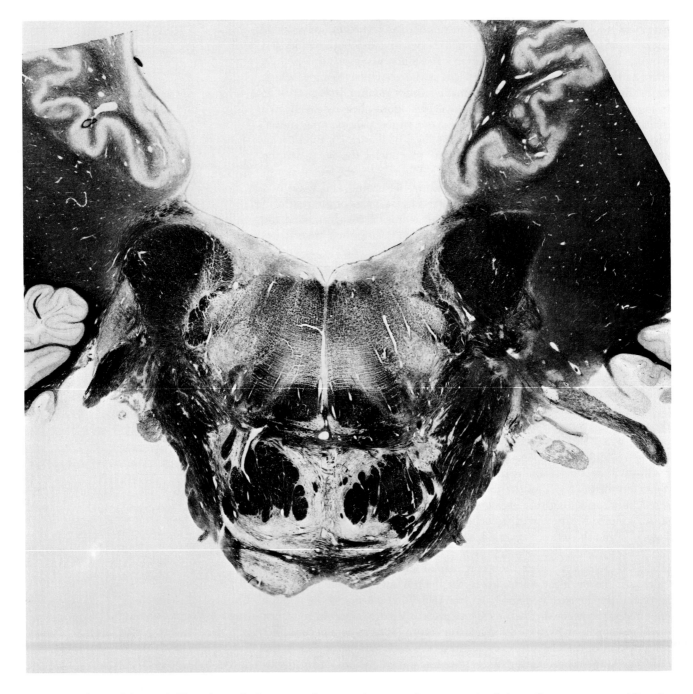

Figure 78: **Advent of the cerebellum** also marks the metencephalon. The core of the organ consists largely of the white matter of the cerebellar peduncles. In addition it includes the four deep cerebellar nuclei. Here the largest, most lateral of the four can be seen: the dentate nucleus, a convoluted sheet of gray matter resembling the inferior olive. Fibers attaining the cerebellum from the vestibular nuclei join with primary sensory fibers from the vestibular nerve to form the juxtarestiform body, at the dorsomedial side of the resti-

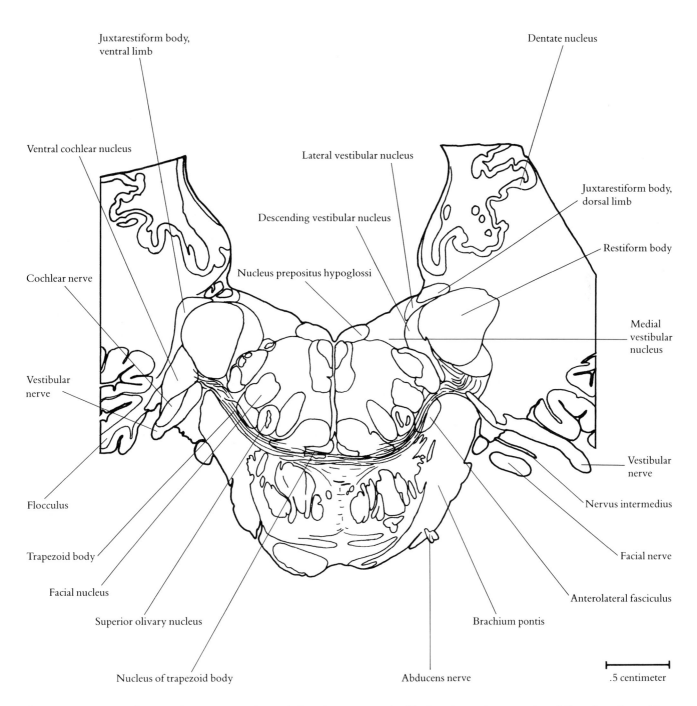

Juxtarestiform body, ventral limb

Dentate nucleus

Ventral cochlear nucleus

Lateral vestibular nucleus

Juxtarestiform body, dorsal limb

Descending vestibular nucleus

Restiform body

Cochlear nerve

Nucleus prepositus hypoglossi

Medial vestibular nucleus

Vestibular nerve

Vestibular nerve

Nervus intermedius

Flocculus

Trapezoid body

Facial nerve

Facial nucleus

Anterolateral fasciculus

Superior olivary nucleus

Brachium pontis

Nucleus of trapezoid body

Abducens nerve

.5 centimeter

form body. The rest of the vestibular nerve is also medial to the restiform body. In contrast, the cochlear nerve (visible on the left side of the figure) stays lateral to the restiform body. In the more ventral part of the section the border of the pons is drawn by the trapezoid body, a decussation consisting of fibers from the cochlear nuclei. The lateral tip of the trapezoid body includes the superior olive, an auditory way station. The lateral lemniscus begins at the lateral tip of the body.

fiber bundle. It is nearing its destination, the inferior colliculus (Figure 83). From there a final link, the brachium of the inferior colliculus, extends the auditory lemniscus rostralward along the lateral side of the superior colliculus (Figure 84) to the auditory relay nucleus of the thalamus, the medial geniculate body (Figure 85). The lemniscus is notable for the way stations in its path. The inferior colliculus intercepts essentially all the lemniscal traffic; three further cell groups, all caudal to the colliculus, intercept rather less. The superior olive, a multipartite gray mass, is embedded in the lateral lemniscus at the place where the lemniscus emerges from the trapezoid body (Figures 78 and 79); a second way station lies in the trapezoid body itself and so is termed the nucleus of the trapezoid body (Figure 79); a third way station, the nucleus of the lateral lemniscus, is an elongated mass of gray matter in the mesencephalic stretch of the lemniscus (Figures 82 and 83). For the most part the fibers emitted by the way stations rejoin the lateral lemniscus. That is not to say reflex channels and cerebellar channels do not exist. They are simply not prominent among the central auditory connections. For example, reflex arcs lead inconspicuously from the cochlear nuclei, the superior olive, and the nucleus of the trapezoid body to the facial motor nucleus and the trigeminal motor nucleus. The facial motor nucleus innervates not only the facial muscles but also the stapedius, a small muscle in the middle ear whose contraction limits the transmission of sound to the inner ear by reducing the sound-induced excursions of a small middle-ear bone, the stapes, the crucial last link in the chain of the auditory ossicles. The trigeminal motor nucleus innervates not only the masticatory muscles but also the tensor tympani, a further middle-ear muscle, which controls the amplitude of the excursions of the eardrum. Both muscles protect Corti's organ from excessive sound, much as the constrictor pupillae protects the retina from excessive illumination.

The central vestibular channels are much the opposite of the central auditory channels. The lemniscal paths are minimal; on the other hand the cerebellar paths are prodigious, and so are the reflex paths. To that extent the vestibular sense is unlike the other senses, much of whose traffic is directed toward the cerebral cortex. One vestibular reflex path is quite prominent throughout the hindbrain and the midbrain. The four vestibular nuclei all contribute fibers, both ipsilateral and contralateral, both ascending and descending, to the medial longitudinal fasciculus, or MLF, a circumscribed fiber bundle that maintains a dorsal position near the midline. The MLF climbs to the abducens, the trochlear, and the oculomotor nucleus, which innervate the external eye muscles. Beyond them it attains the so-called preoculomotor nuclei: the interstitial nucleus of Cajal and the nucleus of Darkschewitsch (Figures 85 and 86). Presumably both are composed of interneurons serving eye movement. In the opposite, caudal direction the MLF descends into the ventral funiculus of the cervical spinal cord. There, in the form of the medial vestibulospinal tract, it links the vestibular nuclei to motor mechanisms controlling the neck muscles. Overall, the MLF establishes the reflex connections by which pairs of semicircular canals, one canal in the left ear, the other in the right, communicate with motor neurons controlling eye and neck movements in the plane of the pair. The eyes can thus be turned in a way that compensates for changes in the position of the head. The reflex function of the vestibular sense is not, however, expressed in eye and neck movements alone. From the lateral vestibular nucleus comes a second reflex path, the lateral vestibulospinal tract, whose fibers, thick in diameter, descend uncrossed in the spinal cord's ventrolateral quadrant to synapse throughout the length of the cord with interneurons, or even directly with motor neurons. By way of the lateral vestibulospinal tract vestibular impulses triggered by tilt or rotation of the body, or of the head alone, can activate groups of limb muscles, thus counteracting an imminent loss of balance.

The cerebellar channel of the vestibular sense remains to be described. Its prominence should be no surprise: remember, the cerebellum arose in phylogeny as an adjunct to the vestibular apparatus, so that in primitive vertebrates such as the cyclostomes the organ is dominated by vestibular input. In more highly developed vertebrates, and particularly in the mammals, the vestibular cerebellum (the part with vestibular input) includes three small cortical regions at the base of the cerebellum: the uvula and the nodulus, which are both at the caudal end of the median strip of cerebellar cortex called the vermis, and the flocculus, more laterally placed, and visible in Figure 78. In primates the four vestibular nuclei all project to the vestibular cerebellum. In addition they project to the fastigial nucleus, the most medial of the deep cerebellar nuclei, which also receives the output of the vestibular cerebellum. The vestibulocerebellar afferents (both primary sensory, from the vestibular nerve, and secondary sensory, from the vestibular nuclei) form a bundle that enters the cerebellum at the medial side of the restiform body. The bundle is therefore called the juxtarestiform body. Figure 78 shows its ventral limb arching laterally over the restiform body, then ventrally, along the medial side of the restiform body, to enter the flocculus. The remaining, dorsal limb follows the medial side of the restiform body to reach the uvula, the nodulus, and the fastigial nucleus. For its part, the fastigial nucleus emits a return projection to the vestibular nuclei. In addition it projects to the medial rhombencephalic reticular formation: the part of the formation where bilateral lesions render animals unable to balance their trunk over their limbs.

The three metencephalic cross sections beginning with Figure 78 share several features. First, they show the size of the pons: in no animal is it as large as it is in the human brain. But then, the pons is interposed in traffic from the entire expanse of the neocortex to the cortex investing the cerebellar hemisphere. In all three sections the gray matter of the pons is framed laterally by the brachium pontis, or middle cerebellar peduncle: the pontocerebellar highway. In all three sections, moreover, the pontine gray matter itself is permeated by fascicles. Some are transverse; they consist of pontocerebellar fibers, which cross the midline to join the contralateral brachium pontis. Some are longitudinal; they come from the neocortex. Many fibers among the latter will terminate in the pons: they establish the massive — and uncrossed — corticopontine connection. Others will emerge from the caudal border of the pons: they will form the medullary pyramid (that is, the pyrami-

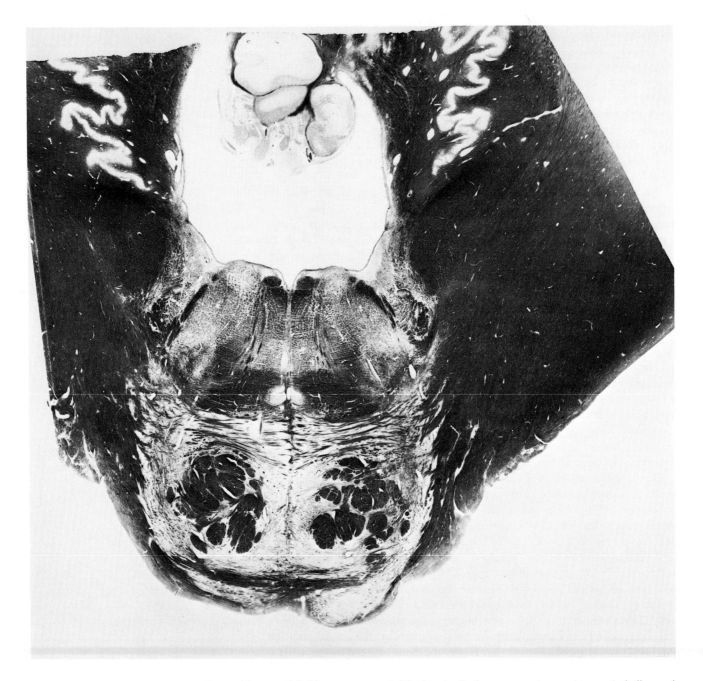

Figure 79: **Pons and tegmentum** are the roughly coequal divisions of this metencephalic cross section. The pons — the ventral division of the section — is framed laterally by the brachium pontis. The pons itself is riddled with fascicles. The transverse ones are pontocerebellar fibers, which cross the midline to join the contralateral brachium pontis. The longitudinal ones are corticopontine, corticobulbar, and corticospinal. The tegmentum — the dorsal division of the section — includes motor nuclei, secondary sensory cell groups, and the reticular core of the section. It also includes nearly all the brainstem's long fiber systems. Within its limits in this section the vestibular

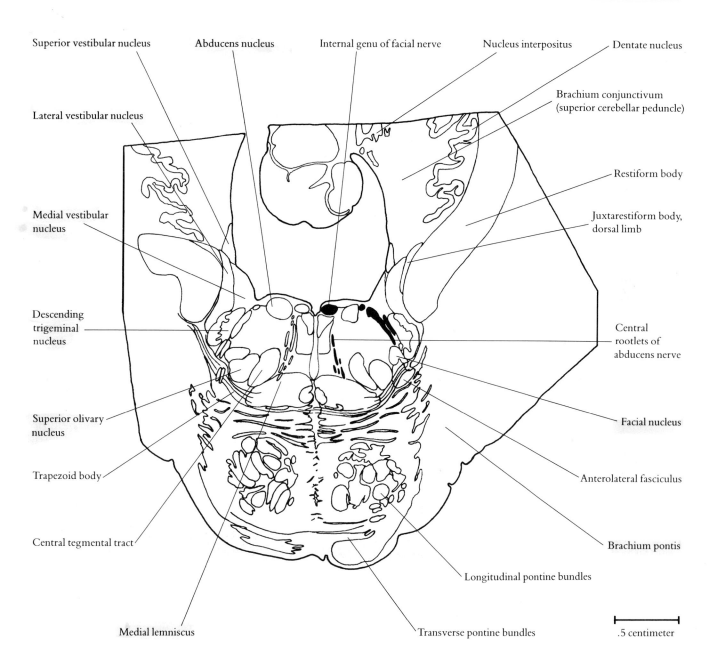

Superior vestibular nucleus

Lateral vestibular nucleus

Medial vestibular nucleus

Descending trigeminal nucleus

Superior olivary nucleus

Trapezoid body

Central tegmental tract

Medial lemniscus

Abducens nucleus

Internal genu of facial nerve

Nucleus interpositus

Dentate nucleus

Brachium conjunctivum (superior cerebellar peduncle)

Restiform body

Juxtarestiform body, dorsal limb

Central rootlets of abducens nerve

Facial nucleus

Anterolateral fasciculus

Brachium pontis

Longitudinal pontine bundles

Transverse pontine bundles

.5 centimeter

triangle comprises two vestibular nuclei, the lateral and the superior. Moreover, the superior olive has been joined by a further auditory way station, the nucleus of the trapezoid body. The somatic motor column is represented by the abducens nucleus; the branchial motor column is represented by the facial nucleus. The latter directs its

efferents around the former, like a rope around a piling, in the internal genu of the facial nerve. In the cerebellum the dentate nucleus is joined on its medial side by the ventralmost tip of the nucleus interpositus, which consists of two deep cerebellar nuclei, the globose and the emboliform.

dal tract). Among these last-named fibers some will terminate in the local motor apparatuses of the hindbrain: they compose the corticobulbar tract, or rather part of the tract, since other corticobulbar fibers have found their targets more rostrally in the rhombencephalon. The rest form the cortico-spinal tract.

Second, the sections include the tegmentum, a term denoting the part of the cross section containing motor nuclei and secondary sensory cell groups as well as the reticular core of the brainstem. The word tegmentum is Latin for cover; in Figures 78 through 80 (and also in Figure 82) the tegmentum "covers" the pons. It is therefore the tegmentum pontis, as distinguished from the pars basilaris pontis, or pons per se. In the midbrain, as later sections will show, the tegmentum "covers" the cerebral peduncles. The border between the tegmentum and the pons is marked first (in Figures 78 and 79) by the trapezoid body; later (in Figures 80 and 82) it is marked by the medial lemniscus. Meanwhile (in Figures 78 through 80) one sees a progressive increase in the dorsoventral dimension of the pons accompanied by a flatten-ing of the tegmentum. All but one of the long fiber systems traveling longitu-dinally through the brainstem nonetheless pass through the tegmental bottle-neck. The sole exception is the pyramidal tract, descending through the pons.

Finally, the three sections beginning with Figure 78 convey some impres-sion of the core of the cerebellum. For the most part the core is formed by the cerebellar peduncles, with their heavy myelination. In addition, however, the core includes the deep cerebellar nuclei, a group of four masses of gray matter in the roof and the lateral wall of the fourth ventricle on each side of the midline. The four are the fastigial nucleus, the globose and emboliform nuclei, together called the nucleus interpositus, and finally, along the lateral wall of the ventricle, the dentate nucleus, which is by far the largest of the four. The ventral part of the dentate nucleus can be seen in several sections (Figures 77 through 79). It is a convoluted sheet of gray matter strongly reminiscent of the inferior olive (except for its greater size). Indeed, it is folded, like the olive, into an ovoid shape with a hilus directed medially, through which its efferents emerge. On the right side of Figure 78 the restiform body enters the core of the cerebellum; in Figure 79, again on the right, it skirts the lateral face of the dentate nucleus before curving inward to reach the medial district of cerebellar cortex in which it makes its chief distribution of fibers. The cerebellar white matter lateral to the restiform body is the brachium pontis, distributing fibers to the cerebellar hemisphere. That leaves the third cerebellar peduncle, the brachium conjunctivum. It is the most medial of the peduncles; it is also the only peduncle almost wholly efferent with respect to the cerebellum. (It consists largely of fibers from the dentate nucleus and the nucleus interpositus.) In Figure 79 it is represented by the white matter separating the dentate nucleus from the lateral wall of the fourth ventricle. In Figure 80 (a rather long rostral jump) it still lies in the lateral wall of the ventricle. Now, however, it is a compact bundle with a roughly oval cross section overarched laterally and dorsally by the brachium pontis. In its further rostralward course it becomes submerged in the tegmentum (Figure 82); then, following a complete decussation in the caudal midbrain (Figure 83), it is distributed to the contralateral red nucleus (Figures 84 and 85) and the thalamus.

The motor nuclei and secondary sensory cell groups appearing in Figure 79 are worth identifying. Among the motor columns the visceral motor is missing. In contrast, the somatic motor column has reappeared: it takes the form of the abducens nucleus, the caudalmost of the motor nuclei governing eye movement. Some central root fascicles emerge from the ventromedial side of the nucleus; they follow an almost directly ventralward course through the tegmentum and the pons to leave the brainstem (at the level of Figure 78) as the abducens nerve, in the quasi-ventral-root position characteristic of the purely motor cranial nerves. The branchial motor column is also represented in Figure 79: the section shows the rostral pole of the facial motor nucleus. On its dorsal side the nucleus abuts the descending trigeminal nucleus; on its ventral side it abuts the superior olive. From both it receives reflex connections. The ones from the trigeminal nucleus close reflex arcs serving (among other trigeminofacial reflexes) the corneal reflex: the forceful closure of the eye in response to mechanical or chemical irritation of the cornea. The connections from the superior olive serve other defensive reflexes, including the auditory blink reflex and the activation of the stapedius muscle. Figure 79 shows much of the remarkable detour the facial nerve makes before leaving the brainstem. From the facial motor nucleus the central root of the nerve first travels dorsomedially; then, immediately under the floor of the fourth ventricle, it turns laterally over the abducens nucleus to begin a hairpin curve around the latter. (The curve is called the internal genu of the nerve.) The curve completed, the root skirts the medial face of the descending trigeminal nucleus, pierces the trapezoid body, and exits (in Figure 78) a short distance medial to the statoacoustic nerve. The sensory fibers and the visceral motor fibers that join the facial nerve (the first arriving from taste buds and destined for the gustatory nucleus, the second directed from the salivary nucleus to the salivary glands, and also the lacrimal gland of the eye) make no such detour. They often, however, form a separate, lateral root of the facial nerve, the nervus intermedius of Wrisberg (again, see Figure 78).

The vestibular triangle completes the identifications in Figure 79. It lies dorsal to the descending trigeminal nucleus, and it comprises two vestibular nuclei, the lateral and the superior. We turn, then, to Figure 80. Here, at an upper pontine level, near the rostral limit of the hindbrain, the somatic motor column has once again disappeared: the section transects the brainstem between the abducens nucleus and the trochlear nucleus. In contrast, the branchial motor column is represented quite prominently by its rostralmost member, the motor nucleus of the trigeminus, also called the masticatory nucleus in recognition of the muscles it governs. In Figure 80 the masticatory nucleus is an oval region of gray matter in the ventrolateral part of the tegmentum, where the nucleus ambiguus and the facial motor nucleus appeared in previous sections. Emerging in a ventrolateral direction from the masticatory nucleus are several central root fascicles, which coalesce as they

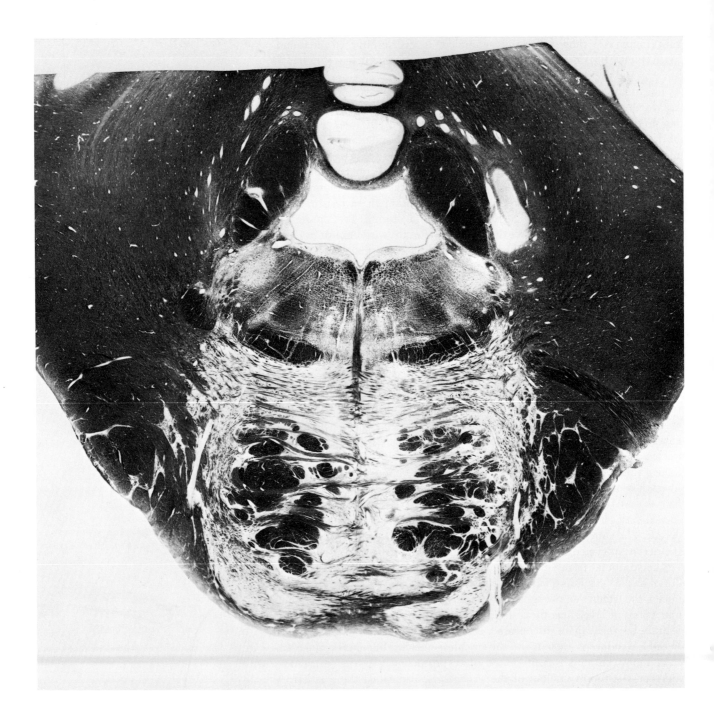

Figure 80: **Final rhombencephalic cross section** includes a tegmentum narrowed dorsoventrally by the great mass of the pons. The dark-staining fiber bundle intervening between the two is the medial lemniscus. Within the tegmentum the branchial motor column now shows its rostralmost constituent, the motor nucleus of the trigeminus. Near it, the main trigeminal sensory nucleus is approached by

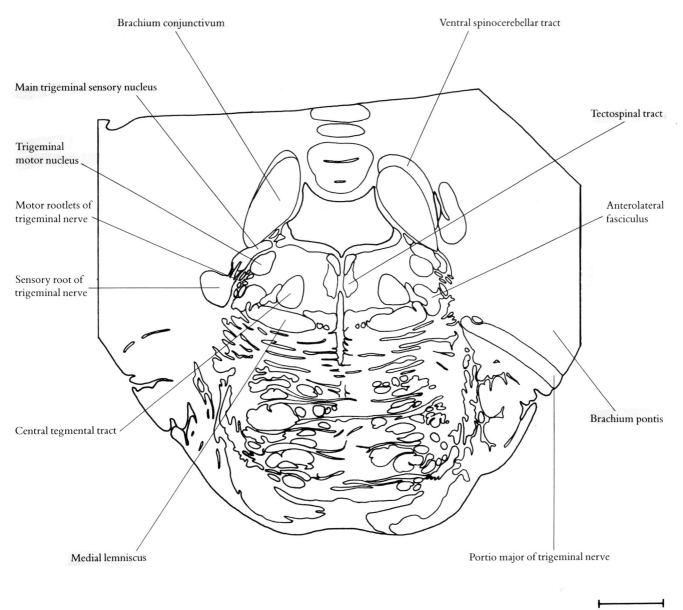

Brachium conjunctivum

Ventral spinocerebellar tract

Main trigeminal sensory nucleus

Tectospinal tract

Trigeminal
motor nucleus

Motor rootlets of
trigeminal nerve

Anterolateral
fasciculus

Sensory root of
trigeminal nerve

Central tegmental tract

Brachium pontis

Medial lemniscus

Portio major of trigeminal nerve

.5 centimeter

the portio major: the sensory contingent of the trigeminus. Dorsal to the tegmentum the brachium conjunctivum, or superior cerebellar peduncle, is an oval bundle in the lateral wall of the fourth ventricle.

It consists almost entirely of cerebellar efferents; the notable exception is the ventral spinocerebellar tract, seen arching over the lateral face of the peduncle.

traverse the brachium pontis to form the motor root, or portio minor, of the trigeminal nerve. The sensory root, or portio major, can also be seen; in Figure 80 it appears on both sides of the section. On the right it is traversing the brachium pontis; on the left it is cut in cross section just as it enters the tegmentum. It consists of the axons directed into the brainstem, just lateral to the portio minor, by the primary sensory neurons in a large neuronal nest, the trigeminal, or semilunar, ganglion; it is directly comparable, therefore, to a dorsal root of the spinal cord. The gray mass lateral and dorsal to the trigeminal motor nucleus is one of its targets: the main, or principal, sensory nucleus of the trigeminus. Some of the portio-major fibers terminate only there. Others bifurcate, sending one branch into the main nucleus while directing the other into the descending trigeminal tract, from which the descending branches invade the descending nucleus, largely in the form of axon collaterals. Still other portio-major fibers join the descending tract without having issued a branch to the main sensory nucleus.

In turn, the general somatic sensory column — that is, the main sensory nucleus and the descending one — emits reflex, cerebellar, and lemniscal channels. The latter presents a complex picture. One would expect to find the lemniscal fibers crossing the midline to join the medial lemniscus and the spinothalamic tract (both of which have decussated), thereby completing for each tract a somatotopic map of the body. Such fibers indeed are known; they originate from both the main and the descending nucleus. The ones augmenting the medial lemniscus terminate, with the lemniscus, in the ventrobasal nucleus of the thalamus. The ones augmenting the spinothalamic tract terminate in part in the ventrobasal nucleus. Many of the rest ascend no farther than the brainstem reticular formation. Still others ascend beyond the ventrobasal nucleus to several thalamic nuclei. Yet in addition to this pair of trigeminal lemnisci, for which analogies to the spinal lemnisci offer themselves so readily, the secondary sensory apparatus of the trigeminal nerve emits a third lemniscal channel. Called the dorsal trigeminal tract, it originates largely, perhaps entirely, in the dorsal part of the main sensory nucleus. It ascends, uncrossed, through dorsal parts of the midbrain tegmentum and distributes itself to the ventrobasal nucleus.

One more detail in Figure 80 should be described. On the right side of the section a conspicuous fiber bundle arches from the tegmentum dorsalward over the lateral face of the brachium conjunctivum. It is the ventral spinocerebellar tract. Its departure from the tegmentum leaves two substantial tracts ascending through the anterolateral corner of the tegmentum: the spinothalamic tract and the lateral lemniscus. A few millimeters rostral to the level of Figure 80 the lateral lemniscus will curve away in the dorsal direction to its mesencephalic destination, the inferior colliculus.

Chapter Twelve

Midbrain

At the transition from rhombencephalon to mesencephalon the internal structure of the brainstem undergoes a number of changes. The most notable change, perhaps, is that secondary sensory cell groups disappear. In other words, the main sensory nucleus of the trigeminus is the highest-placed secondary sensory cell group in the brain. This is not to say the midbrain lacks structures that might be called sensory. The superior colliculus, for example, receives a massive projection from the retina. The superior colliculus, however, is not a secondary sensory cell group. The retina interferes: it embodies a complex circuitry that places several synapses in every conduction path. Though the secondary sensory columns of the rhombencephalon stop short of the mesencephalon, two motor columns do not. The somatic motor column includes, in the mesencephalon, the trochlear nucleus and the oculomotor nucleus. The visceral motor column includes the nucleus of Edinger-Westphal. The cranial nerves emerging from the midbrain are therefore motor nerves. They are two in number. At the caudal limit of the midbrain the trochlear nerve emerges — anomalously — through the brainstem's dorsal midline. It emerges just caudal to the inferior colliculus. To compound the perversity, it decussates completely just before it appears at the surface. Considerably rostral to that level, and in the orthodox ventral position, the oculomotor nerve emerges. It seems surprisingly massive when one considers the small total volume of the extraocular muscles it governs. Muscles vary, however, not only in overall size but in the size of their constituent muscle fibers. Moreover, some motor neurons innervate thousands of muscle fibers, whereas others innervate only a few. That is to say, the "innervation ratio"

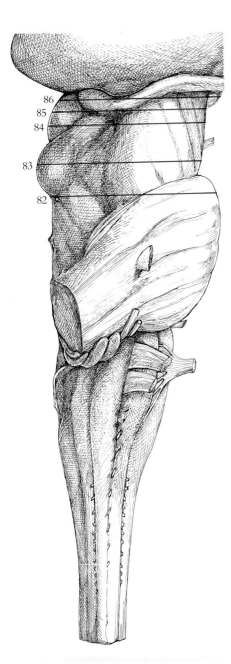

86
85
84
83
82

Figure 81: **Five midbrain cross sections** are displayed in Weigert preparations in the next five illustrations; here their levels are shown on a lateral view of the human brainstem. One section is transitional, one passes through the inferior colliculi, and three pass through the superior colliculi.

varies. (The ratio is generous for the muscles of the hand, more generous still for the extraocular muscles, and most generous of all, it seems, for the muscles of the tongue.) The oculomotor nerve emerges, in any case, through the interpeduncular fossa, the valley between the left and right cerebral peduncle.

Isthmus and Caudal Midbrain

Figure 81 shows the approximate positions of five Weigert-stained cross sections. Then Figure 82 shows the first of those cross sections: it shows the isthmus rhombencephali, the level of transition from the hindbrain to the midbrain. It is indeed an isthmus, a place at which the girth of the brainstem constricts. Again the cross section has two great subdivisions. The ventral one is the uppermost part of the pons; the dorsal one is the tegmentum. In Figure 82 the ventral and lateral borders of the tegmentum are framed by three lemnisci, which form a *V*-shaped rim known as the stratum lemnisci. The ventral limb of the *V*, resting on the pons, is the medial lemniscus. The part of the lateral limb positioned nearest the angle of the *V* is the spinothalamic tract. The remaining, dorsal part of the lateral limb is the lateral lemniscus, which now is quite circumscribed. Its interstices hold the gray matter of the nucleus of the lemniscus. Cupped between the limbs of the *V* is the brachium conjunctivum, or superior cerebellar peduncle, transected a short distance rostral to the level at which it became submerged in the tegmentum after leaving the cerebellum. In Figure 82 the brachium is beginning to make its decussation: one that will lead the entire bundle to the contralateral side of the brainstem. In the midbrain the bundle is targeted on the red nucleus; in the diencephalon it is targeted for the most part on the V.A.-V.L. complex, the rostral part of the ventral nucleus of the thalamus. For now (that is, in Figure 82) the size of the brachium conjunctivum and the packing density of its fibers mask much of the reticular core of the isthmus. On its lateral side, however, between it and the lateral lemniscus, the brachium avoids a prominent zone of gray matter that nonetheless sends fingerlike extensions into the midst of the bundle. The gray matter composes the parabrachial nuclei: the synaptic way stations, as we have noted, for two lemniscal pathways, the gustatory lemniscus, ascending to the thalamus from the rostral third of the nucleus of the solitary tract, and the visceral sensory lemniscus, ascending to the hypothalamus from the caudal two-thirds of the nucleus. Medial to the brachium conjunctivum in the reticular core of the isthmus is the central tegmental tract. We noted it first in Figure 77. Its name is admittedly vague; it specifies only the bundle's position and is silent on where the bundle begins and ends. But then, neither is known for certain. The central tegmental tract is well matched to the reticular formation: it is extremely heterogeneous. Its cells of origin lie not only in the reticular tegmentum and elsewhere in the midbrain but also farther rostrally, in the subthalamus, a region amounting to a continuation of the midbrain tegmentum into the diencephalon. Evidently the tract includes most of the descending fibers that synapse with neurons of the inferior olivary nucleus.

Two regions in Figure 82 command attention because of their dearth of myelin, meaning, of course, their poverty in fibers thick enough to be well myelinated. Both stain only lightly in a Weigert preparation; both span the midline; both are considered constituents of the reticular formation. One of them, the nucleus centralis tegmenti superior of Bechterew (the 19th-century Russian neurologist V. M. Bechterew), is a pale-staining median band that divides the tegmentum into symmetric halves. (The band, however, is breached in the middle third of its height by the decussation of the brachia conjunctiva.) The band is part of a median district of the caudal midbrain tegmentum now known as the raphe nuclei. (*Rhaphe* is Greek for suture or seam; the term here designates the midline.) The band itself is often called the median raphe nucleus. We shall have more to say about the raphe nuclei shortly. The second pale-staining region is called the central gray substance. It is a closed and prominent ring of gray matter surrounding the cerebral aqueduct: the mesencephalic canal connecting the fourth ventricle, the ventricle of the rhombencephalon, with the third ventricle, the ventricle of the diencephalon. The central gray substance has long been known as a destination for fibers that travel with the spinothalamic tract but do not attain the thalamus. It also receives projections from the cerebral cortex, the hypothalamus, and the reticular formation. Its outputs are no less heterogeneous: it projects upward to the hypothalamus and the superior colliculus, radially outward to the surrounding reticular formation, and downward to the rhombencephalic reticular formation, the nucleus of the solitary tract, and the dorsal motor nucleus of the vagus. Its diverse associations seem not to suggest a particular functional role. Nevertheless, the central gray substance has emerged as a structure crucially involved in the perception of pain, and perhaps discomfort in general. For one thing, the electrical stimulation of the central gray substance in experimental animals can elicit behavior indicating that the animal is undergoing agonizing discomfort. Stimulation of lesser intensity is reported to have the opposite effect: it raises the animal's nociceptive threshold. The hypalgesia, however, could signify the inhibition of spinal cord neurons engaged in the processing of nociceptive inputs. The central gray substance could exert such inhibition by way of reticulospinal pathways descending from the medulla oblongata. Moreover, pharmacological studies have now identified the central gray substance as a place in the brain where morphine is preferentially adsorbed by specialized cell-surface receptors: the so-called opiate receptors.* (Another such place is the amygdala.) Perhaps the analgesic effect of morphine and other opiates results when

---

*Presumably evolution did not engender opiate receptors so that morphine would have actions in the brain. Current hypotheses propose that the opiate receptors bind neuropeptides whose actions resemble those of morphine. Endorphins are an example. Indeed, the word endorphin was coined as a contraction of "endogenous morphine."

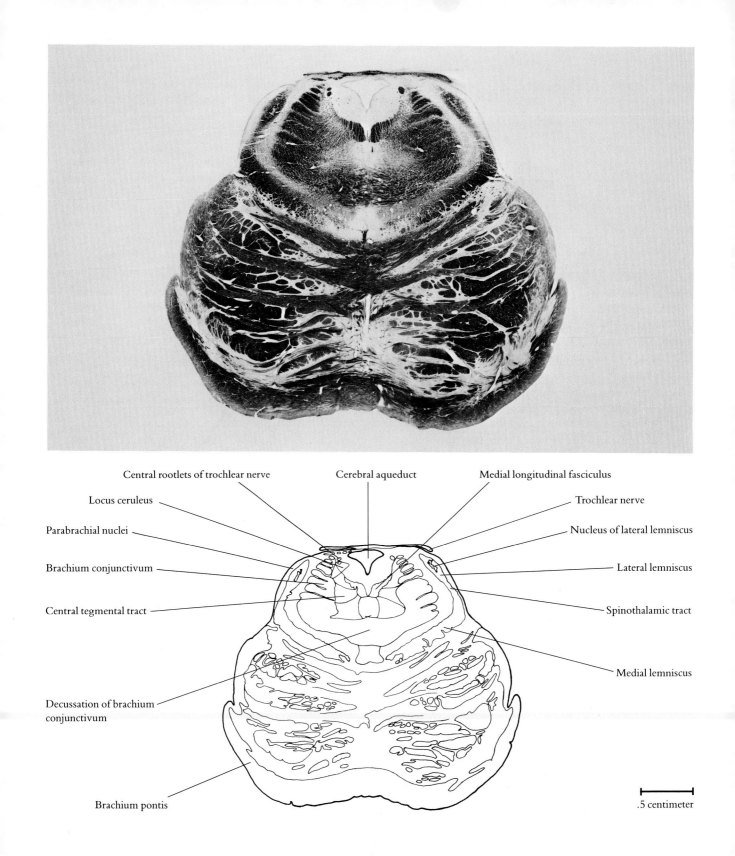

Central rootlets of trochlear nerve

Cerebral aqueduct

Medial longitudinal fasciculus

Locus ceruleus

Trochlear nerve

Parabrachial nuclei

Nucleus of lateral lemniscus

Brachium conjunctivum

Lateral lemniscus

Central tegmental tract

Spinothalamic tract

Medial lemniscus

Decussation of brachium conjunctivum

Brachium pontis

.5 centimeter

the drug modifies neural activity in the central gray substance, where fibers of the spinothalamic tract — the brain's nociceptive lemniscus — end.

Figure 83 shows a midbrain cross section some four millimeters rostral to the level of Figure 82. The dorsum of the section includes on each side of the midline the oval cross section of the inferior colliculus, approached from below by the lateral lemniscus, at the dorsal tip of the stratum lemnisci. The next link in the auditory lemniscus — the brachium of the inferior colliculus, directed to the medial geniculate body — is already marshaling fibers at the lateral surface of the colliculus. The opposite, ventral side of the section now shows not principally the pons (only a small triangle of pontine gray matter remains) but instead, on each side of the midline, the cerebral peduncle: the massive bundle of corticofugal fibers here seen descending toward the hindbrain and the spinal cord. The middle third of the bundle's cross section is occupied by the pyramidal tract; the inner and outer thirds are occupied by corticopontine fibers. Again the ventricle system is represented by the cerebral aqueduct, and again the aqueduct is surrounded by a ring of central gray substance. In the ventral part of the ring the caudal pole of the trochlear nucleus appears, partially embedded in the medial longitudinal fasciculus, from which it gets much of its input. (The bundles of myelinated fibers cut in cross section in the dorsolateral part of the central gray substance in Figure 82 are the central roots of the trochlear nerve, about to decussate in the roof of the cerebral aqueduct and emerge from the dorsal surface of the midbrain, just under the inferior colliculus.) Lateral to the MLF is the triangular part of the tegmentum occupied by the central tegmental tract. Ventral to the triangle a large, nodal patch of white matter straddles the midline. It is the decussation of the brachia conjunctiva. Protruding ventrally from the decussation, a short distance lateral to the midline, is the rubrospinal tract, whose fibers decussate almost immediately after their emergence from the red nucleus, higher in the midbrain. In the course of their further descent the fibers shift laterally, join the spinothalamic tract and the ventral spinocerebellar tract, and enter, alongside those bundles, the lateral funiculus of the spinal cord.

Figure 83 is notable for its wealth of cell groups employing a monoamine neurotransmitter, specifically norepinephrine, serotonin, or dopamine. We shall take each one in turn. The transmitter norepinephrine is employed by the locus ceruleus, a group of roughly 20,000 neurons extending from the ventrolateral corner of the central gray substance some distance into the

Figure 82: **Isthmus rhombencephali** is a local constriction of the girth of the brainstem at the transition from hindbrain to midbrain. Here the tegmentum is framed by the lateral lemniscus, the spinothalamic tract, and the medial lemniscus, which form the stratum lemnisci. Between the limbs of the stratum is the brachium conjunctivum, now accompanied by the parabrachial nuclei. The ventral fibers in the brachium are making their decussation; the rest will follow more rostrally. The midline of the tegmentum is notably lacking in myelin, both ventrally, in a band called the median raphe nucleus, and dorsally, in the central gray substance, which surrounds the cerebral aqueduct. In the dorsalmost part of the central gray substance the trochlear nerves make their decussation.

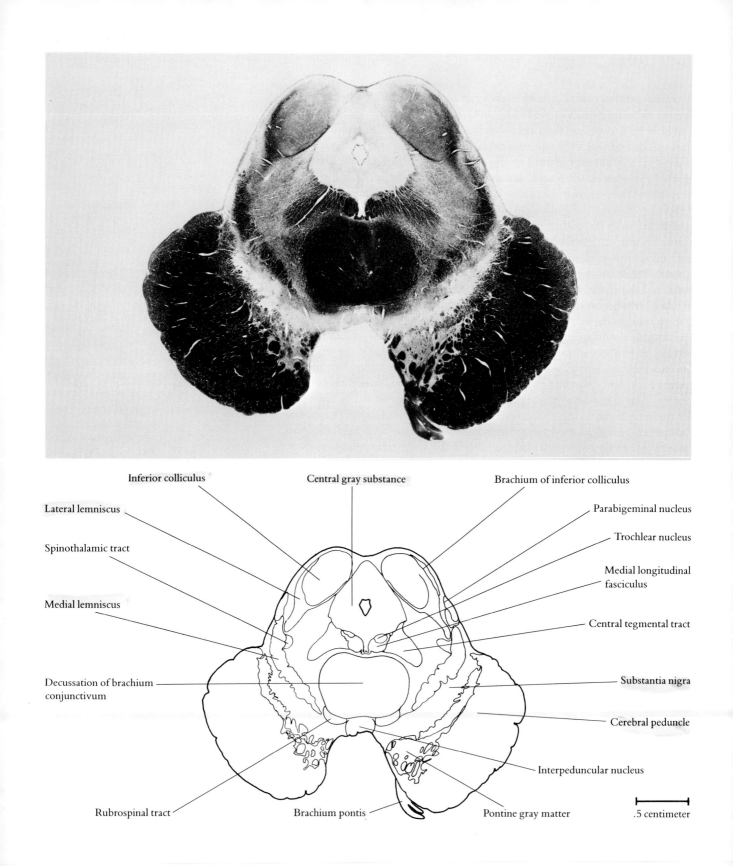

Inferior colliculus

Central gray substance

Brachium of inferior colliculus

Lateral lemniscus

Parabigeminal nucleus

Spinothalamic tract

Trochlear nucleus

Medial longitudinal fasciculus

Medial lemniscus

Central tegmental tract

Decussation of brachium conjunctivum

Substantia nigra

Cerebral peduncle

Interpeduncular nucleus

Rubrospinal tract

Brachium pontis

Pontine gray matter

.5 centimeter

adjacent tegmentum in Figure 83, and also (more visibly) in Figure 82. The region indeed is cerulean, or distinctly dark blue in color, both in fresh brains and in brains fixed in formaldehyde. The blueness reflects the region's content of neuromelanin, a pigment synthesized by most of the neurons of the locus. The pigment is a polymer of dihydroxyphenylalanine, or DOPA, the precursor of the catecholamine neurotransmitters. Apart from its chemical properties, the locus ceruleus is remarkable anatomically: its efferents are distributed to all the main divisions of the central nervous system. On average, then, its 20,000 neurons must each influence a very great number of neurons elsewhere in the brain. In that respect the locus ceruleus is a caricature of the reticular formation: it embodies the extreme expression of a prominent reticular trait, an apparent diffuseness and nonspecificity of synaptic connections.

The monoamine neurotransmitter serotonin is employed by the raphe nuclei. Indeed, it now appears that the brain deploys its serotonergic neurons chiefly at the raphe of the midbrain and to a certain extent the hindbrain. Two of the raphe nuclei are in Figure 83: the median raphe nucleus, which we encountered in Figure 82, and the dorsal raphe nucleus, a fountain-shaped region in the ventral part of the central gray substance, distinguishable by dint of its slightly greater degree of myelination. Both project to the forebrain. The dorsal raphe nucleus sends fibers mainly to the striatum, the median raphe nucleus mainly to limbic structures and to the neocortex. The projections travel upward in the medial forebrain bundle; the projection to neocortex is the one mentioned in Part I that appears to terminate, at least in part, without making orthodox synapses. In Figure 83 a major source of input to the midbrain raphe nuclei occupies the most ventral part of the tegmentum: it is the interpeduncular nucleus, a small node of gray matter in the roof of the interpeduncular fossa. In spite of its smallness the nucleus consists of several cell groups that differ markedly in the details of their inputs and outputs. The inputs, however, come mostly from two places: the central gray substance and the habenula, a structure on the dorsum of the thalamus.

Finally, the monoamine neurotransmitter dopamine is employed by the substantia nigra, which makes its first appearance in Figure 83 and extends upward from there through the levels of Figure 84 and Figure 85. Fundamentally, it is a large, somewhat lens-shaped mass immediately dorsal to the cerebral peduncle. For the most part it is markedly poor in myelin. Also, it is

Figure 83: **Caudal midbrain** shows a number of changes from pontine levels. The dorsal face of the section is now formed by the inferior colliculi, each approached from below by the lateral lemniscus. The ventral face of the section is formed by the cerebral peduncles. The section is notable for its content of monoamine cell groups. The locus ceruleus, a pigmented cell group positioned in part in the central gray substance, employs as its neurotransmitter the monoamine norepinephrine. The raphe nuclei (here the median raphe nucleus and also the dorsal raphe nucleus, in the central gray substance) employ the monoamine serotonin. The pigmented cells of the substantia nigra, a lens-shaped mass immediately dorsal to the cerebral peduncle, employ the monoamine dopamine.

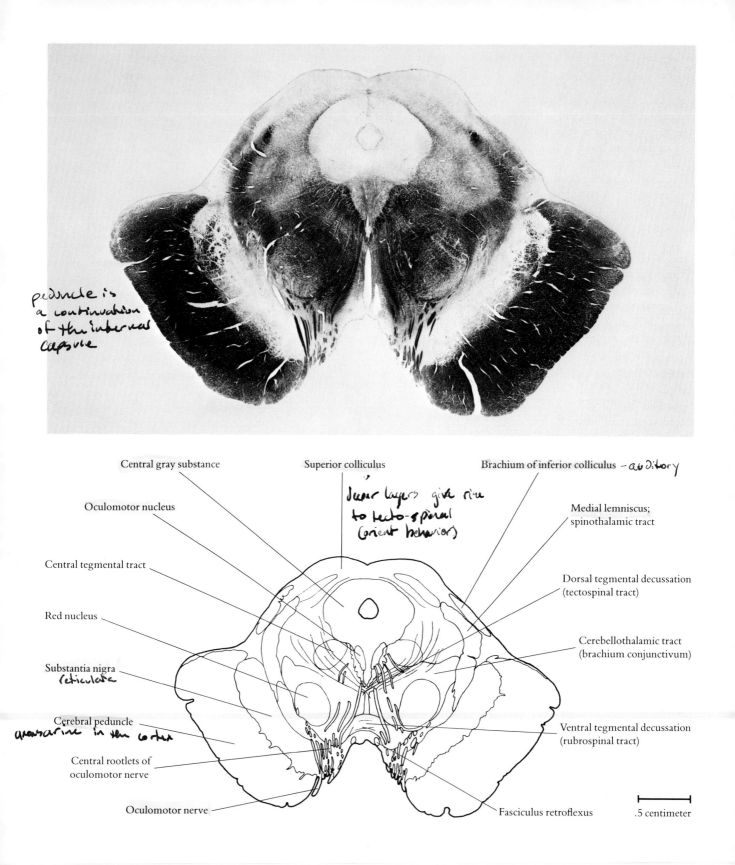

peduncle is a continuation of the internal capsule

Central gray substance

Oculomotor nucleus

Central tegmental tract

Red nucleus

Substantia nigra
reticulata

Cerebral peduncle
crossarine in the cortex

Central rootlets of
oculomotor nerve

Oculomotor nerve

Superior colliculus

deeper layers give rise
to tecto-spinal
(orient behavior)

Brachium of inferior colliculus — auditory

Medial lemniscus;
spinothalamic tract

Dorsal tegmental decussation
(tectospinal tract)

Cerebellothalamic tract
(brachium conjunctivum)

Ventral tegmental decussation
(rubrospinal tract)

Fasciculus retroflexus

.5 centimeter

two-layered. Its dorsal layer, the pars compacta, consists of large, closely crowded neurons displaying a dark pigmentation; hence the overall name of the structure. The thicker, ventral layer, the pars reticulata, consists of far more widely spaced cells, of which only a relative few are pigmented. The pigment again is neuromelanin; in the nigra, however, the pigmented neurons are dopaminergic. They project to the striatum, largely by way of the medial forebrain bundle; in fact they give the striatum its only known dopaminergic input. The importance of that input for normal bodily movement is demonstrated by Parkinson's disease, with its characteristic symptoms of muscular rigidity, tremor, and hypokinesia, or paucity of intentional movement. It now seems certain that the disease results when a pathological process, itself of unknown origin, brings on the progressive loss of the nigra's pigmented neurons. The substantia nigra does have targets other than the striatum. The unpigmented neurons of the pars reticulata direct nondopaminergic efferent fibers to a medial part of the ventral lateral nucleus of the thalamus, a part called the ventromedial nucleus, which projects in turn to neocortex bordering the motor cortex. Moreover, in the midbrain the nondopaminergic efferents innervate the superior colliculus and also the pedunculopontine nucleus, in the dorsal part of the midbrain tegmentum. Since the input to the substantia nigra comes mostly from the striatum, the nigrofugal projections are pathways by which the nigra could broadcast the influence of the striatum to widespread regions of the forebrain and the midbrain, and ultimately to the lower motor system of the hindbrain and spinal cord.

Rostral Midbrain

Figure 84 is a cross section made high enough in the midbrain so that some crucial changes have taken place. The trochlear nucleus has given way to the oculomotor nucleus; thus the stout central root bundles fanning widely through the tegmentum belong to the oculomotor nerve.

In addition, at the dorsum of the section, the superior colliculus now appears on each side of the midline. Unlike the inferior colliculus it is conspicuously laminated. Its superficial gray layers receive fibers from the retina and from the primary visual cortex. The fibers from the retina course past the

Figure 84: **Superior colliculus and red nucleus** dominate a section made at roughly the middle of the mesencephalon. The colliculus, at the dorsal face of the section, is a strikingly laminated structure. Its deep layers emit the tectospinal tract, whose decussation, called the dorsal tegmental decussation, lies ventral to the medial longitudinal fasciculus. The red nucleus, at the center of the tegmentum, is an almost spherical mass. The fascicles inside it have arrived from the cerebellum by way of the brachium conjunctivum; the rest of the brachium, bound for the thalamus, skirts the borders of the sphere. From the ventromedial edge of the nucleus comes an efferent bundle, the rubrospinal tract, whose crossing of the midline composes the ventral tegmental decussation. The dark-staining fascicles aggregating ventral to the red nucleus are constituents of the oculomotor nerve.

geniculate bodies, the medial and the lateral, and enter the superior colliculus from the lateral side as the brachium of the superior colliculus, which will be visible in Figure 86. Two deeper gray layers receive fibers from a variety of structures: the spinal cord, by way of spinotectal fibers accompanying the spinothalamic tract; the inferior colliculus; the tegmentum; the pars reticulata of the substantia nigra; the central gray substance; and nearly the full expanse of the neocortex. The identification of the superior colliculus with any one sensory modality is plainly an oversimplification. On the other hand, the electrical stimulation of the superior colliculus in experimental animals elicits conjugate eye movements that turn the gaze toward the contralateral side of the visual world. The stimulation of the superior colliculus on the right side of the brain makes the eyes turn in unison toward the left, and vice

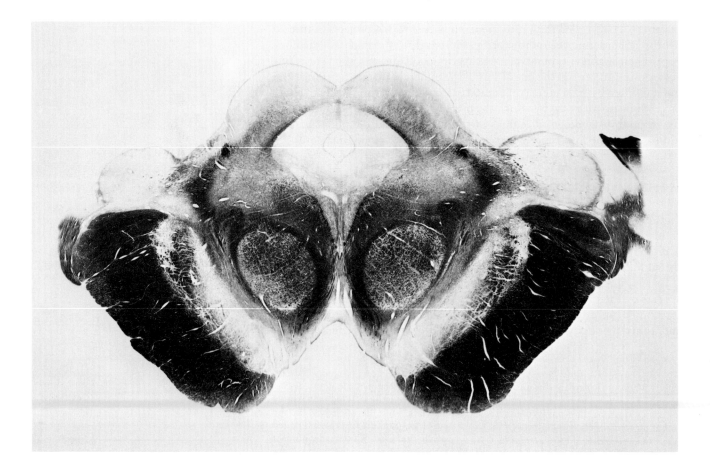

Figure 85: **Several transitions** distinguish this cross section, made high in the midbrain, from the section in Figure 84. The medial geniculate body, at the dorsal end of the cerebral peduncle, marks the

first appearance of the thalamus. Conversely, the oculomotor nucleus, immediately ventral to the central gray substance, marks the last appearance of the somatic motor column, and the Edinger-

versa. In fact, the stimulation of the rostral half of a superior colliculus makes the eyes turn not only horizontally but downward. The stimulation of the caudal half makes the eyes turn horizontally and upward.

By what outgoing paths could the superior colliculus evoke such movements? Large neurons in the two deep gray layers of the colliculus emit a prominent fiber system, the tectospinal tract, which sweeps through the tegmentum and promptly crosses the midline. The crossing, known as the dorsal tegmental decussation or the fountain decussation of Meynert, is plainly visible in Figure 84 immediately ventral to the medial longitudinal fasciculus. The crossing completed, the fibers assemble into a fairly circumscribed bundle that hugs the midline in its descent. (We encountered it in that position in the medulla oblongata, just dorsal to the medial lemniscus.) The

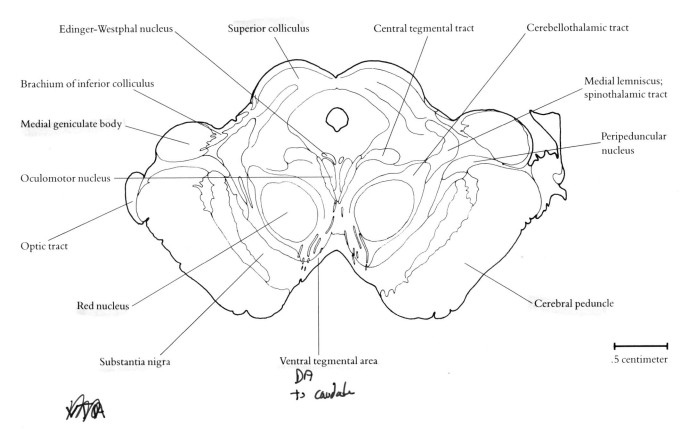

Edinger-Westphal nucleus

Superior colliculus

Central tegmental tract

Cerebellothalamic tract

Brachium of inferior colliculus

Medial lemniscus; spinothalamic tract

Medial geniculate body

Peripeduncular nucleus

Oculomotor nucleus

Optic tract

Red nucleus

Cerebral peduncle

Substantia nigra

Ventral tegmental area

DA
to caudate

.5 centimeter

Westphal nucleus, a pale-staining cap of the oculomotor nucleus, marks the last appearance of the visceral motor column. Indeed, the two motor nuclei are the final appearance of motor neurons. The region between the red nucleus and the substantia nigra is the ventral tegmental area of Tsai. It is remarkable for pigmented, dopaminergic neurons that project to limbic forebrain structures.

bundle makes no direct connections with the motor neurons controlling eye movement. But in its descent through the brainstem it issues fibers to the medial reticular formation, and there, at middle and upper pontine levels near the abducens nucleus, the brainstem includes the paramedian pontine reticular formation, or, to use a less anatomical term, the lateral-gaze control center, a "function generator" mentioned in Part II that coordinates conjugate, horizontal eye movements. It, too, is not directly connected with motor neurons; its output goes instead to interneurons, some in the abducens nucleus, others in gray matter near the abducens nucleus (in particular the nucleus prepositus hypoglossi). Evidently a command to adjust the lateral gaze, issuing from the superior colliculus, can reach motor neurons only by a succession of at least two subaltern stations. A similar succession affecting vertical gaze appears to involve the so-called accessory oculomotor nuclei, high in the midbrain: the nucleus of the posterior commissure, the interstitial nucleus of Cajal, and the nucleus of Darkschewitsch.

The tectospinal tract continues into the spinal cord, where it positions itself in the ventral funiculus but gets no farther than cervical segments. Both of these facts are suggestive: the ventral funiculus is the path followed by fiber systems attaining the medial part of the ventral horn, where motor neurons and interneurons serving axial muscles are found, and in the case of the cervical spinal cord the axial muscles are those of the neck. The question thus becomes: Why should the superior colliculus selectively influence eye and neck movements? The answer, evidently, is that the eyes and the neck are often in collusion. When your attention is attracted by a sudden sound, for instance, your eyes typically turn first. Then your neck turns, and with it your head. The eyes almost always overshoot; an interplay between eye and neck musculature is required before the gaze is steadied. It seems, then, that the superior colliculus should be termed a tracking mechanism. And since vision is emphatically a receptor of distant events, the heavy investment of retinofugal fibers in the mechanism can hardly be surprising. Still, one tracks with several senses. When one is set on in the dark by a flying, buzzing insect, one's head knows where to turn to confront the enemy. The superior colliculus, perhaps correspondingly, is multisensory.

The center of the tegmentum in Figure 84 is dominated, on each side of the midline, by the red nucleus, or nucleus ruber, a structure termed red because in unfixed brain tissue it has a distinctive pinkish hue. It is a spherical mass, more sharply defined than almost any other cell group in the tegmentum and large enough to deflect the path of the tegmental fiber bundles, including the ones in the stratum lemnisci. The nucleus itself is filled with fascicles; they represent the part of the brachium conjunctivum (that is, the cerebellar outflow) directed into the nucleus. A second input, not as easy to discern, arrives from the motor cortex. The remainder of the brachium, the part destined for the thalamus, skirts the nucleus on its lateral, dorsal, and medial sides. From the ventromedial corner of the nucleus the rubrospinal tract emerges. Its fibers cross the midline in the ventral tegmental decussation; then they descend, initially grouped in the circumscribed fiber bundle we encountered near the base of the tegmentum in Figure 83. The sight of the tract is disturbing: it seems rather small, especially in comparison with the combined volumes of the two connections afferent to the nucleus. Further circumstances only heighten one's perplexity. For one thing, the red nucleus markedly augments in size in the higher primates. The rubrospinal tract seems to dwindle. Perhaps some fundamental aspect of the associations of the red nucleus has so far escaped detection.

Figure 85 shows a midbrain cross section that cuts through the middle of the superior colliculus. It is a section much like the preceding one. Still, there are some noteworthy additions. First, the thalamus has appeared: the oval structure at the dorsal end of the cerebral peduncle is the medial geniculate body. On its medial side it is entered by the brachium of the inferior colliculus. A short distance lateral to the medial geniculate body, the optic tract sweeps dorsally around the lateral margin of the cerebral peduncle in its approach to the lateral geniculate body, which is not yet in view. Second, each oculomotor nucleus, in the *V*-shaped trough between the medial longitudinal fasciculi, has been joined by its visceral motor component, the Edinger-Westphal nucleus, a circumscribed, pale-staining cap on the somatic motor cell group. The Edinger-Westphal nucleus consists of the preganglionic, parasympathetic motor neurons that govern two internal eye muscles: the ciliary muscle and the constrictor pupillae muscle. The nucleus marks the rostral end of the visceral motor column; the oculomotor nucleus marks the rostral end of the somatic motor column. The branchial motor column ended much farther caudally, with the masticatory nucleus, at upper pontine levels. We shall encounter no further motor neurons in either the diencephalon or the cerebral hemisphere.*

Between the red nucleus and the substantia nigra in Figure 85 is a third addition to the cross section: a region called the ventral tegmental area of Tsai. The region continues dorsally a short distance along the midline. In all the quadruped animals studied so far, it contains a multitude of fairly large, dark-looking neurons, which is probably the reason why Chan-Nao Tsai (at the University of Chicago in the early 1920's) distinguished the region from its rostral continuity with the lateral hypothalamus. What Tsai could not have known is that the large, dark-looking neurons synthesize dopamine and employ it as their neurotransmitter. In fact, the neurons are indistinguishable

---

*The statement refers to motor neurons in the conventional sense of neurons with motor axons that leave the central nervous system to animate peripheral effector tissues, either directly or through the intervention of ganglionic neurons. A different conclusion must be drawn if a motor neuron is more broadly defined as the final element in a neural sequence affecting peripheral tissues. The definition would then include forebrain neurons: for example, the hypothalamic neurons that themselves emit a hormone (say, the neurons of the supraoptic nucleus) or the hypothalamic neurons that trigger an endocrine effector chain by shedding a releasing factor into the hypothalamopituitary portal system. Charles Sherrington's phrase "the final common path" may ultimately prove applicable to a wide range of brain neurons.

from the dopaminergic neurons of the substantia nigra's pars compacta. Perhaps they arise in ontogeny as a dorsomedial extrusion from the pars compacta. In any event they have a specific name. Annica Dahlström and Kjell Fuxe of the Karolinska Institute in Stockholm, who undertook in the early 1960's the first systematic study of monoamine cell groups in the brainstem, called them dopamine cell group A10, thus distinguishing them from cell group A9: the dopaminergic neurons of the pars compacta proper. Two

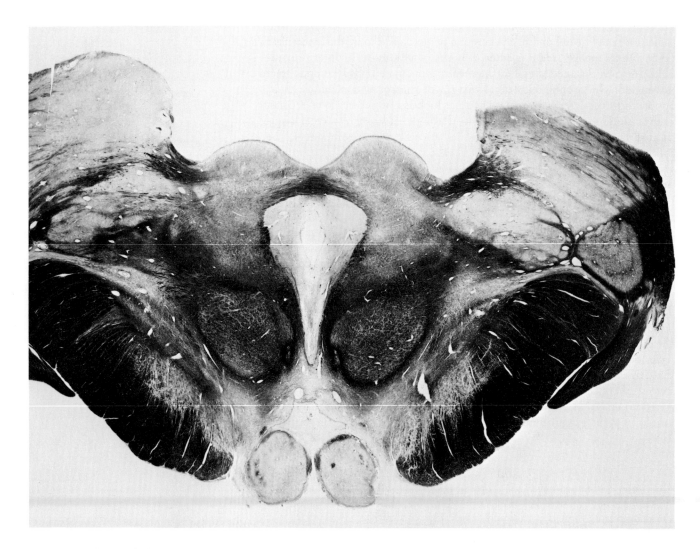

Figure 86: **Advent of the diencephalon** is apparent at several places in a final midbrain cross section. The ventral part of the central gray substance, expanding along the midline, is really the medial hypothalamus: pale-staining gray matter surrounding the third ventricle. The ventral tegmental area of Tsai, between the red nucleus and the interpeduncular fossa, is really the lateral hypothalamus: a mass of more darkly staining gray matter traversed by the medial forebrain bundle. The tegmentum dorsal and lateral to the red

things about the ventral tegmental area make it special. For one, the medial forebrain bundle passes through it. Indeed, the grayness of the ventral tegmental area in Figure 85, or any other Weigert preparation, is due largely to the presence of the medial forebrain bundle. Furthermore, the ventral tegmental area emits a remarkable dopaminergic adjunct to the projection from the substantia nigra to the striatum. The adjunct projects in part to the striatum: a large, ventromedial sector of the striatum. (More about that in

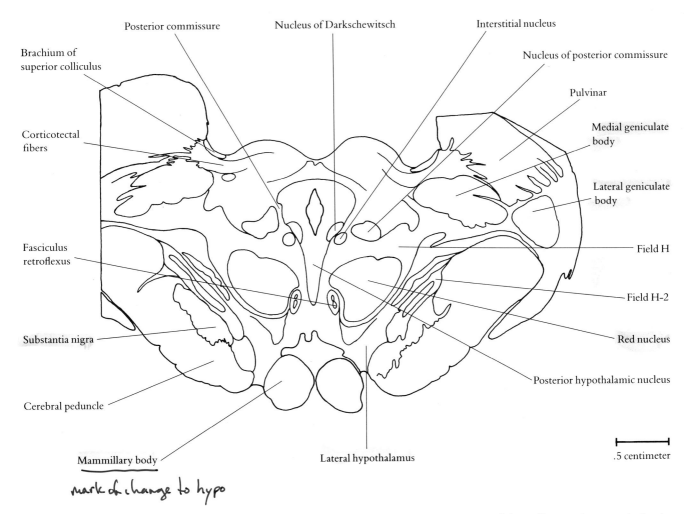

Posterior commissure

Nucleus of Darkschewitsch

Interstitial nucleus

Brachium of superior colliculus

Nucleus of posterior commissure

Pulvinar

Corticotectal fibers

Medial geniculate body

Lateral geniculate body

Fasciculus retroflexus

Field H

Field H-2

Substantia nigra

Red nucleus

Posterior hypothalamic nucleus

Cerebral peduncle

Mammillary body

Lateral hypothalamus

.5 centimeter

mark of change to hypo

nucleus is really the subthalamus. The two round bodies in the interpeduncular fossa are hypothalamic cell groups: the mammillary bodies. Finally, in lateral parts of the section, three thalamic cell groups appear: the geniculate bodies and the pulvinar. The superior colliculus betokens the last of the midbrain. It is approached at its lateral side by two of its principal afferents: retinotectal fibers occupy the surface of the midbrain, and under them lie corticotectal fibers.

Chapter 14.) In addition it projects to components of the limbic system: the amygdala, the entorhinal area, and the septum. Its longest efferents are the dopaminergic fibers that invade the frontal association cortex. In recognition of this limbic affinity the ventral tegmental area and its dopaminergic efferents are called the mesolimbic system; the prefix *meso-* alludes to the mesencephalic origin of the projection. The dopaminergic projection to frontal cortex is sometimes given a separate name: the mesocortical system.

Figure 86 shows a final midbrain cross section, a section best described as a slice through the transition from midbrain to diencephalon. The center of the section still looks mesencephalic: it exhibits, in dorsal-to-ventral sequence, the superior colliculus, then the central gray substance, in juxtaposition with the tegmentum (the latter includes the red nucleus), and finally the cerebral peduncle. First comes the colliculus, cut here through the rostral third of its height. On both sides of the section, but more clearly on the left, two of its principal afferent systems enter its lateral side. Retinotectal fibers compose the brachium of the superior colliculus, at the surface of the midbrain. Just under them one sees a substantial bundle of corticotectal fibers. The ventral border of the colliculi is formed by the tectal commissure, which interconnects the deep gray layers of the colliculi. Then comes the central gray substance. Here the oculomotor nucleus has disappeared from view. It is replaced by an accessory oculomotor nucleus: the nucleus of Darkschewitsch (the Russian neurologist L. O. Darkschewitsch). Just lateral to it, but outside the central gray substance, are the other accessory nuclei: the interstitial nucleus of Cajal and the nucleus of the posterior commissure. For its part the central gray substance seems to be making a ventralward expansion along the midline. There, however, the section is turning diencephalic: the expansion is really the first appearance of the medial hypothalamus, a zone of poorly myelinated gray matter that will surround the third ventricle much as the central gray substance surrounded the cerebral aqueduct. (In fact Figure 86 grazes the caudal limit of the third ventricle.) The lateral hypothalamus, a more myelinated region traversed by the medial forebrain bundle, appears farther ventrally: it occupies the space between the red nucleus and the interpeduncular fossa, where it replaces the ventral tegmental area of Tsai. More ventrally yet, the hypothalamus shows a frank token of its presence: the round cross sections of the mammillary bodies (the hypothalamic end stations for the fornix bundles) occupy the interpeduncular fossa.

In more lateral parts of Figure 86 the midbrain tegmentum is becoming the subthalamus. The mass of fibers extending laterally and dorsally from the red nucleus comprises thalamic afferents in the brachium conjunctivum and, more laterally, the somatic sensory lemnisci: the medial lemniscus and the spinothalamic tract. The three are forming field H-1 of Forel, a fiber stratum defining the ventral border of the thalamus. A more ventral fiber stratum is called field H-2; in contrast to field H-1 it consists mostly of descending fibers, including ones directed to the midbrain tegmentum from the globus pallidus. The pale-staining gray matter intervening between the fields, which it invades from the lateral side, is called the zona incerta. It stops short of a node of white matter known as field H of Forel. The most lateral part of the cross section is the thalamus itself, or rather the caudal thalamus, with its characteristic triad of cell groups. The lateral geniculate body, showing its six gray layers, protrudes ventrally to meet the incoming optic tract; the medial geniculate body is closer to the midline. Above them both is the thalamic cell group called the pulvinar.

Chapter Thirteen

Forebrain

By the end of the third week of human ontogeny the cervical flexure and the cephalic flexure are conspicuous in the embryo. The prosencephalon remains far from conspicuous. Still, an evagination has just begun to develop near its rostral end on each side of the neural tube. Each is an optic vesicle, from which a retina and its stalk, the optic tract, will develop. At the end of the fifth week a second, more domelike evagination appears on each side of the tube, but in a more dorsal position. It will become a cerebral hemisphere. At this point the prosencephalon has assumed its basic shape: the central part of the forebrain (the prospective diencephalon) now has a pair of side chambers (the prospective cerebral hemispheres). The lumen of each cerebral hemisphere is the lateral ventricle; the lumen of the diencephalon is the third ventricle. Throughout the development of the brain the two will retain their connection, by way of a short passage, the interventricular foramen of Monro (named for the 18th-century Scottish anatomist Alexander Monro, Jr.). In turn, the third ventricle will retain its connection with the fourth ventricle by way of the cerebral aqueduct. Then, too, the cerebral hemisphere will remain broadly footed in the central, unpaired part of the prosencephalon. Through this footing — this cerebral pedestal — the complex circuitry connecting the cerebral hemisphere with the diencephalon and lower levels of the central nervous system will pass. The circuitry will include the great fiber complex called the internal capsule, whose caudal extension we have encountered in the mesencephalon as the cerebral peduncle and in the rhombencephalon and spinal cord as the pyramidal tract.

Among the difficulties bedeviling the internal structure of the forebrain, two are fundamental. The first is a matter of orientation. In the brain of a quadruped mammal the forebrain, the brainstem, and the spinal cord are more or less colinear. In the human brain this is not the case: the long axis of the forebrain and the long axis of the brainstem make an angle of roughly 60 degrees (Figure 87). The difference, which corresponds to the difference in posture between bipeds and quadrupeds, entails a number of complications in establishing uniform meanings for terms of spatial reference. In the forebrain of any vertebrate, the term rostral means toward the frontal pole (the most forward tip of the brain). Caudal means toward the occipital pole (the rearmost tip of the brain). Thus the terms preserve their alignment with the long axis of the central nervous system. In addition they apply to both quadruped and biped. In the former, their orientation is unchanging (or nearly so) from brainstem to forebrain. In the latter, they make an abstraction of the angle between the two. That leaves dorsal and ventral. In the forebrain, dorsal means toward the crown of the skull. Ventral means toward the base of the skull. They, too, apply to quadrupeds and bipeds. The terms dorsal and ventral, rostral and caudal are better, therefore, than the older, persistent terminology involving anterior and posterior. After all, a biped carries its face and its abdomen anteriorly, so that the term anterior, applied to a vertical structure such as the spinal cord, refers most naturally to the forward-facing aspect of the structure. A quadruped carries only its face anteriorly. Is the term anterior thus to signify the top end of the spinal cord, but only in quadrupeds?

Inside the Hemisphere

The second difficulty concerns the human cerebral hemisphere. In the course of evolution the cerebral hemisphere of the mammal forsakes the earlier, simpler shape whose descendant is found today in the brain of an amphibian: it forsakes the shape of a cylinder. Specifically, the cerebral cortex enlarges, and as if to accommodate its enlargement in the volume of the cranium, the cerebral cortex arches into a horseshoe: it comes increasingly to curve from the frontal lobe, the most forward part of the hemisphere, through the parietal lobe to the occipital lobe, the rearmost part of the hemisphere, and then underneath itself into the temporal lobe, which advances beneath the rest of the hemisphere, reaching around the side of the brainstem and then far enough forward so that it appears in the human brain under the caudal half of the frontal lobe (Figure 88). The evolutionary process by which the cerebral hemisphere conduplicates — the process by which it assumes a horseshoe shape — might well be termed the temporalization of the hemisphere. After all, the plainest result of the process is the formation of the temporal lobe. Yet the consequences of temporalization are apparent not only at the surface of the brain. Temporalization causes structures within the human cerebral hemisphere to be in essence a set of nested horseshoes. The intricacies of the nesting will display themselves in the cross sections that accompany Chapter 14. For now, as a preface to those sections, we shall describe the nesting globally.

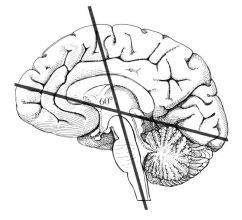

Figure 87: **Angle of 60 degrees** is made in the human brain by the axes of the forebrain and the brainstem; thus a forebrain cross section is oblique to a brainstem cross section. The obliqueness can make it difficult to preserve one's sense of direction when transferring one's attention from the brainstem to the forebrain. In quadrupeds such as the carnivores, the spinal cord, the brainstem, and the forebrain are more or less aligned.

In Figure 89 we construct the cerebral hemisphere of a human brain, proceeding from inside out. One step in the construction is to position the lentiform nucleus: the somewhat lens-shaped cell mass formed by the globus pallidus and the putamen. It is the only structure in the cerebral hemisphere essentially unaffected by temporalization: it lies on the axis of the hemisphere's conduplication and is therefore the structure about which the nested horseshoes revolve. Another step is to position the internal capsule. Let us begin with its forerunner, the cerebral peduncle. In Chapter 12 we found the peduncle at the base of the midbrain's cross section, beginning with Figure 83. The bundle consists exclusively of corticofugal fibers bound for the midbrain, the hindbrain, and the spinal cord. Followed upward into the forebrain (against the direction of impulse flow), the cerebral peduncle rapidly widens. For the most part it courses dorsally, so that the majority of its fibers compose a thick, almost vertical plate of white matter skirting the lateral side of the thalamus. It is now the internal capsule. As it passes the thalamus it is joined by fibers that connect the thalamus with the cerebral cortex and fibers that have come the other way, from the cortex to the thalamus. Thus the internal capsule contains not only the descending fibers that compose the cerebral peduncle but also the massive fiber traffic between thalamus and cortex.

Anatomically, however, the capsule is more than a thick, almost vertical plate. Its fibers course not only upward, between the thalamus and the lentiform nucleus, but also sideways (that is, in the lateral direction), under the lentiform nucleus, and caudalward, behind the lentiform nucleus. In other words, the capsule curves under itself, and around the lentiform nucleus, so as to distribute fibers to all parts of the neocortex: the rind of the cerebral hemisphere. As a result the internal capsule assumes the shape of a hollow cone, one that encloses the lentiform nucleus. The apex of the cone points caudally, medially, and ventrally, into the diencephalon. There it becomes continuous with the cerebral peduncle. The base of the cone opens laterally and rostrally, into the cerebral hemisphere. There it sends fibers flowing toward all of the neocortex. The cone is incomplete: there is a large, triangular gap in the anterior part of its ventral wall. The gap corresponds to the gap between the prongs of the cerebral hemisphere — that is, the deep crease between the frontal lobe and the temporal lobe. The cone can be divided into three districts, if only arbitrarily and for topographic purposes. The massive part of the cone passing dorsal to the lentiform nucleus is the supralenticular limb of the internal capsule; it includes the pyramidal tract and, immediately behind it, the somatic sensory radiation (the fibers directed to or from the somatic sensory cortex). The much smaller part of the cone passing under the lentiform nucleus (the caudal fourth or so of the nucleus) is the sublenticular limb of the capsule; it includes the auditory radiation and the ventral part of the optic radiation. The latter courses forward far into the temporal lobe, then curves back to visual cortex on the medial face of the occipital lobe, thus describing what is called the loop of Meyer-Archambault. Finally, the massive part of the cone intermediate between the supralenticular limb and the sublenticular limb, skirting the caudal face of the lentiform nucleus, is the retrolenticular limb of the capsule; it comprises the greater part of the optic radiation and much of the parietal radiation. Where the cone of the internal capsule expands far enough into the cerebral hemisphere to emerge from around the margin of the lateral base of the lentiform nucleus (specifically the putamen), it assumes a new name — a final name that joins with "internal capsule," "cerebral peduncle," and "pyramidal tract" to signify four stretches of the great axonal continuum linking the neocortex with the thalamus, the brainstem, and the spinal cord. In particular, its many millions of fibers, now streaming toward neocortical origins or destinations from around the lentiform nucleus, join the white matter under the cortex. On account of their fanlike arrayal they are called the corona radiata.

The remaining details of Figure 89 complete the construction of a cerebral hemisphere. Examine the caudate nucleus (Figure 89*b*). It clings to the outer face of the cone of the internal capsule. Specifically, its rostral part, the head, or caput, of the nucleus, bends ventralward over the rostral wall of the cone. The deepest part of the head fuses with the putamen through the triangular gap in the cone. (Recall that the caudate nucleus and the putamen are divisions of the striatum and are histologically indistinguishable. In the human brain the internal capsule cleaves them apart, except at the gap in the cone.) Followed the other way, the head of the caudate nucleus extends caudalward over the surface of the internal capsule. It diminishes in girth; the locus of diminution is called the corpus, or body, of the nucleus. Next comes the cauda, or tail, of the nucleus, which passes ventralward behind the retrolenticular limb of the internal capsule and then rostralward under the sublenticular limb. In the temporal lobe, the tail of the caudate nucleus is continuous with the amygdala, the deep gray matter under the uncus of the temporal lobe. In turn the amygdala is dorsally contiguous with the putamen. We have thus described a ring; it consists of the caudate nucleus, the amygdala, the putamen, and then again the caudate nucleus. The important point, however, is that the caudate nucleus describes a horseshoe around the internal capsule, just as the internal capsule (or rather its longitudinal cross section) describes a horseshoe around the lentiform nucleus.

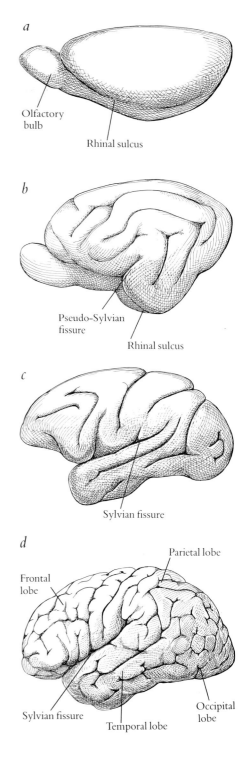

Figure 88: **Temporalization** is a one-word characterization of the evolutionary sequence by which the cerebral hemisphere arches into a horseshoe shape. The most apparent result of the process (apparent, that is, at the surface of the brain) is the temporal lobe's emergence. The illustration shows the brain of a rat, a cat, a monkey, and man. In the rat (*a*) no horseshoe is found. In the cat (*b*) the horseshoe is incipient: the caudal end of the cerebral hemisphere extends slightly downward. In the monkey (*c*), and especially in man (*d*), the horseshoe is pronounced: the cerebral hemisphere curves from one prong, the frontal lobe, through the parietal lobe and a vertex, the occipital lobe, and finally into a second prong, the temporal lobe, which reaches forward around the brainstem. Comparisons such as the ones in this illustration cannot establish the actual progression of evolution; the species alive today have individual histories of evolutionary modification. In one metaphor, they are leaves of a tree that has vanished.

Next examine the thalamus (again, Figure 89*b*), already mentioned with regard to the internal capsule. Like the caudate nucleus, it lies outside the cone of the capsule. Its position, however, is medial and ventral to that of the caudate nucleus. The thalamus extends along a curve much like that of the caudate nucleus, although not nearly as far. Still, the caudal end of the thalamus probes downward and somewhat forward.

Next examine the corpus callosum (Figure 89*b* and *e*). Anatomically it is a massive fiber plate spanning the fissure between the two cerebral hemispheres as a canopy over the thalamus and the head and body of the caudate nucleus of the left and right side. Functionally it is a commissure connecting homotopic fields of the neocortex for all but the temporal fields. (The temporal fields have their own connection, the anterior commissure.) The rostral end of the corpus callosum bends double under itself. The bend is called the genu, meaning knee; the underfold is called the rostrum. The opposite, caudal end of the callosum is called the splenium, meaning bandage. It is a thick part of the callosum. Its millions of fibers course largely between the left and right occipital cortex; the splenium is therefore a commissure mostly for cortex serving vision. Slung under the splenium (but not visible in Figure 89) is a further commissure, one that has no direct association with the neocortex. It is the commissure of the hippocampi, also called the commissura fornicis, the lyra Davidis, or the psalterium. (The last two names reflect the harplike shape of the structure when it is viewed from the dorsal side.) In the human brain the corpus callosum does not resemble a horseshoe, nor does the hippocampus. But if it were not for the corpus callosum, the hippocampus might have kept a horseshoe shape. In rodents, and insectivores, and especially in marsupials, the hippocampus does look like a horseshoe, with a dorsal limb slung over the thalamus. Then the enlargement of the neocortex and the concordant enlargement of the corpus callosum drives the hippocampus into

Figure 89: **Constructing a cerebral hemisphere** from the inside out is one way to master the basics of the hemisphere's internal structure. The construction is done in five steps. First (*a*) the internal capsule is positioned. It is in essence a hollow cone consisting of axons coursing to or from the neocortex. The cone is incomplete: a gap facing forward and downward corresponds to the gap between the prongs of the cerebral hemisphere's horseshoe shape. Well into the cerebral hemisphere the internal capsule becomes the corona radiata; in the brainstem it becomes the cerebral peduncle. Next (*b*) two forebrain structures are positioned dorsal and medial to the capsule. (In this lateral view they lie behind the capsule.) They are the caudate nucleus and the thalamus. Each has a horseshoe shape, although the thalamic horseshoe is not pronounced. Two further forebrain structures, the amygdala and the hippocampus, occupy the temporal lobe. Next (*c*) the lentiform nucleus is positioned in the hollow of the capsule. In this view its lateral part, the putamen, hides its medial part, the globus pallidus. Fourth (*d*), the insula, a deep expanse of the cerebral cortex, is positioned outside the lateral face of the lentiform nucleus. At the same time several bundles of neocortical association fibers take their positions; they, too, are superficial to the corona radiata. A final drawing (*e*) includes all the neocortex, thus completing the construction.

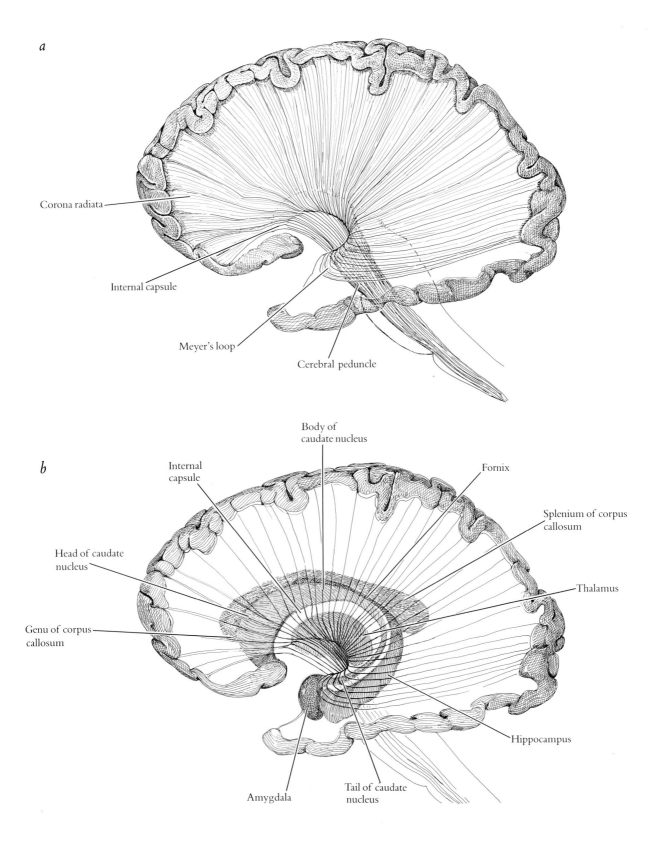

a

Corona radiata

Internal capsule

Meyer's loop

Cerebral peduncle

b

Body of
caudate nucleus

Internal
capsule

Fornix

Splenium of corpus
callosum

Head of caudate
nucleus

Thalamus

Genu of corpus
callosum

Hippocampus

Amygdala

Tail of caudate
nucleus

c

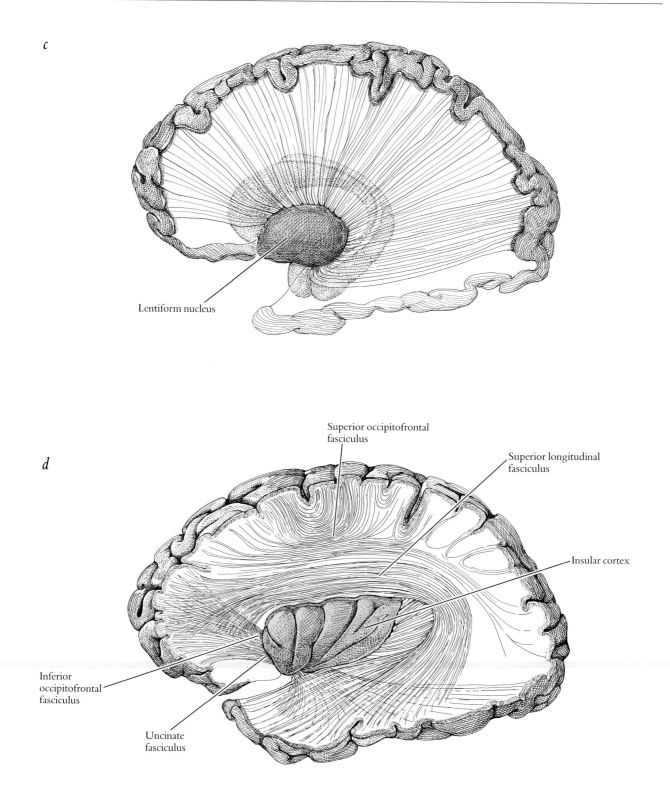

Lentiform nucleus

d

Superior occipitofrontal fasciculus

Superior longitudinal fasciculus

Insular cortex

Inferior occipitofrontal fasciculus

Uncinate fasciculus

the temporal lobe. In Figure 89*b* it has the shape of half a horseshoe. The position of its dorsal, suprathalamic limb remains marked by the fornix, the principal efferent bundle of the hippocampus.

There is, however, a complication not apparent in Figure 89; we show it in Figure 90. In all mammalian species with a platelike corpus callosum (which is to say all mammalian species except the marsupials, in whose brain an enormous anterior commissure is the only neocortical commissure) the fornix, and sometimes part of the hippocampus itself, is found under the corpus callosum. In all such species, however, a thin, inconspicuous sheet of hippocampal gray matter called the indusium griseum or the supracallosal hippocampal rudiment covers the upper — not the lower — surface of the callosum. It is positioned between the callosum and the overarching cingulate gyrus, on the medial face of the cerebral hemisphere. In its caudal extent, the hippocampal rudiment courses around the splenium of the callosum, where it takes on the shape of a slender, somewhat rounded band. Indeed, it becomes a

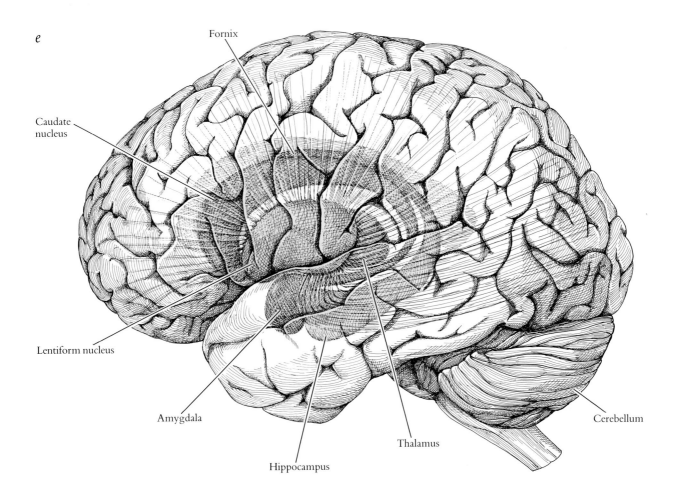

e

Fornix

Caudate nucleus

Lentiform nucleus

Amygdala

Hippocampus

Thalamus

Cerebellum

miniature gyrus. In that form it extends ventralward, then forward, first on the underside of the splenium, then on the medial face of the temporal lobe, as the gyrus fasciolaris or fasciola cinerea. (The second name means the little gray bundle.) Finally it merges into the dentate gyrus, which caps the hippocampus and marks the true edge of the cerebral cortex. The dentate gyrus gets its name because a fairly regular spacing of transverse grooves etching the gyrus makes it resemble a row of teeth. In its opposite, rostral extent, the hippocampal rudiment curves around the genu of the corpus callosum. Then, after following the underside of the rostrum, it descends vertically on the medial face of the cerebral hemisphere. In this last part of its course it is called the taenia tecta—the hidden (covered) band. What hides it is a shallow groove, the sulcus parolfactorius posterior, which marks the border between the frontal cortex anterior to it and the subcortical tissue of the base of the septum behind it. The hippocampal rudiment marks throughout its extent the true edge of the cerebral cortex. The question arises: If the hippocampal rudiment is above the corpus callosum and the fornix is underneath it, where was the hippocampus before the enlargement of the corpus callosum drove it wholly (except for its supracallosal rudiment) into the temporal lobe? Perhaps there was a time before the current evolutionary arrangements were complete when the corpus callosum cleaved the hippocampus, placing the larger part of it ventral and a smaller part dorsal.

A further question arises: If the hippocampal rudiment marks the cortical edge, where is Broca's great lobe of the hem? Figure 90 shows it. In Figure 90 the brainstem has been removed, exposing the hilus of the hemisphere, a region bordered dorsally by the curvature of the corpus callosum and ventrally by the temporal lobe. Through the hilus the hemisphere is anchored to the diencephalon and beyond that to the brainstem. Surrounding the hilus are the gyrus cinguli, its forward bend around the genu and rostrum of the corpus callosum to form the subcallosal gyrus, and its rearward bend around the splenium of the callosum to form first the retrosplenial area, then the hippocampal gyrus (or parahippocampal gyrus; the two are synonymous), and finally, on the medial face of the temporal lobe, the uncus. The whole of this

Figure 90: **Edge of the cerebral cortex** can be seen in this dissection, which shows the medial face of the human cerebral hemisphere. The brainstem has been removed, exposing the pedestal through which the hemisphere links itself to the diencephalon. The edge encircles the pedestal but is rather hard to find. Above the corpus callosum it is the indusium griseum, a thin remnant of hippocampal gray matter. Followed caudally, it curves around the splenium of the corpus callosum, then comes forward on the medial face of the temporal lobe, where it becomes the dentate gyrus, a part of the hippocampus. Followed rostrally, it curves around the genu of the corpus callosum, then descends the medial face of the cerebral hemisphere. The almost annular cortical region nearest the edge of the cerebral cortex is the gyrus fornicatus; it consists of the subcallosal gyrus, the cingulate gyrus, the retrosplenial area, the hippocampal gyrus, and the uncus. The massive fiber bundle positioned under the corpus callosum and curving downward toward the hypothalamus, specifically the mammillary body, is the fornix.

almost annular cortical locus is Broca's great limbic lobe, or rather the part of the lobe exposed on the medial wall of the cerebral hemisphere. It is called the gyrus fornicatus because of its arciform shape. (*Fornix* is Latin for arch.) The other use of "fornix" has a related explanation. Early anatomists saw that the vertical part of a massive, circumscribed fiber bundle in the medial wall of the cerebral hemisphere had the look of a column supporting the gyrus fornicatus from under the corpus callosum. They called it the columna fornicis: the

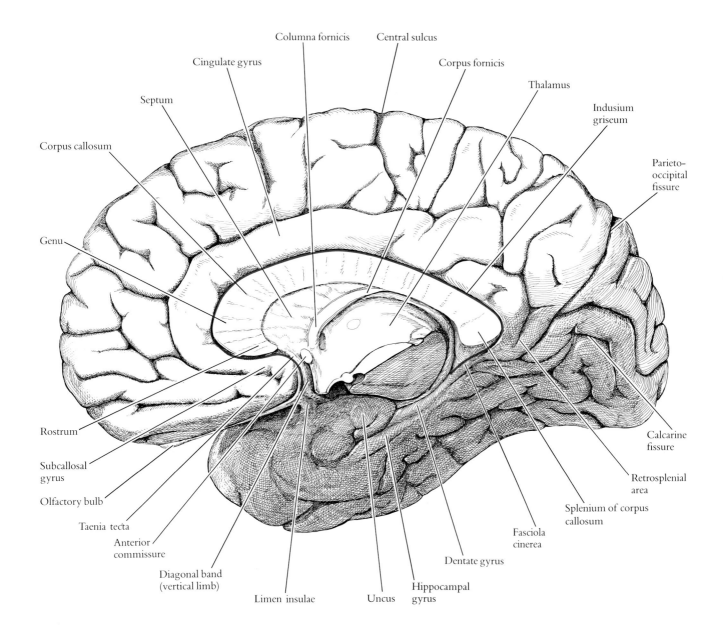

pillar supporting the arch. The name persists. Indeed, the entire fiber bundle has claimed the name of fornix. But then, it, too, is an arch: the full extent of its curve from the hippocampus to the hypothalamus is visible in Figure 90.

Lateral Ventricle

A final horseshoe in the forebrain is described by the ventricle of the cerebral hemisphere, the lateral ventricle (Figure 91). Some things about it are basic. First, the lateral ventricle has only the narrow passage called the interventricular foramen through which to meet the third ventricle. That meeting, however, is essential, because the choroid plexus of the lateral ventricle is far larger than that of the third ventricle or that of the fourth, and accordingly it is thought to be the brain's major site of production for cerebrospinal fluid. Second, the lateral ventricle is lateral mostly with reference to the rest of the ventricle system. In the cerebral hemisphere it is a decidedly medial chamber. Most of its medial wall is no more than choroid plexus. (In contrast, the third

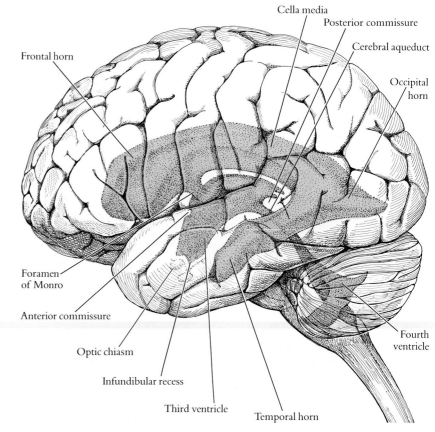

Figure 91: **Lateral ventricle** is the ventricle of the cerebral hemisphere; it gets its name not because it is notably lateral (in fact it is quite medial within the cerebral hemisphere) but because it is lateral to the rest of the ventricle system. Like much else in the cerebral hemisphere, it has the shape of a horseshoe. Its upper prong is the ventricle's frontal horn and cella media; the frontal horn's caudal limit is marked by the interventricular foramen of Monro, through which the lateral ventricle communicates with the third ventricle, at the diencephalic midline. Its apex is a clawlike caudal pocket, the occipital horn. Its lower prong is the ventricle's temporal horn.

ventricle and the fourth ventricle have a choroid roof.) The most rostral part of the medial wall (the part rostral to the interventricular foramen) is formed by true brain tissue. But even there the wall is no more than a thin vertical plate, the septum.

The anatomy of the lateral ventricle is best described in stages. First: The district of the lateral ventricle rostral to the interventricular foramen is the frontal horn of the ventricle. Its shape is determined largely by the genu of the corpus callosum, which forms its roof and anterior wall, and by the rostrum of the corpus callosum, which forms part of its floor. Its sloping lateral wall is the head of the caudate nucleus. Its medial wall is the septum. It has no choroid plexus.

Second: The district of the lateral ventricle behind the frontal horn completes the upper limb of the ventricle's horseshoe shape. It is called the cella media, from *cella,* the Latin for storeroom or compartment. Here the roof of the ventricle is still the corpus callosum. The medial wall, however, is formed by the fornix and choroid plexus. It happens that the plexus folds deeply into the lumen of the ventricle. The explanation is straightforward. At an early stage of ontogeny, the plexus walling the ventricle is more or less tautly stretched. Then its dorsal and ventral (upper and lower) lines of attachment to the tissue of the forebrain draw together. Concomitantly, and perhaps in part as a consequence, the plexus crumples. The dorsal line of attachment remains fixed on the fornix. All such lines are known as taeniae; this one is the taenia fornicis. The ventral line of attachment shifts. Originally it follows the medial border of the tail of the caudate nucleus. As the brain develops, however, a ventral part of the choroid plexus gets pushed down onto the dorsum of the thalamus, perhaps by the increasing pressure of cerebrospinal fluid accumulating in the lateral ventricle. Ultimately, this pushed-down part of the plexus becomes bonded to the thalamus; in the fully formed brain it is called the lamina affixa. It slightly thickens the surface of the thalamus and renders it somewhat whiter in appearance. The medial margin of the lamina affixa is the shifted line of attachment, which is called the taenia thalami. The original line of attachment stays visible in the brain. Its course is marked — fortuitously, one supposes — by the stria terminalis, a slender bundle of efferents from the amygdala on their way to the hypothalamus.

Third: From the caudally directed vertex of the horseshoe shape of the lateral ventricle a blind, clawlike extension tunnels into the white matter of the occipital lobe. It is variably developed from one brain to another. It is called the occipital horn. Like the frontal horn, it is enclosed on all sides by brain tissue; hence it lacks a choroid plexus. Then comes the temporal horn, which represents the lower prong of the ventricle's horseshoe shape. It is simply a long, narrow slit. The explanation, no doubt, is that the hippocampus, the rolled-in free edge of the cerebral cortex, bulges deeply into its lumen. By now the lateral ventricle has completed a turn of nearly 180 degrees. It is logical, therefore, that the tail of the caudate nucleus, which forms part of the floor of the cella media, should form part of the roof of the temporal horn. After all, it has completed a similar turn: it, too, has rotated about the cerebral hemisphere's axis of conduplication. Several further aspects of temporal architecture can be understood in a similar way. In the cella media, the stria terminalis coincides—or rather, it would have coincided but for the aforementioned vagary of ontogeny—with the ventral line of attachment for the choroid plexus of the lateral ventricle. In the temporal horn, it coincides with the dorsal line of attachment. In the cella media, the fornix coincides with the dorsal line of attachment for the choroid plexus of the lateral ventricle. In the temporal horn, it coincides with the ventral line. There, however, the fornix is represented by the fimbria fornicis, the marshaling ground for fibers of the fornix on the surface of the hippocampus.

Arterial Portals

Temporalization also shapes the ventral surface of the brain, as shown in Figure 92. We begin with a curious characteristic of how the cerebral hemisphere is supplied with arterial blood. Basically, three arteries bring blood to the forebrain. One of them, the basilar artery, arises from the confluence of the vertebral arteries on the ventral surface of the hindbrain. The other two, the internal carotid arteries, arrive by serpentine routes. On the ventral surface of the diencephalon the three form the circle of Willis, an arterial shunting network. There the basilar artery gives rise to the posterior cerebral arteries. Meanwhile each internal carotid artery gives rise to a middle cerebral artery and an anterior cerebral artery. Together the cerebral arteries nourish the cerebral hemisphere. The posterior cerebral artery sends blood to the cerebral cortex investing the occipital lobe and the underside of the temporal lobe; the far-spreading trunks of the middle cerebral artery and the anterior cerebral artery send blood to all of the rest of the cerebral cortex. In addition, in the early part of their course, the middle and the anterior cerebral artery

Figure 92: **Ventral surface** of the human brain incorporates a number of structures whose positions can be described with reference to blood vessels. Three vessels—the basilar artery and the internal carotid arteries—form the circle of Willis, which emits the cerebral arteries: the anterior, the middle, and the posterior. The circle surrounds the elevations raised by the hypothalamus. Rostral to one such elevation (the stalk of the pituitary complex) the optic nerves meet at their hemidecussation, the optic chiasm. Lateral to the circle of Willis are the cerebral peduncle and the uncus. Rostral to the circle (toward the pole of the frontal lobe) are the olfactory bulb and its stalk, the olfactory peduncle. The site of their connection to the base of the frontal lobe is the olfactory trigone. There the lateral olfactory stria (the main olfactory tract) veers laterally along the caudal margin of the orbitofrontal cortex. Then, at the limen insulae (the base of the insula), the tract describes a sharp medial turn that takes it into the primary olfactory cortex, on the rostral and medial face of the uncus. The turn cannot be seen: it is concealed by the temporal lobe, which folds the tract into the crease that becomes (on its lateral side) the Sylvian fissure. In the right half of the drawing the tip of the temporal lobe is resected, exposing much of the hidden part of the tract.

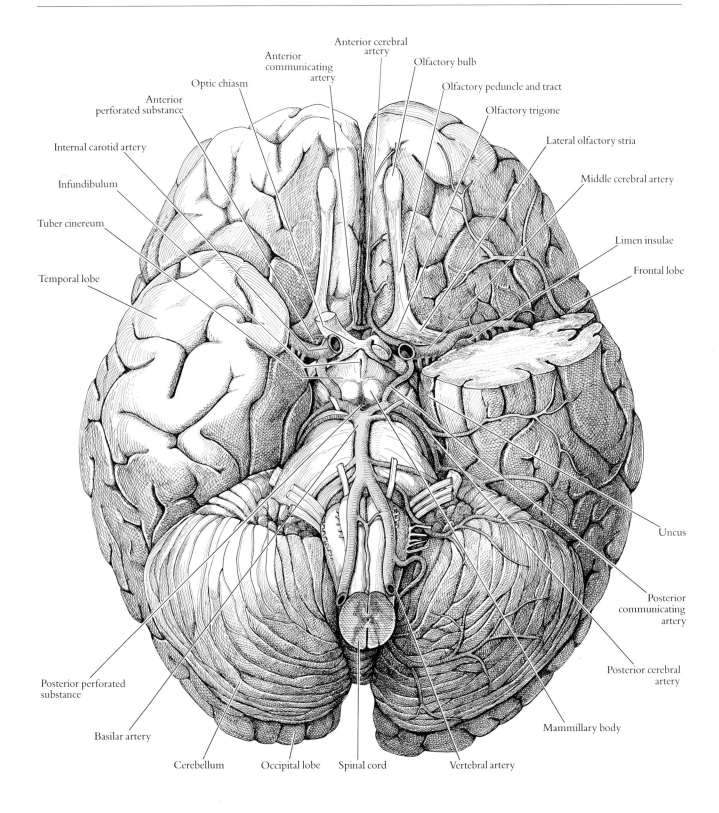

Anterior cerebral artery

Anterior communicating artery

Olfactory bulb

Optic chiasm

Olfactory peduncle and tract

Anterior perforated substance

Olfactory trigone

Lateral olfactory stria

Internal carotid artery

Middle cerebral artery

Infundibulum

Limen insulae

Tuber cinereum

Frontal lobe

Temporal lobe

Uncus

Posterior communicating artery

Posterior cerebral artery

Posterior perforated substance

Mammillary body

Basilar artery

Cerebellum

Occipital lobe

Spinal cord

Vertebral artery

emit a series of small branches, the lenticulostriate arteries, also known as the perforating arteries, which promptly enter the brain. The tissue shot through by their entrance is called the anterior perforated substance. (A site of similar perforation under the head of the basilar artery on the ventral surface of the midbrain is the posterior perforated substance; it occupies the depth of the interpeduncular fossa.) The anterior perforated substance accounts for no more than, say, two square centimeters on the surface of the brain. Yet the arteries entering there are responsible for the supply of arterial blood to nearly all the deep structures of the cerebral hemisphere, including the corpus striatum and the internal capsule. In contrast, the venous channels draining blood from the cerebral hemisphere take a number of directions — every conceivable direction, it seems. Why should the supply of arterial blood to the core of the cerebral hemisphere come through so small a region? In general the well-localized arterial portal for a given organ is at the part of the organ's surface least affected by the mechanical consequences of the organ's development: the part, in other words, that remains most nearly stable

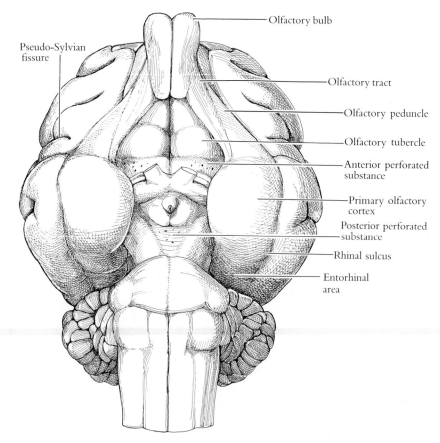

Olfactory bulb

Pseudo-Sylvian
fissure

Olfactory tract

Olfactory peduncle

Olfactory tubercle

Anterior perforated
substance

Primary olfactory
cortex

Posterior perforated
substance

Rhinal sulcus

Entorhinal
area

Figure 93: **Ventral surface of the cat brain** makes a useful contrast to the ventral surface of the human brain because temporalization is only incipient in the cat and so has not yet placed olfactory structures behind the thrust of the temporal lobe. In the cat the olfactory bulb juts ahead of the frontal pole. Its output bundle, the olfactory tract, forms the whitish surface of the olfactory peduncle; then, veering laterally, the tract distributes its fibers to the primary olfactory cortex, visible in its entirety on the rostral part of the piriform lobe. The caudal part of the piriform lobe is entorhinal cortex, which is the neocortical gateway to the hippocampus. The rhinal sulcus delimits much of the olfactory continuity.

throughout the organ's growth. A vascular hilus — that is to say, a well-localized arterial portal — lies, for example, on the medial aspect of the kidney. Another is on the ventral aspect of the liver. The anterior perforated substance makes no exception to this pattern. Of all the places on the surface of the cerebral hemisphere it is the one positioned closest to the axis about which the cerebral hemisphere conduplicates.

An inspection of Figure 92 establishes that the region encompassing the anterior perforated substance and the posterior perforated substance on the ventral surface of the brain is a roughly quadrilateral depression. Its rostral border is the orbital face of the frontal lobe; its caudal border is the brainstem, specifically the rostral margin of the pons. Its lateral border is in part the cerebral peduncle, in part the olfactory cortex investing the uncus, the medial bulge of the hippocampal gyrus. Its floor exhibits a number of structures. The caudal fourth of the floor is the posterior perforated substance. Then, from the rest of the floor, the hypothalamus rises, producing a sequence of elevations. First are the mammillary bodies, a pair of nearly spherical prominences marking the caudal boundary of the hypothalamus. Then comes the tuber cinereum (Latin for gray bulge), an unpaired, funnel-shaped, median prominence whose ventral extension, the infundibulum (Latin for funnel), produces the hypophyseal or infundibular stalk. The end of the stalk is a terminal swelling, the posterior lobe of the pituitary complex. Immediately rostral to the infundibulum is the optic chiasm, the hemidecussation of the visual pathways. From its caudal end the optic tracts extend in a caudal and lateral direction, each passing over the ventral aspect of a cerebral peduncle. In Figure 92 the full trajectory of the optic tract cannot be seen; the hippocampal gyrus hides it. Just lateral to the optic chiasm on each side of the midline is the anterior perforated substance. It is a roughly triangular area, partly hidden in a deep notch that intervenes between the caudal border of the frontal lobe and the uncus of the temporal lobe. The notch is the medial entrance to the lateral (or Sylvian) fissure.

Olfactory Structures

Our intent at this point is to describe the olfactory structures at the base of the cerebral hemisphere. The problem is that the arrayal of those structures in the human brain and the brains of other primates is affected by temporalization to such an extent that their continuity is partly concealed. It becomes useful, then, to consult Figure 93, which shows the ventral aspect of the brain of the cat. Note first the olfactory bulb, a more or less ovoid protuberance that juts ahead of the frontal pole. Its surface is a cortex in which mitral cells receive primary olfactory fibers. Caudal to the olfactory bulb is the olfactory peduncle. In mammals other than primates, it, too, has a cortex, but of a type so inconspicuously laminated that its accepted name is simply the anterior olfactory nucleus. The axons emitted by the mitral cells in the olfactory bulb pass caudalward in the plexiform layer of the inconspicuous cortex. They compose the olfactory tract, a substantial, ribbonlike bundle, plainly visible on the ventral aspect of the brain because it is whiter than its surroundings. Some of the axons terminate in the anterior olfactory nucleus. The majority extend farther caudally; then, veering laterally past a little-understood circle of paleocortex called the olfactory tubercle, they distribute themselves to the rostral part of the piriform lobe, a pear-shaped region that forms the larger part of the base of the cerebral hemisphere in the brain of the cat and other nonprimate mammals. (Remember that *pirus* is Latin for pear.) The rostral part of the piriform lobe is the primary olfactory cortex, also called, in light of its position, the piriform cortex. It has a three-layered architecture. That is, two cell-containing layers are under its plexiform layer. The caudal half of the lobe is the entorhinal area, a more multilayered cortex. The entorhinal area is known to receive some of its input from the olfactory bulb. It also gets input from the neocortex flanking it laterally. It is of particular interest because its major projection is to the hippocampus: it is a portal for traffic passing from the neocortex into the limbic system.

Note in Figure 93 that the olfactory bulb, the olfactory peduncle, and the primary olfactory cortex are smooth in the cat: neither gyri nor sulci ripple their surface. Note, too, that a groove called the rhinal sulcus delimits the olfactory peduncle and the piriform lobe from the neocortex beyond their lateral margin. Projecting laterally from the sulcus is a shorter groove, the pseudo-Sylvian fissure. It marks the incipient fold between the temporal lobe and the frontoparietal cortex. Thus it marks the modest progress of temporalization. In other species, notably primates, the corresponding fold is longer and more pronounced: it is the Sylvian fissure, which intervenes between the frontoparietal cortex and the well-developed, forward-jutting temporal lobe.

In the brain of a primate the olfactory bulb is small compared with the rest of the brain. In the human brain, moreover, it lies entirely under the frontal lobe's orbital surface; that is to say, it does not jut out ahead. Still, its cytoarchitecture is much the same as it is in the cat. In the olfactory peduncle, the changes are more radical. First, the cell content of the peduncle is greatly diminished. As a result, the peduncle becomes in essence a fiber tract. It is a long, white stalk made up almost exclusively of the axons of mitral cells. True, some gray matter remains. Even in the human brain the anterior olfactory nucleus is present as a modest trickle of cells under the fiber bundle proper. Here, in other words, the designation "nucleus" seems quite appropriate: the gray matter no longer shows the organization of a cortex. Second, the peduncle loses its broad binding to the overlying cerebral hemisphere. In the cat it joins the hemisphere at a point where the orbital surface of the frontal lobe reflects onto the dorsal aspect of the peduncle. In a primate it is free-floating, except at its caudal end. Little wonder that early anatomists mistakenly considered it the most rostral cranial nerve.

The olfactory peduncle finally joins the primate's cerebral hemisphere at the olfactory trigone, which lies just rostral to the olfactory tubercle. The trigone is peculiar to the brain of a primate. The reason is plain: the trigone is simply the triangular prominence that marks the site of attachment. As in the cat, the olfactory tract swings laterally on the ventral surface of the brain. Thus it becomes the lateral olfactory stria, which follows the caudal margin of the orbital face of the frontal lobe. In the primate, however, the lateral turn means that the tract soon disappears under the forward thrust of the temporal cortex. It disappears, then, toward the Sylvian fissure. The groove that marks the turn can be considered the beginning of the rhinal sulcus, which also disappears from view. A dissection demonstrates that the hidden part of the olfactory tract overlies the most rostral part of the primary olfactory cortex. In particular, the olfactory tract and the subjacent paleocortex are part of the insula, literally the island, a term denoting a large, oval expanse of cortex hidden at the bottom of the Sylvian fissure. The most rostral part of the primary olfactory cortex is thus the limen insulae: the threshold of the insula. The limen insulae marks a sharp medial turning of the olfactory continuity —a hidden turning by which the olfactory tract and the olfactory cortex reflect from the base of the insula onto the upper surface of the uncus.

Association Cortex

Neocortex now claims our attention. Part *a* of Figure 94 gives a lateral view of the brain. It is, however, the brain of a rat. Two aspects of its anatomy are immediately apparent. First, the olfactory bulb is prominent: it protrudes boldly beyond the frontal pole of the cerebral hemisphere. In the human brain, the homologous structure is hidden at the base of the hemisphere. Second, the brain of the rat is lissencephalic: it has neither gyri nor sulci, except for a marked rhinal sulcus and a hippocampal fissure, not visible in the figure. These furrows delimit the piriform lobe. The dearth of gyri and sulci means that the functional subdivisions of the animal's neocortex must be mapped without the assistance of landmarks. In Figure 94 the mapping is shown. The visual cortex occupies the upper rear of the cerebral mantle; below it is the auditory cortex, and in front of the two lies a somatic cortex in which the distinction between somatic sensory and somatic motor areas is problematic because the architecture characteristic of somatic sensory cortex widely overlies the architecture characteristic of motor cortex. Little space

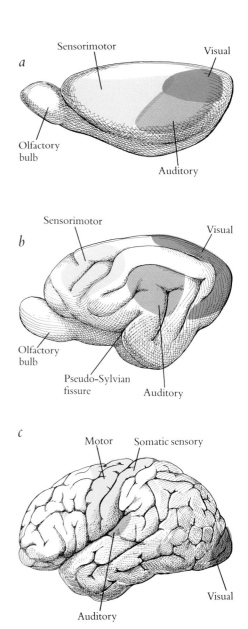

Figure 94: **Lateral views of three brains** aid the effort to mark off association areas on the neocortical sheet. The rat (*a*) has almost no gyri and sulci. Visual cortex, auditory cortex, and somatic sensorimotor cortex cover most of the cerebral hemisphere's surface. The cat (*b*) has numerous gyri and sulci. Visual cortex, auditory cortex, somatic sensory cortex, and somatic motor cortex occupy much of the hemisphere's surface, but unidentified expanses are appreciable as well. They are association areas. The human brain (*c*) is furrowed to such a degree that the extent of a cortical field is often hard to determine. In the human brain association cortex falls into two great zones termed the anterior and posterior association cortex.

remains on the cerebral mantle when these districts have been marked off.

Part *b* of Figure 94 gives a lateral view of the brain of a cat. The olfactory bulb remains visible, even prominent, yet the horseshoe shape of the cerebral cortex is beginning to develop: the piriform lobe now is flanked on its lateral side by a modest outthrust of temporal neocortex. The entorhinal area is large, but it is hidden almost entirely by the incipient temporal lobe. Note that the cerebral cortex is marked by a pattern of gyri and sulci. The pattern is hardly less impressive than the one in the brain of a monkey. Among the sulci is the pseudo-Sylvian fissure, which delineates the incipient temporal region. When visual, auditory, and somatic sensorimotor areas are marked off on the cerebral mantle of the cat, large unidentified spaces remain; they occupy a far larger proportion of the mantle than they did in the brain of the rat. They are association areas, and our method of finding them is not at all nonchalant. In truth, the association areas are the districts of neocortex that remain when one has eliminated the fields whose modality can be named. To put the matter baldly, the term association cortex distinguishes areas whose function is hard to formulate, or simply is unknown.

In the human brain a great proportion of the cerebral mantle is association cortex, but it is difficult to judge just how much by inspecting part *c* of Figure 94, which gives a lateral view of the human brain, because a large fraction of the cortical expanse — probably the greater part of it — is hidden in the walls and floors of the numerous sulci. Only a tiny part of the visual cortex, for example, lies on the lateral surface of the cerebral hemisphere. Most of it lies on the medial surface and in the walls of the calcarine fissure, which deeply incises the medial surface. Likewise, most of the auditory cortex lies in the depth of the Sylvian fissure. (It forms part of the lower wall of the fissure.) True, somatic sensory cortex is visible on the convexity of the postcentral gyrus and somatic motor cortex is visible on the convexity of the precentral gyrus. Yet much of the somatic sensory cortex is hidden on the posterior wall of the central sulcus and much of the somatic motor cortex is hidden on the anterior wall of that sulcus. All of the neocortex in the human brain not shown in color in Figure 94 is association cortex; thus it is not surprising that the thalamic nuclei projecting to those areas are large. In the brain of most primates, including man and the great apes, association cortex falls into two vast zones, one anterior, the other posterior to the complex formed by the precentral and postcentral gyri, or, in functional terms, the somatic motor area and the somatic sensory area. The anterior association cortex (to employ the terminology introduced by A. R. Luria of the University of Moscow) forms nearly all of the primate's frontal lobe; it is the region to which the mediodorsal nucleus of the thalamus projects and from which the mediodorsal nucleus receives corticofugal fibers in return. The posterior association cortex forms the larger, posterior part of the parietal lobe. (The smaller, anterior part is the somatic sensory cortex.) In addition, it includes a broad band of the occipital lobe and nearly all of the temporal lobe. It is the region to which the lateral nucleus of the thalamus projects and from which the lateral nucleus receives corticofugal fibers in return.

Chapter Fourteen

Frontal Sections

Here we shall describe the anatomy of the forebrain on a series of frontal sections: that is, sections perpendicular to the long axis of the forebrain. It is a dangerous thing to do. Structures one wants to discuss together turn out to be far apart. Structures one never thinks of together turn out to be close neighbors. Structures of which there is much to say turn out to look unimpressive. Structures about which little is known turn out to dominate the landscape. The dissector's knife is indifferent. But perhaps that is an advantage. In a purely conceptual treatment of the nervous system a fiber bundle has only an origin and a destination. Its tortuous trajectory need not be acknowledged. Also, a cell group need not exist — not if its function, or its alliances in the circuitry of the brain, are confusing or unknown. On cross sections everything shows. We shall therefore be compelled to point out things we have had no occasion to mention, along with the structures prominent in the current understanding of the central nervous system. One frontal section from now, the striatum will take on some curious complexities. Two and three sections from now, the base of the forebrain will do the same. Five sections from now, a tangled anatomy will turn out to underlie the assertion that the globus pallidus projects to the thalamus. And so it goes.

Here, then, is a 10-slice atlas of the human forebrain. Eight slices are photographed in color. The slices are Weigert stained. Thus myelin is black; gray matter is bright yellow. Different degrees and patterns of myelination yield varying textures, by which different regions are distinguished. It all begins simply enough. The first cut through the brain shown in Figure 95 passes through the frontal lobes. No temporal lobes are beneath them; we are too far forward for that. The gray matter exposed at the cut is frontal association cortex. The white matter is frontal, too. In part it consists of fibers passing through the corpus callosum to connect homotopic frontal fields across the midline. In part it consists of fibers projecting to frontal association cortex from the mediodorsal nucleus of the thalamus. In part it consists of corticofugal fibers returning that projection. The latter two classes of fibers are constituents of the frontal radiation of the corona radiata. The node of white matter at the center of the section is the genu of the corpus callosum. The genu is flanked on each side by the frontal horn of the lateral ventricle.

Nucleus Accumbens

The second cut in Figure 95 exposes the frontal section shown photographically in Figure 96. Already the pattern is more complex. For one thing, the cut transects the tips of the temporal lobes, which show up as crescents of cortex, each with a core of white matter. Moreover, the frontal horn of the lateral ventricle is no longer just a cavitation of the corpus callosum. Its roof remains the callosum. Its medial wall, however, is now formed by the septum, and its lateral wall is formed by the head of the caudate nucleus. The lateral edge of the caudate nucleus is marked by the internal capsule, which separates the caudate nucleus from the putamen. Two circumstances suggest that the separation is fortuitous, thus helping to confirm that the caudate nucleus and the putamen form a single entity: the striatum. First, the caudate nucleus and the putamen are joined by gray bridges that perforate the internal capsule. Second, the caudate nucleus and the putamen meet at the ventral limit of the capsule. (In fact they meet through the triangular gap in the cone of the internal capsule.) The zone of confluence is called the nucleus accumbens, or, more elaborately, the nucleus accumbens septi: the nucleus leaning against the septum. It does that quite markedly in the rat or the cat.

To an extent the nucleus accumbens is typical of the striatum as a whole. It receives input from the neocortex, and it projects, with the rest of the striatum, to the globus pallidus and to the substantia nigra. In short, it participates in the circuitry of the extrapyramidal motor system. On the other hand, the nucleus accumbens, along with much, perhaps even all, of the caudate nucleus, receives input from the limbic system. Indeed, it receives substantial direct projections from both of the limbic "head ganglia," the hippocampus and the amygdala. Thus there is reason to divide the striatum into a region under multiple limbic influence and a region receiving much sparser limbic input. The neocortical afferentation of the striatum obeys this parcellation in a curious way. The nucleus accumbens and the rest of the "limbic striatum" get their neocortical input from frontal association cortex — from the most nearly limbic part of the neocortex, one might say. The "nonlimbic striatum" gets its neocortical input from all the rest of the neocortex, including the motor cortex. The fibers leaving the "limbic striatum" are equally curious. For one thing, the nucleus accumbens projects, by way of the medial forebrain bundle, to the midbrain reticular formation and to the hypothalamus.

Then, too, the nucleus accumbens projects to the most ventral part of the globus pallidus, a zone not even known to be part of the globus pallidus until 1975, when it was intensively examined by Lennart Heimer and Richard Wilson at the Massachusetts Institute of Technology. They named it the ventral pallidum. (It will be visible in Figure 97.) The ventral pallidum participates in the characteristic extrapyramidal circuitry by projecting in turn to the subthalamic nucleus. In addition, however, the ventral pallidum projects to the mediodorsal nucleus of the thalamus. Moreover, it projects to limbic structures, including the amygdala. One begins to see that limbic influences loop into the corpus striatum, first to the "limbic striatum," a locus for which the nucleus accumbens, the most ventral and medial part of the striatum, is an emblem, then to the "limbic pallidum," the most ventral part of the globus pallidus, and finally back to the limbic system. Put even more broadly: the limbic system and the neocortex both direct part of their output through the striatum, then the pallidum, and finally back to the output's place of origin. One begins to find it strange that the corpus striatum is taken merely to be motoric.

The frontal cortex in Figure 96 shows the beginnings of complex infoldings. Perhaps the pattern is more apparent in Figure 95. There the cortex investing the convexity of the cerebral hemisphere becomes a pair of wavelike folds that meet like lips at the Sylvian fissure, and in the brain of a primate these folds, or opercula (the word means "lid" or "cover"), conceal a large, more or less oval expanse of cortex at the bottom of the fissure. This hidden expanse is the insula: the island. It can be seen as a striking example of cortex hidden at the fundus of a deep fissurization. (Three ovals of gray matter appearing in the subcortical white matter on the left side of Figure 96 are also the bottoms of sulci.) In Figure 96 the insula is continuous with the rearward extent of the orbitofrontal cortex. The white matter subjacent to the insula —that is, the cable basement of the insular cortex—is called the capsula extrema; its ventral half is thickened by fibers streaming between orbitofrontal cortex and temporal cortex. Together these fibers form the uncinate fasciculus, a cortical association bundle establishing reciprocal connections between the frontal lobe and the temporal lobe. Under the capsula extrema is a thin sheet of gray matter, the claustrum, meaning "wall." The claustrum in turn is superficial to a well-defined sheet of white matter, the external capsule, which marks the lateral margin of the putamen. The external capsule is thought to consist largely of fibers projecting from the neocortex to the putamen in the first link of the funneling of neocortical data that typifies the extrapyramidal motor system.

Diagonal Band; Substantia Innominata

The third cut in Figure 95 exposes the frontal section shown photographically in Figure 97. It exhibits further complexities. The black bow tie floating under the section is the optic chiasm, the hemidecussation of the optic nerves on their way to the lateral geniculate body in the thalamus and the superior colliculus in the midbrain. Above it, on both the left side and the right, a much smaller, darkly staining bundle, the olfactory peduncle, becomes attached to the rest of the brain. (In Figure 96 it was unattached to the brain: it floated freely in the mouth of a deep orbitofrontal groove known as the olfactory sulcus.) Here, then, we see the olfactory trigone; we have arrived at olfactory cortex. On the right a curve can be seen that reflects the olfactory cortex from the base of the frontal lobe onto the uncus, which is beginning to appear on the medial face of the temporal lobe. The curve encloses the middle cerebral artery, which is about to enter the subarachnoid cistern of the Sylvian fissure. A similar reflection has not yet happened on the left; the section is slightly asymmetrical. Still, the artery is visible. The curve occupies the medial face of a pedestal by which the temporal lobe connects to the rest of the brain. On the opposite, lateral face of the pedestal the temporal neocortex connects to the insular cortex. Inside the pedestal, fibers of the uncinate fasciculus stream into the white matter of the temporal lobe at the base of the capsula extrema.

The single most notable visual hallmark of Figure 97 is a prominent fiber bundle looking rather like a mustache under the internal capsule and then the ventral margin of the globus pallidus. A small part of the pallidum stays under the fiber bundle. It is the ventral pallidum of Heimer and Wilson: the chief target of the extrapyramidal lines from the nucleus accumbens. The bundle is the anterior commissure. In primates the bulk of its fibers interconnect temporal neocortex on the left and right cerebral hemisphere. It is in essence a private corpus callosum for a large rostral part of the temporal lobes. Under the anterior commissure, especially on the left, is striatal tissue: the nucleus accumbens. Medial to that, and more heavily myelinated, is a gray and white structure called the diagonal band of Broca. It draws us into a region of the brain that is little known even today. Beginning in a medial part of the septum, the diagonal band descends the medial face of the cerebral hemisphere, passing vertically in front of the anterior commissure. Then, at the base of the hemisphere, it makes a caudal and lateral turn that directs it along the lateral side of the optic tract on a trajectory toward the amygdala. Figure 97 catches it at the bend between these two limbs of its course. Its fibers lay down a whitish band on the surface of the brain: hence the name of the structure. They do not quite attain the amygdala. Instead the diagonal band loses its identity in the substantia innominata, another structure we have not had occasion to mention, which is incipient on the right side of Figure 97, where its rostral pole usurps the place of the nucleus accumbens. The substantia innominata will be prominent on both sides of the brain in Figures 98 and 99. The term substantia innominata appears to derive from a hoax. It is thought that a jokester whose identity can no longer be traced had been reading the published work of Karl Reichert, a Berlin anatomist who in the 1860's systematically examined the cell groups at the base of the forebrain. Reichert had unaccountably neglected to supply a name for the tissue under the globus pallidus. To rectify the omission the wag provided a term: the substantia innominata of Reichert. It is in truth the substance Reichert left unnamed. It is best defined as the gray and white matter separating the globus pallidus from the ventral surface of the forebrain.

The status of the diagonal band and the substantia innominata in the circuitry of the brain is readily summarized. The diagonal band is a gray and white bridge that carries reciprocal links between the septum and the substantia innominata; in turn the substantia innominata is a gray and white bridge that carries reciprocal links between the amygdala and the hypothalamus. (It carries the ventral amygdalofugal path and the reciprocating fibers, and it taps into both those lines.) Beyond that, there is much that makes the substantia innominata and the diagonal band well worth considering together. For one thing, they both include constellations of large neurons. The substantia innominata includes the nucleus basalis of Meynert — the 19th-century Viennese neurologist Theodor Meynert. It is the largest magnocellular cell group found at the base of the forebrain. The diagonal band includes along its limbs the nucleus of the band, a smaller but equally magnocellular group. Both have limbic connections. The nucleus basalis maintains reciprocal links with the amygdala; the nucleus of the diagonal band maintains reciprocal links with the hippocampus. In addition, the nucleus basalis projects to the neocortex — the entire neocortex, in a fairly orderly topologic fashion. It can therefore be said that the nucleus basalis and the nucleus of the diagonal band both project to cerebral cortex. It is reported that the nucleus basalis and the nucleus of the diagonal band are impoverished of their magnocellular neurons in victims of the rapidly progressive dementia known as Alzheimer's disease. Such patients lose their memory and become confused and disoriented; they are incapable of abstract thought, and in advanced stages of the disease they become unable to recognize their closest friends and relatives. No other dementia ever attains such proportions. Current views of the nucleus basalis and the nucleus of the diagonal band conceive of them, accordingly, as a mechanism crucial for intellectual function. Perhaps they exercise a set-point modulation of the hippocampus and neocortex. One final thing about them is rather more firmly established. They are cholinergic: their magnocellular neurons employ acetylcholine as their neurotransmitter. In fact, they have emerged as the only known source of cortical afferentation employing acetylcholine. It is an impressive attribute for parts of the brain so long ignored.

The part of the cross section above the anterior commissure is somewhat less unsettling. Note first the internal capsule. To its lateral side is the lentiform nucleus, which plainly has two divisions. The lateral, light-staining part is the putamen; the medial, more darkly staining part is the globus pallidus. The latter in turn shows two divisions, but in Figure 97 the divisions are only beginning; they will be plainer later on. Closest to the midline are the columns of the fornices. Each marks the descent of the fornix toward the hypothalamus at the end of its arc from the hippocampus. The column on the left is cut behind its vertex; thus it appears in two unconnected fragments. The column on the right is whole. The somewhat triangular space between

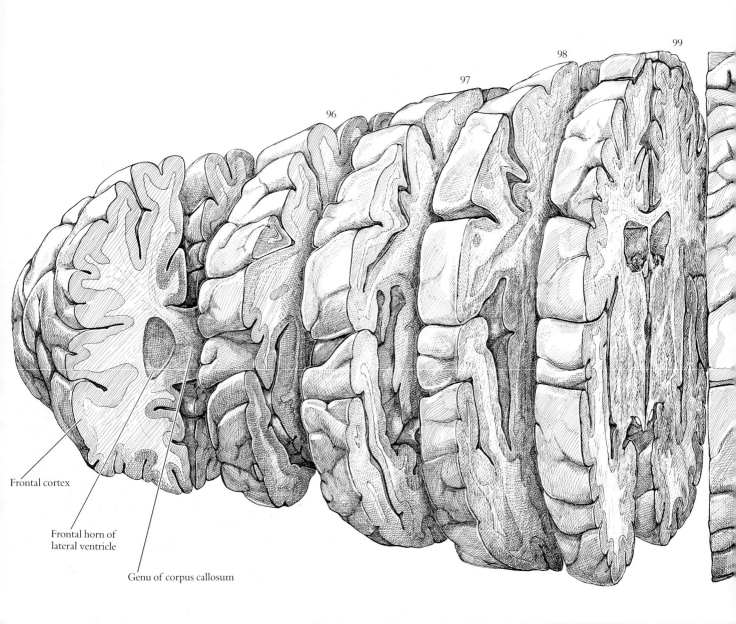

Frontal cortex

Frontal horn of
lateral ventricle

Genu of corpus callosum

Figure 95: **Atlas of cross sections** of a human brain begins with this drawing, which
displays ten cuts through a brain. The cuts are all frontal: that is, they are perpendicular to
the long axis of the forebrain. The pattern exposed at the first cut is relatively simple: it
includes only cortex and white matter near the tip of the frontal lobes. The central node of
white matter is the genu of the corpus callosum, which is flanked by the frontal horn of the
lateral ventricle. The pattern exposed at the tenth cut again is relatively simple. There, too,

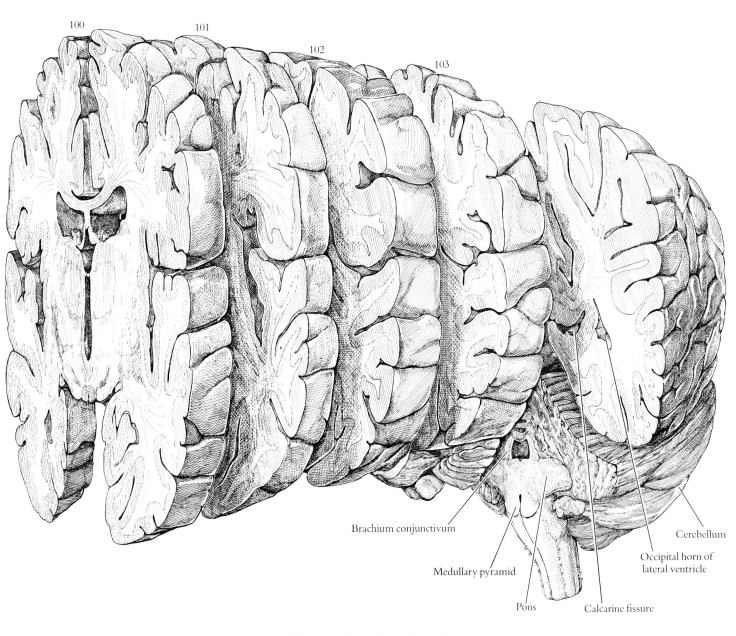

100   101   102   103

Brachium conjunctivum

Medullary pyramid

Pons

Calcarine fissure

Cerebellum

Occipital horn of
lateral ventricle

the pattern is dominated by cortex: that of the occipital lobes, in the broad folds called gyri, and that of the cerebellum, in the narrow folds called folia. The white matter of each occipital lobe is cavitated by the occipital horn of the lateral ventricle. In turn the occipital horn is pressed inward by visual cortex in the walls of the calcarine fissure. The patterns exposed at cuts two through nine are rendered photographically and accompanied by maps in the next eight illustrations.

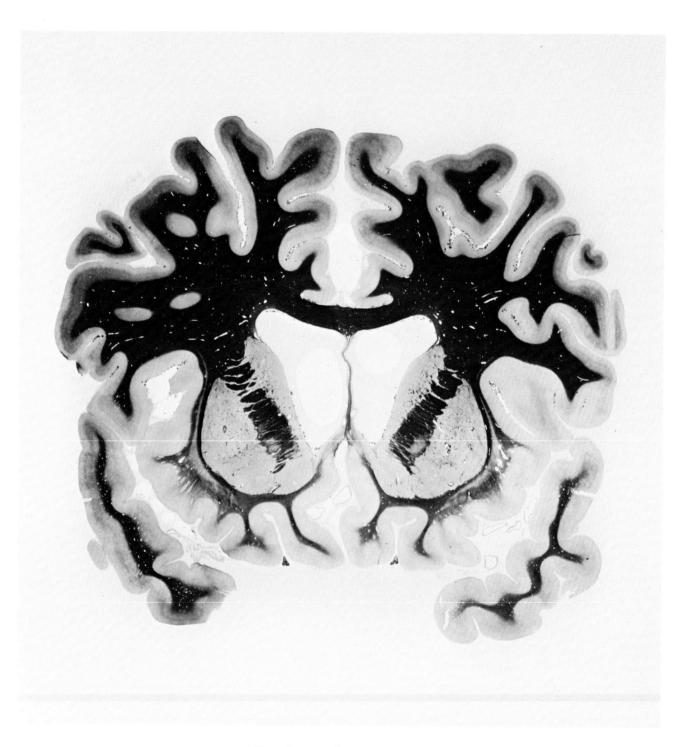

Figure 96: **Second section** in the atlas begins to show details of the forebrain's internal structure. Within each frontal lobe the frontal horn of the lateral ventricle is bounded medially by the septum and laterally by the head of the caudate nucleus. In turn the caudate nucleus is flanked by the internal capsule, which cleaves the striatum into two districts, the

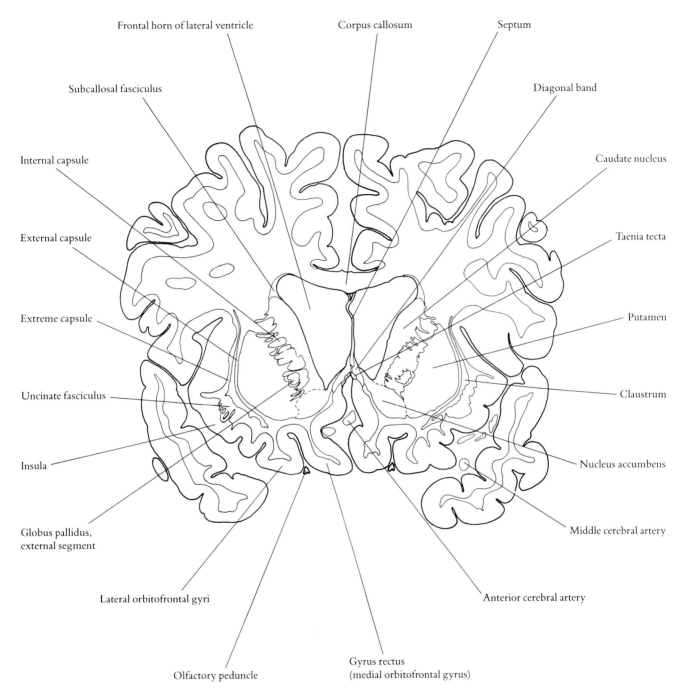

Frontal horn of lateral ventricle

Corpus callosum

Septum

Subcallosal fasciculus

Diagonal band

Internal capsule

Caudate nucleus

External capsule

Taenia tecta

Extreme capsule

Putamen

Uncinate fasciculus

Claustrum

Insula

Nucleus accumbens

Globus pallidus,
external segment

Middle cerebral artery

Lateral orbitofrontal gyri

Anterior cerebral artery

Olfactory peduncle

Gyrus rectus
(medial orbitofrontal gyrus)

caudate nucleus and the putamen. The cleavage is incomplete: through the ventral gap in the capsule the caudate nucleus and the putamen meet at what is called the nucleus accumbens. It is a part of the striatum with connections to the limbic system. The section is Weigert stained; thus white matter is black, gray matter is yellow.

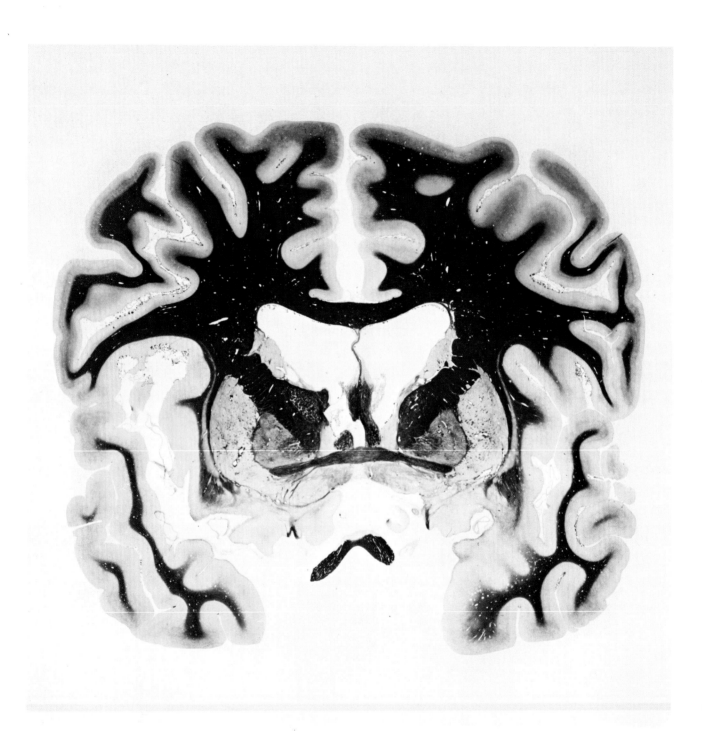

Figure 97: **Third section** in the atlas shows further complexities. Again the internal capsule divides the caudate nucleus from the putamen. Now, however, the capsule is invaded by patches of gray matter; they compose what is called the reticular nucleus, which thinly covers much of the thalamus. (Here the patches mark the rostral pole of the thalamus.) For its part, the putamen is joined by the globus pallidus, or pallidum, completing the

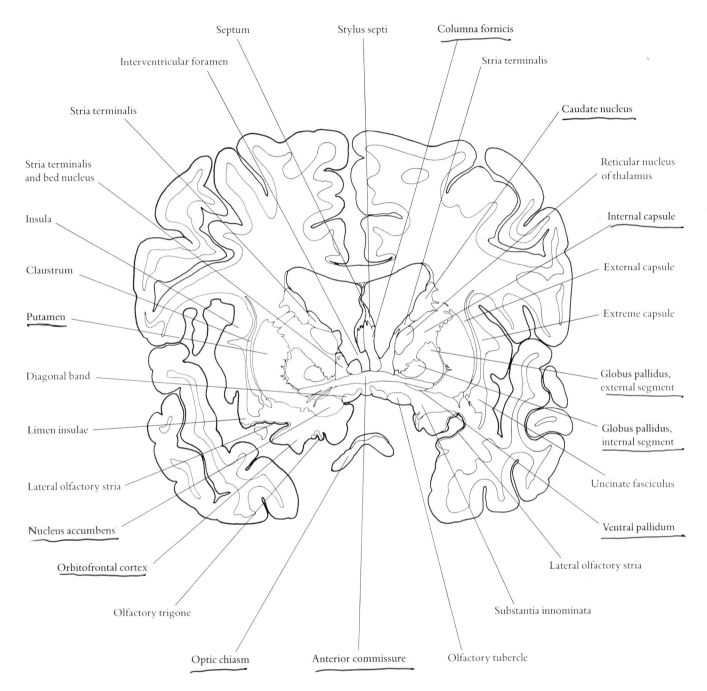

Septum

Stylus septi

Columna fornicis

Interventricular foramen

Stria terminalis

Stria terminalis

Caudate nucleus

Stria terminalis
and bed nucleus

Reticular nucleus
of thalamus

Insula

Internal capsule

Claustrum

External capsule

Putamen

Extreme capsule

Diagonal band

Globus pallidus,
external segment

Limen insulae

Globus pallidus,
internal segment

Lateral olfactory stria

Uncinate fasciculus

Nucleus accumbens

Ventral pallidum

Orbitofrontal cortex

Lateral olfactory stria

Olfactory trigone

Substantia innominata

Optic chiasm

Anterior commissure

Olfactory tubercle

lentiform nucleus. The broad avenue of white matter under the pallidum is the anterior commissure. The section is slightly asymmetric: on the left side of the section the commissure overlies the nucleus accumbens; on the right it overlies two little-known regions at the base of the cerebral hemisphere, the diagonal band of Broca and the substantia innominata. Both project to the cerebral cortex.

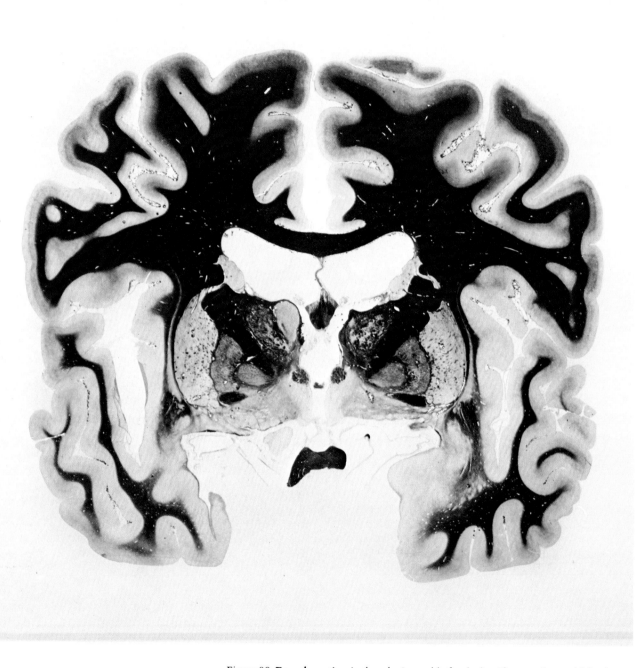

Figure 98: **Fourth section** in the atlas is notable for the lentiform nucleus, which takes on its characteristic appearance. In the medial part of the nucleus, the globus pallidus shows two segments called internal and external, or inner and outer. Meanwhile, in the lateral part of the lentiform nucleus, the putamen shows stipples known as the pencil bundles. They are striatal efferents bound in part for the globus pallidus, in part for the striatal satellite, the substantia nigra. The gray matter (here a pale yellow) surrounding the third

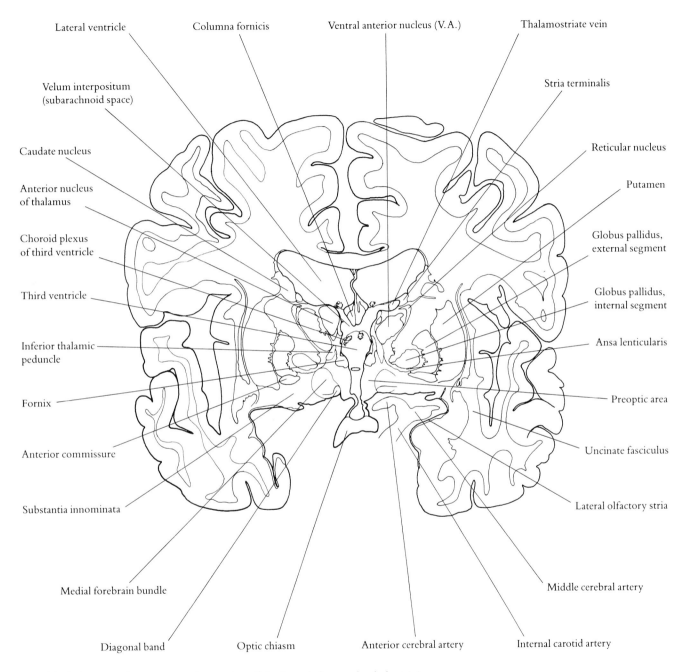

Lateral ventricle

Columna fornicis

Ventral anterior nucleus (V.A.)

Thalamostriate vein

Velum interpositum
(subarachnoid space)

Stria terminalis

Caudate nucleus

Reticular nucleus

Anterior nucleus
of thalamus

Putamen

Choroid plexus
of third ventricle

Globus pallidus,
external segment

Third ventricle

Globus pallidus,
internal segment

Inferior thalamic
peduncle

Ansa lenticularis

Fornix

Preoptic area

Anterior commissure

Uncinate fasciculus

Substantia innominata

Lateral olfactory stria

Medial forebrain bundle

Middle cerebral artery

Diagonal band

Optic chiasm

Anterior cerebral artery

Internal carotid artery

ventricle is the preoptic area, a rostral extension of the hypothalamus; the dark-staining circle inside it is the fornix, cut in cross section. The variegated gray matter dorsal and medial to the internal capsule is the thalamus. On the left side of the section the reticular nucleus and the ventral anterior, or V.A., nucleus are joined by the anterior nucleus, a far more uniform mass of gray matter. The anterior nucleus is the thalamic participant in the loop of limbic projections called the Papez circuit.

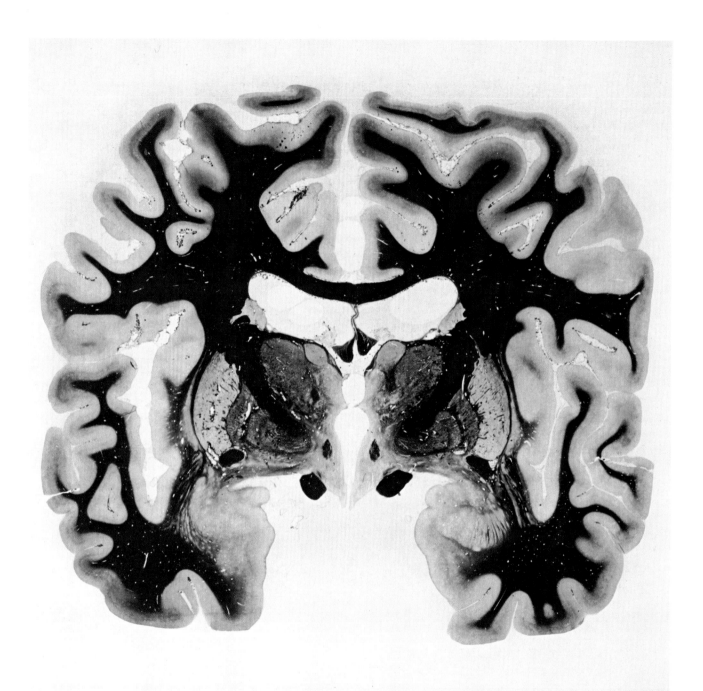

Figure 99: **Fifth section** in the atlas shows a number of forebrain structures not yet at their most telling. On the right side of the section the anterior nucleus is approached by its afferent bundle, the mammillothalamic tract. To the medial side of the tract is a large thalamic cell group, the mediodorsal nucleus; to the lateral side of the tract is a further thalamic cell group, this one darkened by heavier myelination: the V.A.-V.L. complex. Lower in the section the medial face of the temporal lobe covers the amygdala. Striations of white matter inside the latter (more easily seen on the right side of the section) comprise its

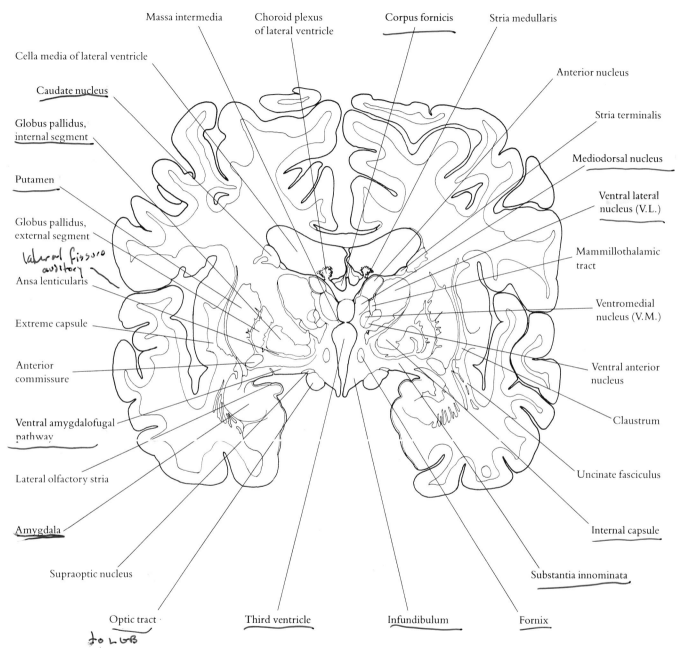

Massa intermedia

Choroid plexus
of lateral ventricle

Corpus fornicis

Stria medullaris

Cella media of lateral ventricle

Caudate nucleus

Globus pallidus,
internal segment

Putamen

Globus pallidus,
external segment

lateral fissure
auditory

Ansa lenticularis

Extreme capsule

Anterior
commissure

Ventral amygdalofugal
pathway

Lateral olfactory stria

Amygdala

Supraoptic nucleus

Optic tract

to LGB

Anterior nucleus

Stria terminalis

Mediodorsal nucleus

Ventral lateral
nucleus (V.L.)

Mammillothalamic
tract

Ventromedial
nucleus (V.M.)

Ventral anterior
nucleus

Claustrum

Uncinate fasciculus

Internal capsule

Substantia innominata

Third ventricle

Infundibulum

Fornix

reciprocal links to temporal neocortex. The amygdala abuts the substantia innominata, which in turn abuts the hypothalamus, cut just anterior to the stalk of the pituitary complex. The white matter inside the hypothalamus is the fornix, descending toward the mammillary bodies. Lateral to the fornix the hypothalamus is occupied by a more disseminated fiber system, the medial forebrain bundle. Still farther laterally, a band of white matter under the inner pallidal segment is the contingent of pallidal outflow called the ventral division of the ansa lenticularis.

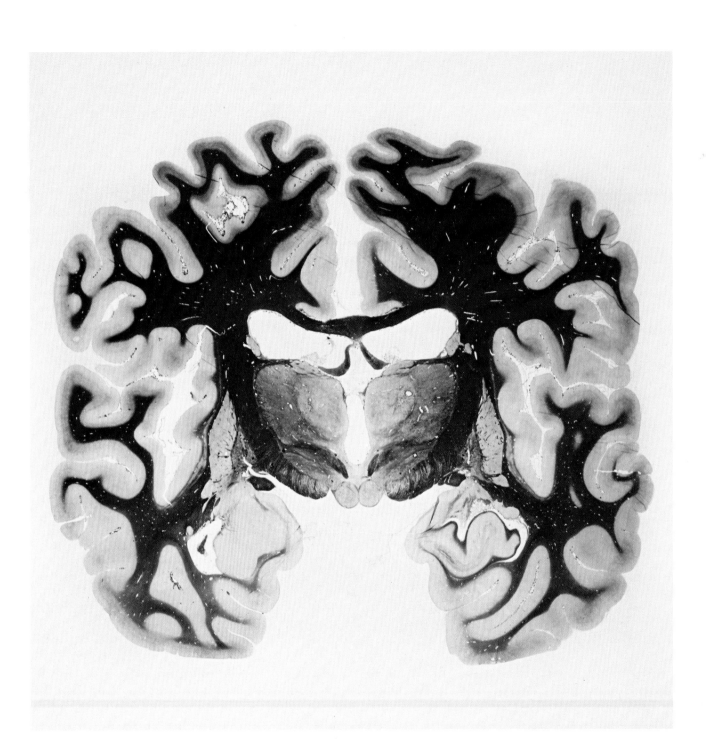

Figure 100: **Sixth section** in the atlas reveals complexities in the anatomy of the extrapyramidal motor system. At the heart of the section the internal capsule extends toward the midline, where it becomes the cerebral peduncle. The peduncle is pierced by multitudinous fascicles: the comb system, consisting of striatal and pallidal efferents. Overlying the peduncle is the subthalamus: first the subthalamic nucleus, and then a fiber plexus called

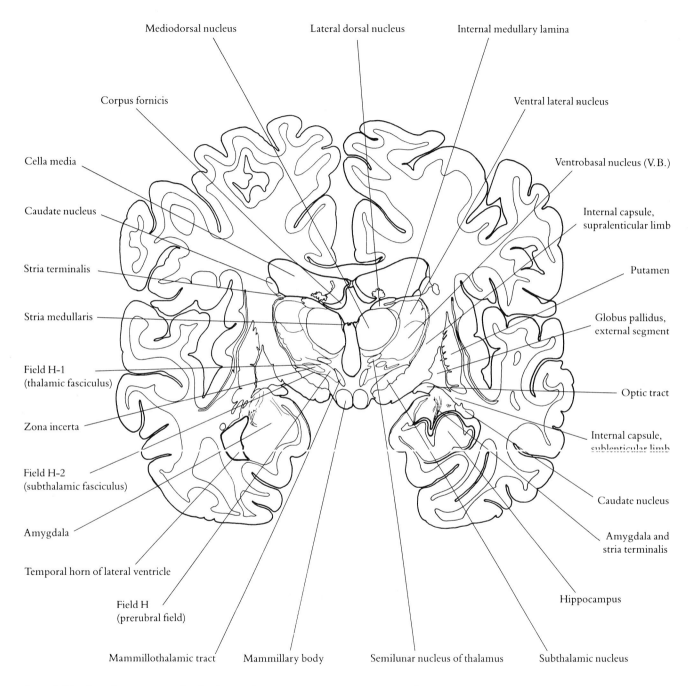

Mediodorsal nucleus

Lateral dorsal nucleus

Internal medullary lamina

Corpus fornicis

Ventral lateral nucleus

Cella media

Ventrobasal nucleus (V.B.)

Caudate nucleus

Internal capsule, supralenticular limb

Stria terminalis

Putamen

Stria medullaris

Globus pallidus, external segment

Field H-1
(thalamic fasciculus)

Optic tract

Zona incerta

Internal capsule, sublenticular limb

Field H-2
(subthalamic fasciculus)

Caudate nucleus

Amygdala

Amygdala and stria terminalis

Temporal horn of lateral ventricle

Hippocampus

Field H
(prerubral field)

Mammillothalamic tract

Mammillary body

Semilunar nucleus of thalamus

Subthalamic nucleus

the H fields of Forel, comprising chiefly the ansa lenticularis—that is, the pallidal efferents—interwoven with two ascending systems, the medial lemniscus and the cerebellothalamic projection. Overlying the H fields is the thalamus. It shows a pale-staining inner
zone, here consisting mostly of the mediodorsal nucleus, a dark-staining outer zone, here
the ventral lateral and ventrobasal nuclei, and between them the internal medullary lamina.

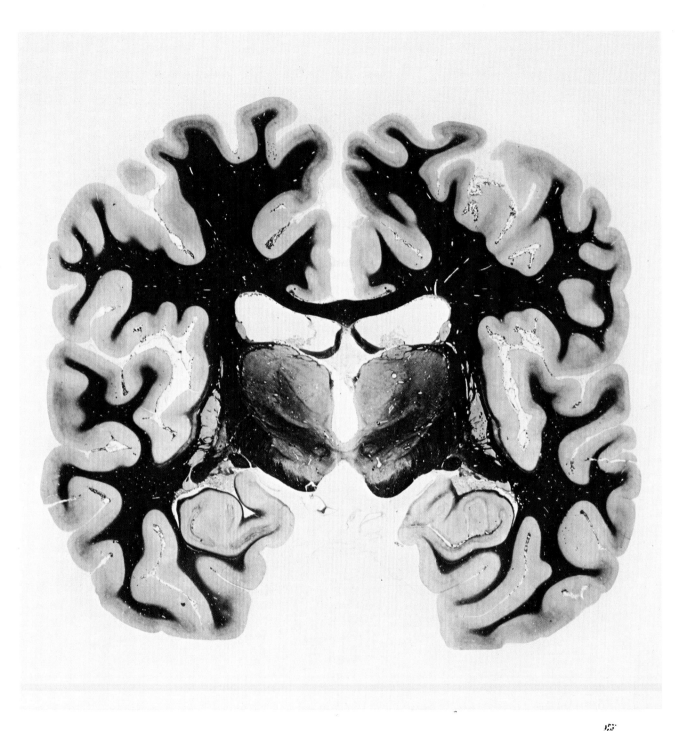

Figure 101: **Seventh section** in the atlas marks the middle of the forebrain: it is the frontal section equidistant from the frontal pole and the occipital pole of the cerebral hemisphere. In token of its position, it includes the centrum medianum, the largest of several thalamic nuclei enclosed by the internal medullary lamina. The light-staining, medial part of the thalamus is again the mediodorsal nucleus; the dark-staining, lateral part is two nuclei, the

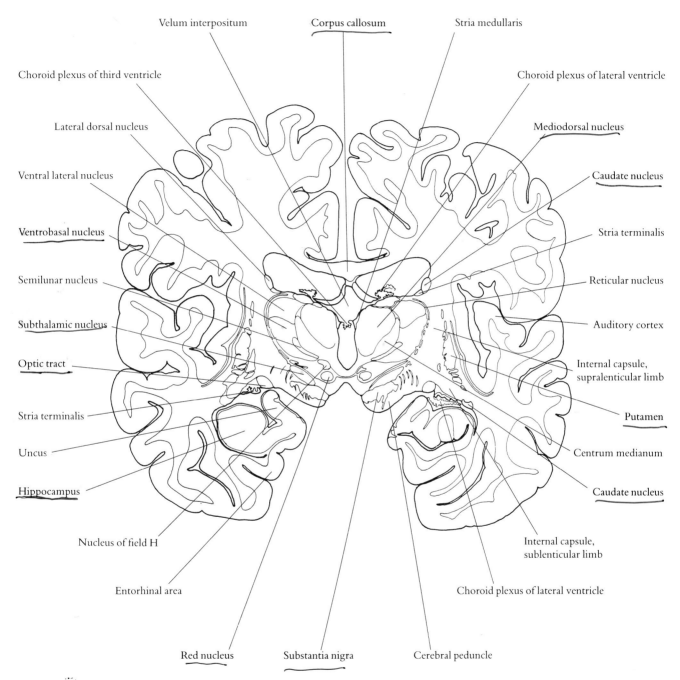

Velum interpositum

Corpus callosum

Stria medullaris

Choroid plexus of third ventricle

Choroid plexus of lateral ventricle

Lateral dorsal nucleus

Mediodorsal nucleus

Ventral lateral nucleus

Caudate nucleus

Ventrobasal nucleus

Stria terminalis

Semilunar nucleus

Reticular nucleus

Subthalamic nucleus

Auditory cortex

Optic tract

Internal capsule, supralenticular limb

Stria terminalis

Putamen

Uncus

Centrum medianum

Hippocampus

Caudate nucleus

Nucleus of field H

Internal capsule, sublenticular limb

Entorhinal area

Choroid plexus of lateral ventricle

Red nucleus

Substantia nigra

Cerebral peduncle

ventral lateral nucleus, and below it the ventrobasal nucleus. A light-staining crescent inside the latter is the thalamic gustatory nucleus, which processes taste sensation. Under the thalamus, the subthalamus is giving way to the midbrain. The cerebral peduncle is overlain by the substantia nigra. Moreover, the rostral pole of the red nucleus occupies the medial part of the H fields.

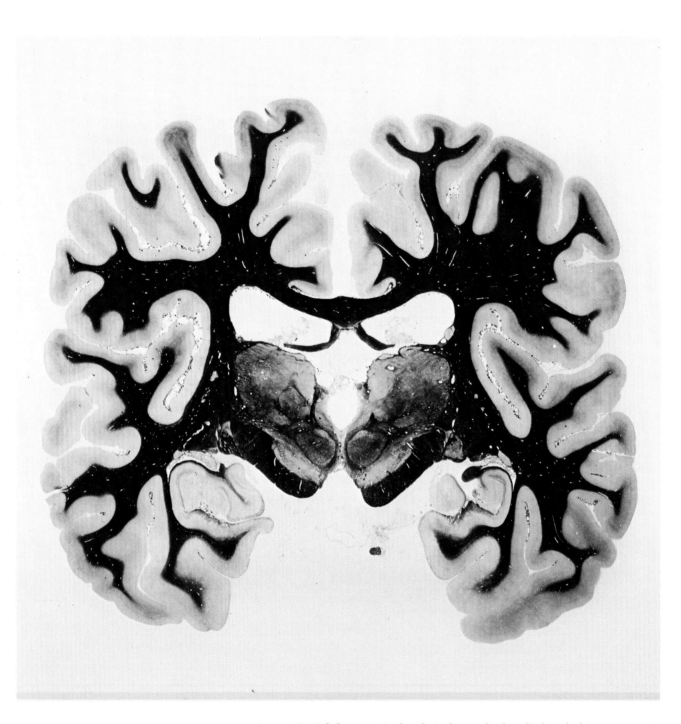

Figure 102: **Eighth section** in the atlas is the one that best displays the hippocampus. On both sides of the section the cortical sheet investing the medial face of the temporal lobe folds laterally, then medially (that is, over itself), then under the second fold and into the mouth of the *U*-shaped dentate gyrus. (The pattern is shown at greater magnification in Figure 104.) The white matter forming the hippocampal cable basement is the fimbria fornicis: the marshaling ground of the fornix. The hippocampal folds evert it, so that it

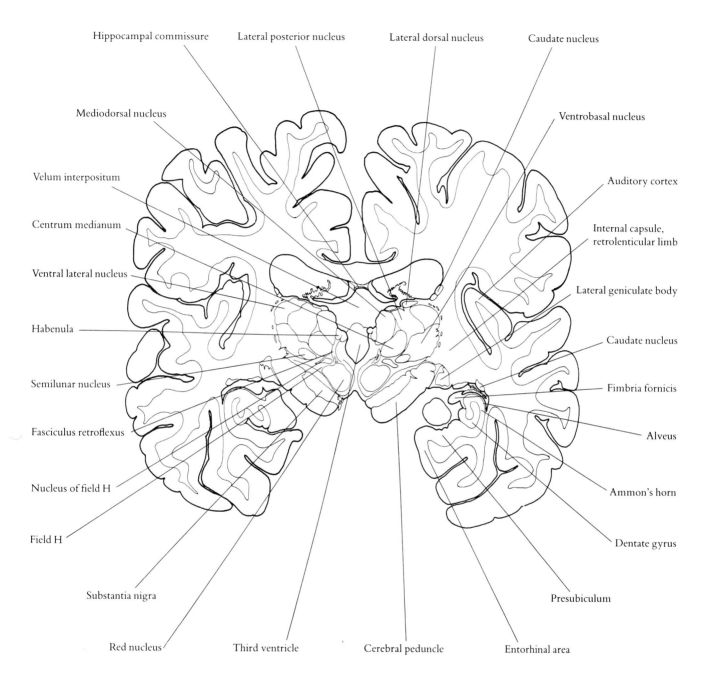

Hippocampal commissure

Lateral posterior nucleus

Lateral dorsal nucleus

Caudate nucleus

Mediodorsal nucleus

Ventrobasal nucleus

Velum interpositum

Auditory cortex

Centrum medianum

Internal capsule, retrolenticular limb

Ventral lateral nucleus

Lateral geniculate body

Habenula

Caudate nucleus

Semilunar nucleus

Fimbria fornicis

Fasciculus retroflexus

Alveus

Nucleus of field H

Ammon's horn

Field H

Dentate gyrus

Substantia nigra

Presubiculum

Red nucleus

Third ventricle

Cerebral peduncle

Entorhinal area

occupies the surface of the brain. On the left side of the section the thalamus is notable for the fasciculus retroflexus, a prominent fiber bundle projecting from the thalamic cell groups called the habenular nuclei to the serotonergic cell groups of the midbrain raphe. On the right side of the section the retrolenticular limb of the internal capsule is invaded from behind by the lateral geniculate body, which composes the caudal, slightly recurving tip of the thalamus.

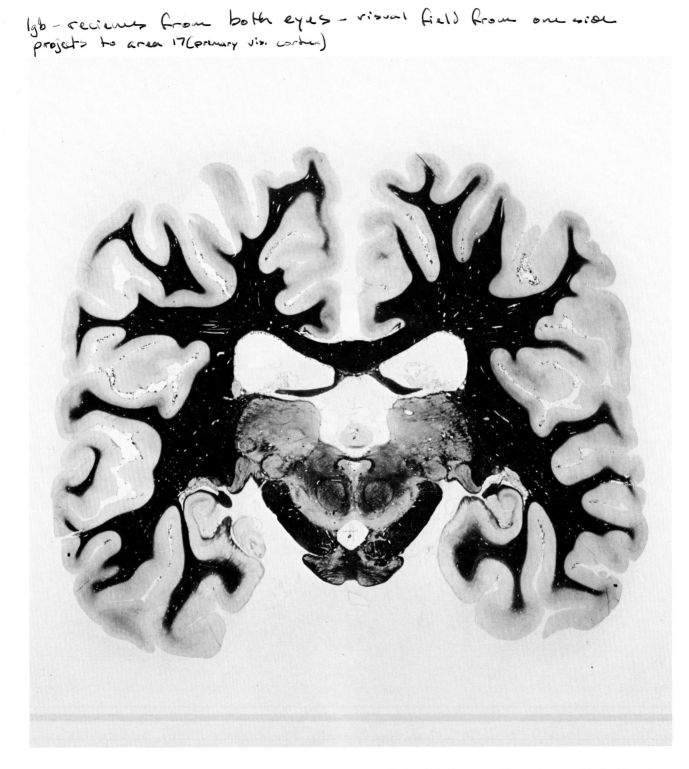

Figure 103: **Ninth section** in the atlas is the last one shown photographically. (A tenth cut, however, is shown in Figure 95.) The thalamus, seen here near its caudal limit, displays three nuclei: the pulvinar (the largest thalamic nucleus) and underneath it the geniculate bodies, the medial and the lateral. The latter shows laminations. Below the thalamus the

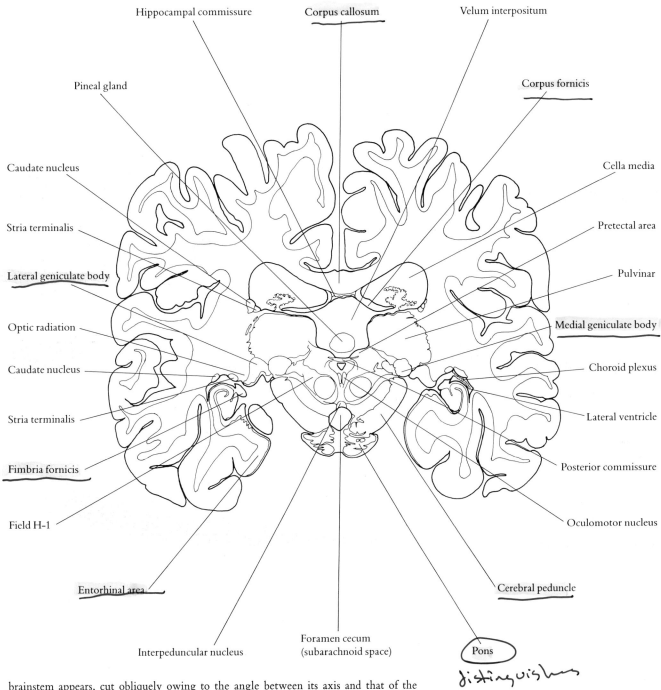

Hippocampal commissure

Corpus callosum

Velum interpositum

Pineal gland

Corpus fornicis

Caudate nucleus

Cella media

Stria terminalis

Pretectal area

Lateral geniculate body

Pulvinar

Optic radiation

Medial geniculate body

Caudate nucleus

Choroid plexus

Stria terminalis

Lateral ventricle

Fimbria fornicis

Posterior commissure

Field H-1

Oculomotor nucleus

Entorhinal area

Cerebral peduncle

Interpeduncular nucleus

Foramen cecum
(subarachnoid space)

Pons

distinguishes

brainstem appears, cut obliquely owing to the angle between its axis and that of the forebrain. In ventral-to-dorsal sequence the cut exposes the rostral tip of the pons, then the cerebral peduncles, then the substantia nigra, then the red nucleus, then the central gray substance, and finally the pretectal area, which includes the posterior commissure.

the columns is part of the third ventricle; on the left the foramen of Monro establishes its continuity with the frontal horn of the lateral ventricle. For its part the frontal horn is framed medially by the septum, which broadens at its base atop the fornix columns to produce what is called the stylus septi. The stylus contains most of the septum's neurons. Meanwhile the lateral wall of the frontal horn is formed first by the caudate nucleus and then by a cascade of gray matter ending in a gray triangle between the fornix and the internal capsule. On the left one sees the triangle; on the right one sees the cascade. Either way, the gray matter is the bed nucleus of the stria terminalis, which accompanies the stria on its descent toward the hypothalamus at the end of its arc from the amygdala.

There is at least one neural curiosity above the anterior commissure in Figure 97. At the medial side of the internal capsule (particularly the one on the left side of the section) the dark-staining mass of the capsule is invaded by patches of gray matter that give the capsule a mottled appearance. The patches mark the rostral pole of the thalamus. Specifically, they mark the reticular nucleus, a sheet of gray matter that covers not only the rostral pole of the thalamus but also its ventral and lateral margins. The reticulation arises because the nucleus intervenes between the thalamus and the internal capsule; hence it is pierced by fascicles consisting of fibers that enter the capsule to establish reciprocal connections between the thalamus and the neocortex. Such fascicles compose groups called the thalamic peduncles; here we have encountered the anterior thalamic peduncle. The main afferents to the reticular nucleus appear to be the collaterals of thalamic-peduncle fibers; thus in 1966 Arnold and Madge Scheibel of the University of California at Los Angeles characterized the reticular nucleus as a cell group screening the two-way traffic that passes between thalamus and cortex. Strangely, the output of the reticular nucleus is directed exclusively back to the thalamus, and not forward to the cortex.

Rostral Corpus Striatum

The fourth cut in Figure 95 exposes the frontal section shown photographically in Figure 98. Again the temporal lobe is linked to the rest of the cerebral hemisphere by what amounts to a pedestal. Here, however, the pedestal is apparent on both sides of the brain. Through it the uncinate fasciculus courses toward temporal cortex from its marshaling ground at the base of the capsula extrema. Medial to the pedestal (and lateral to the optic chiasm) the internal carotid artery branches into two subsidiary vessels at the forward end of the circle of Willis. They are the anterior cerebral artery, which takes a medial course at first, and the middle cerebral artery. Each emits numerous smaller arteries, which perforate the base of the forebrain, producing the anterior perforated substance. We see now that what they perforate is the substantia innominata, the gray and white bridge connecting the amygdala to the hypothalamus. The right side of Figure 98 comes close to showing the full span of the bridge. In lateral-to-medial order it shows the rostral tip of the amygdala (Figure 99 will show it better); then the substantia innominata, whose heterogeneity of textures in this Weigert preparation confirms that it harbors a variety of cell groups, including the nucleus basalis; and finally, toward the margin of the third ventricle, the preoptic area, named solely for its position: much of it is rostral to the place where the optic chiasm attaches itself to the base of the forebrain. The preoptic area is in essence the anterior hypothalamus. For its part, the anterior cerebral artery courses forward toward the anterior pole of the cerebral hemisphere. Meanwhile the middle cerebral artery swings laterally, then backward around the pedestal of the temporal lobe, thus arriving on the face of the insula in the depth of the Sylvian fissure. There it ramifies into an extensive "candelabra" of vessels. Most of the candelabra ramifications hook back over the lips of the fissure to supply a large region of cortex on the convexity of the hemisphere.

Above the substantia innominata in Figure 98 one finds the anterior commissure, or more precisely the temporal limb of the commissure, cut obliquely on its course toward temporal cortex. The figure thus displays the fundamental model of how connections are established between neocortical regions. In Figure 98 the temporal neocortex on each side of the brain receives fibers from homotopic cortex across the midline by means of a commissural bundle. Here the bundle is the anterior commissure; elsewhere it would be the corpus callosum. In addition the temporal neocortex on each side of the brain links itself to ipsilateral cortex by means of cortical association bundles. Here the bundle is the uncinate fasciculus. This general pattern — emission and receipt of both ipsilateral and contralateral corticocortical fibers — is true for nearly all neocortical fields. Above the anterior commissure is the globus pallidus. It is plainly bipartite: a thin sheet of white matter, the lamina medullaris interna, divides it into segments called medial and lateral, internal and external, or simply inner and outer. On average the cells of the inner segment are slightly larger than those of the outer segment. (The ventral pallidum is part of the outer segment.) Next to the outer segment is the putamen, which completes the lentiform nucleus. The putamen stains quite lightly. It is stippled, however, by a wealth of slender, wispy fascicles, each consisting of thin fibers that nonetheless have myelin sheaths. In an unfixed brain the fascicles produce the striation that early dissectors could see in striatal tissue; early in this century the English neurologist S. A. K. Wilson named them the pencil bundles. They are striatal efferents with two main destinations. Some of the fibers composing the pencil bundles project to the substantia nigra, thus reciprocating the dopaminergic projection from the nigra to the striatum. The rest converge on the globus pallidus, both the inner and the outer segment, thus extending the extrapyramidal "funnel" of data.

Above the lentiform nucleus is the internal capsule. On both the left and the right of the section, but especially on the left, it is invaded by a gray bridge joining the putamen to the caudate nucleus. Then comes the thalamus, in its characteristic position medial and dorsal to the capsule. On the right side of Figure 98 it looks much as it did in Figure 97: one sees the reticular nucleus, a dappled, oval field. Here, however, at the center of the oval, the ventral anterior, or V.A., nucleus has appeared. On the left a further, light-staining nucleus appears. It is the anterior nucleus, the thalamic representative of the Papez circuit. Recall that the circuit runs from the hippocampus to the mammillary body, then to the anterior nucleus, next to the gyrus fornicatus, and finally back to the hippocampus. In Figure 98 a shortcut in the Papez circuit is visible. The fornix appears twice on each side of the section: once in the base of the septum, accompanied by the gray matter of the stylus septi, and again atop the bed nucleus of the stria terminalis, which here becomes continuous with the preoptic area. (The stria and the fornix are nearing the end of their spiraling course.) From the second fornix transection fibers rise dorsolaterally. The anterior nucleus is one of their main destinations. The mammillary body is thereby avoided.

Transitions

The fifth cut in Figure 95 exposes the frontal section shown photographically in Figure 99. It is notable chiefly for aspects of the forebrain's anatomy not yet at their most telling. The thalamus, for instance, has not quite taken on the cross-sectional appearance that typifies the thalamus throughout much of its length. Still, the thalamus shows three distinct nuclei. One of them, the anterior nucleus, was present in Figure 98. Now, however, a heavily myelinated fiber bundle enters it from below, especially on the right side of the section. The bundle, called the mammillothalamic tract, is part of the Papez circuit: it ascends to the anterior nucleus from the mammillary body. Just below the anterior nucleus is the mediodorsal nucleus, or at least its rostral pole. The mediodorsal nucleus projects to the frontal association cortex. As we have noted, its inputs are remarkable. In addition to receiving a reciprocation of its frontal projection it receives fibers from the primary olfactory cortex and from limbic structures such as the amygdala. Together the anterior nucleus and the mediodorsal nucleus compose a medial, light-staining district of the thalamus. The larger, darker-staining region is the V.A.-V.L. complex: the terminus for the brachium conjunctivum, from the cerebellum, and the ansa lenticularis, from the globus pallidus.

The amygdala, too, is not yet at its best. Nevertheless, its principal relations with the rest of the brain are apparent. The dark striations in the ventral part of the amygdala on the right side of the section represent reciprocal connections between the amygdala and the inferior temporal gyri. Here, then, is a visible sign of the limbic system's participation in neocortical activity. In addition, the anatomical relation of the amygdala to the substantia innominata is quite plain, especially on the right side of the section. There the amygdala forms the lower limb of a C-shaped gray arc. Inside it the thinly myelinated fibers of the ventral amygdalofugal path traverse the substantia innominata on their way to the hypothalamus, which lies at the medial end of the upper limb of the C. Some longer amygdalofugal fibers curve dorsally around the medial margin of the internal capsule and thus attain the thalamus; for the most part they end in the mediodorsal nucleus. Above the part of the *C* in which the dorsal neck of the amygdala becomes continuous with the substantia innominata, the temporal limb of the anterior commissure joins the uncinate fasciculus on a communal course to the white core of the temporal lobe. (Here, of course, the Weigert stain blackens the core.) Also above the *C*, on both the left and the right, the globus pallidus is prominent. In Figure 99 it does not quite show the full array of its output lines. But one efferent trajectory is visible. On both the right and left of the section, the base of the globus pallidus is accentuated by a fairly thick black band. It is a stratum of white matter representing a ventral contingent of thick, heavily myelinated fibers leaving the internal pallidal segment. They course toward the midline; then, on both sides of Figure 99, they can be seen looping around the medial margin of the internal capsule. Thus they get their name: they form the ansa lenticularis. In Figure 99 the ansa can be followed only onto the dorsum of the internal capsule; a discussion of its subsequent trajectory is best deferred until the next section is in view.

One item first. A feature of Figure 99 is difficult to see, but it would be no plainer on any other section. It is the medial forebrain bundle. To find it, note that as before the fornix shows up twice on each side of the section: once at the base of the septum and again in the hypothalamus. Examine its surroundings in the latter. To its ventral side, the hypothalamus makes a funnel-like downward protrusion between the optic tracts. The funnel is cavitated by the infundibular recess of the third ventricle; the section is just anterior to the beginning of the infundibular stalk (that is, the stalk of the posterior lobe of the pituitary gland). To the lateral side of the fornix is the medial forebrain bundle. Its fibers are thin and tend not to aggregate; they are nonetheless responsible for the reticulated texture of the lateral hypothalamus, through which they are passing longitudinally. (They pass through a region bordered medially by the fornix and laterally by the internal capsule.) One thing about the bundle is apparent on the section. The name medial forebrain bundle survives from a nomenclature introduced by Ludwig Edinger in which the bundle was contrasted with a far more massive fiber system, which Edinger called the lateral forebrain bundle. Today it is called the internal capsule, or rather the internal capsule plus the cerebral peduncle, the extension of the capsule into the brainstem. The medial forebrain bundle is in essence a limbic traffic artery; its medial placement suits the medial placement of the limbic structures it serves. The lateral forebrain bundle is in essence a neocortical traffic artery; its lateral placement suits the lateral placement of most of the neocortex.

Thalamus; Amygdala; Fields of Forel

The sixth cut in Figure 95 exposes the frontal section shown photographically in Figure 100. Here the hypothalamus is represented by the mammillary bodies, a pair of spherical elevations flanking the midline at the base of the forebrain. They are the only closed parts of the hypothalamus. That is, they alone are sharply circumscribed from the rest of the hypothalamus (the lateral hypothalamus, and also the supramammillary region, dorsal to the mammillary bodies in Figure 100), and they alone have little communication with other hypothalamic cell groups. Instead they receive about half the fornix (much of the rest ends in the septum) and project to two targets: the anterior nucleus of the thalamus (as part of the Papez circuit), and a group of small nuclei medially situated near the caudal limit of the midbrain tegmentum. Remarkably, the mammillofugal projections leave each mammillary body in a single fiber bundle directed anterodorsally (forward and upward) in the forebrain. The bundle bifurcates into the mammillothalamic tract (visible in Figure 99) and the smaller mammillotegmental tract.

Figure 100 represents a large caudal jump; thus it makes explicit three aspects of forebrain anatomy that were only incipient in Figure 99. The thalamus now shows its characteristic cross section. The amygdala shows its remaining relations to the rest of the forebrain. The ansa lenticularis (that is, the efferent bundle emerging from the globus pallidus) shows hints of its course beyond the point where it arrived (in Figure 99) atop the dorsum of the internal capsule.

First, the thalamus. Its internal composition is readily summarized. Throughout much of its length it has a pale-staining (hence myelin-poor) inner segment, medial and dorsal on the cross section, and a more dark-staining outer segment, which flanks the inner segment on its ventral and lateral side. Between the two is a fairly conspicuous fiber layer called the internal medullary lamina. The inner segment consists primarily of a single, very large cell mass, the mediodorsal nucleus, and rostral to it a smaller but nonetheless prominent mass, the anterior nucleus. (The former dominates in Figure 100; the latter dominated Figure 98 and Figure 99.) The outer segment includes the ventral nucleus, which has three divisions designated ventral anterior, ventral lateral, and ventral posterior or ventrobasal. (In Figure 99 the first two are visible; then, in Figure 100, the ventral anterior nucleus is gone, replaced by the ventrobasal nucleus.) The outer segment also includes the lateral nucleus. It, too, has three divisions. In rostral-to-caudal sequence they are the lateral anterior or lateral dorsal, then the lateral posterior, and then the pulvinar. In Figure 100 the first of them, the lateral anterior, is visible on the dorsum of the thalamus atop the internal medullary lamina. Finally, the internal medullary lamina has embedded in its meshes a number of nuclei, of which the centrum medianum, not yet visible, is the largest. Several small thalamic nuclei defy this tripartite schematization. An example appeared in Figure 99. It is the massa intermedia, a slender bridge between the left and right thalamus. The massa intermedia is formed by two cell groups, the periventricular nucleus and the nucleus reuniens, which abut the wall of the third ventricle. A further example in Figure 99 is medial to the mammillothalamic tract. It is the ventromedial nucleus. Still another example, the habenula, will appear in Figure 102.

Why call this collection the thalamus? That is, why give so varied a set of cell groups a single, encompassing name? The attempts to find commonalities among them have managed at best to place them in five distinct functional classes. The specific sensory relay nuclei of the thalamus are interposed in sensory conduction lines ascending toward primary sensory fields of the neocortex. They are the lateral geniculate body, the medial geniculate body, and the ventrobasal nucleus — thalamic processing stations for vision, hearing, and the somatic sense. All but the last are still to come in this series of frontal sections. The secondary relay nuclei of the thalamus are interposed in conduction lines leading from the globus pallidus and the cerebellum not to sensory fields of the neocortex but instead to the motor cortex and to fields closely associated with the motor cortex. They are the ventral anterior nucleus and the ventral lateral nucleus, which compose the V.A.-V.L. complex. The association nuclei of the thalamus are the third thalamic class. They were long thought to be associated only with neocortex. That is, they were known to project to neocortex and to get corticofugal fibers in return. They are the mediodorsal nucleus, which "associates" with the frontal association cortex, and the lateral nucleus, which "associates" with a second great field of association cortex encompassing large parts of the parietal, occipital, and temporal lobes. Both are now known to get other, noncortical input. To give only two examples: the mediodorsal nucleus receives fibers from the amygdala; the lateral nucleus (specifically the lateral posterior nucleus) receives fibers from the superior colliculus. The anterior nucleus of the thalamus is alone in the fourth thalamic class. It participates in the Papez circuit; it is thus a "limbic nucleus." Specifically, it receives fibers from the mammillary body and some from the fornix directly and in turn has reciprocal connections with limbic cortex: the cingulate gyrus. Finally, the nonspecific nuclei of the thalamus are the intralaminar nuclei, which are enmeshed by the internal medullary lamina, and the midline nuclei such as the periventricular nucleus and the nucleus reuniens. They receive a bewildering array of inputs; some of the smaller ones (there is only one large one, the centrum medianum) get input, for example, from the motor cortex, the cerebellum, and the reticular formation. That alone is a reason to call them nonspecific. In addition, the ones that project to the neocortex ignore the boundaries between neocortical fields. In contrast, a specific sensory relay nucleus projects only to a primary sensory field. Further still, the nonspecific nuclei that project to the neocortex make synapses in all cortical layers, but preferentially in the outermost, plexiform layer, among the end branches of apical dendrites emitted by neurons in all the cell-containing cortical layers. It is as if they were giving the cortex a bias: a baseline excitation. In contrast, the neocortical afferents from "specific" thalamic nuclei (in this usage, the other four categories) tend to terminate preferentially in layer 3 and layer 4, at the middle of the thickness of the cortex.

Five distinct categories! The justification for calling all of it the thalamus is nonetheless both functional and anatomical. In the first place, nearly all the nuclei said to be thalamic maintain reciprocal relations with one or another part of the cerebral cortex. The only exceptions seem to be certain intralaminar nuclei, which can easily, on anatomical grounds, be said to be part of the thalamus. They are enveloped by the thalamus. Second, all of the nuclei said to be thalamic are contained within the ovoid mass that lies, with the caudate nucleus, dorsal and medial to the cone of the internal capsule.

Next, the amygdala. On the right side of Figure 100 one sees its caudal pole, with tributary bundles of the stria terminalis gathering inside it. The tail of the caudate nucleus abuts its lateral margin; the temporal horn of the lateral ventricle lies between it and the hippocampus. For its part, the hippocampus shows a number of dorsal incisures, some of them quite deep. One or two of them are visible in the figure. They are known as the impressiones digitatae because early anatomists were struck by their resemblance to the impressions a potter's fingers might leave in wet clay. On the left side of the figure the amygdala is larger; the hippocampus has not yet appeared. Fundamentally, the amygdala is a mass of gray matter in the medial part of the temporal lobe. On cross section it typically is teardrop shaped, with a massive, rounded, ventral district joined to a narrow, dorsal-ranging neck. A part of its medial side fuses into the overlying olfactory cortex; that is the cortical nucleus. The rest is unarguably subcortical. At its dorsomedial border the neck of the amygdala becomes continuous with the substantia innominata. (The continuity was visible in Figure 99.) Extending dorsally, meanwhile, the neck of the amygdala abuts the putamen. The abutment is interrupted by a thin but appreciable layer of fibers. Nevertheless, early anatomists regarded the amygdala as a part of the striatum and called it the archistriatum, or sometimes even the olfactory striatum, in light of its additional fusion with the primary olfactory cortex. The names no longer serve. After all, the amygdala sends its output chiefly to the hypothalamus; the striatum — with the exception of the nucleus accumbens — does not. Conversely, the striatum sends its output chiefly to the globus pallidus and the substantia nigra; the amygdala does not.

Last, the globus pallidus and its output channel, the ansa lenticularis. Here some preliminaries are necessary. In Figure 100 the globus pallidus is rapidly diminishing. Moreover, the gray matter underneath it — the substantia innominata — is nearly gone. On the right side of the section its place is being taken by a broad avenue of white matter directed medially from the core of the temporal lobe and so passing under the putamen and then the globus pallidus. It is the sublenticular limb of the internal capsule, which here extends far enough ventrally so that it reaches the base of the brain, where its medial expansion forms the cerebral peduncle. Above this ventromedial part of the capsule is a mass of gray matter shaped like a biconvex lens. It is the subthalamic nucleus, the pallidal satellite whose destruction causes hemiballism. The subthalamic nucleus is the ventral half of the subthalamic region, or simply the subthalamus: a part of the caudal diencephalon that inserts itself like a wedge between the cerebral peduncle and the thalamus. The wedge is really a forward extension of the midbrain tegmentum. One frontal section from now, the subthalamic nucleus will begin to yield its position to the substantia nigra. Two sections from now, the red nucleus will fill the center of the wedge.

Overlying the subthalamic nucleus in Figure 100 is the remainder, the dorsal half, of the subthalamic wedge. It is occupied by a fiber network consisting largely of the ansa lenticularis. The anatomy is daunting. The fundamental problem is that the lentiform nucleus — the globus pallidus and the putamen — is lateral and ventral to the supralenticular limb of the internal capsule. In contrast, the targets for fibers leaving the lentiform nucleus — namely the subthalamic nucleus, the thalamus, the substantia nigra, and the midbrain tegmentum — are dorsal to the capsule or, farther caudally, the cerebral peduncle. This means the projections must either traverse the capsule or loop around it. No wonder the ansa lenticularis is complicated; it consists, in fact, of three pallidofugal divisions, which are obscured in several places by their entanglement with the continuum formed by the internal capsule and cerebral peduncle.

Note, to begin, that the cerebral peduncle under the subthalamic nucleus on both sides of Figure 100 is pierced more or less vertically by a multitude of fascicles that give the peduncle the appearance of a palisade. Thus they get their collective name: they are called the comb system. In Figure 100 they incorporate two projections. The more ventral among the comb-system fascicles consist of rather thin fibers. They come from the striatum, and so they form no part of the ansa lenticularis, a term reserved for pallidal outflow. Farther rostrally in the forebrain the striatal fibers were part of the pencil bundles. Then they passed through the globus pallidus, and now they are tunneling through the peduncle in the furtherance of their route to the substantia nigra. Their trajectory is matched by reciprocating, dopaminergic fibers projecting from the substantia nigra to the striatum. The more dorsal among the comb-system fascicles consist of fairly thick fibers. They, too, have passed through the globus pallidus, or rather the internal pallidal segment: they arise in the external segment, and here are seen entering the subthalamic nucleus from below. They compose the middle division of the ansa lenticularis. They, too, are matched in trajectory by a reciprocating projection, which terminates in not only the external pallidal segment but also the internal one. The subthalamic nucleus emerges, therefore, as a neural mechanism astride the globus pallidus, receiving most of the output of the external pallidal segment but affecting both pallidal segments.

The fibers emitted by the internal pallidal segment must now be described. They are among the thickest, most heavily myelinated fibers found anywhere in the forebrain. Somehow they, too, must get to the dorsal side of the internal capsule. One group of them — the dorsal division of the ansa lenticularis — pierce the internal capsule, thus forming a rostral part of the comb system. A second group — the ventral division of the ansa — leave by a different route: the fibers turn downward, not upward, and exit the internal segment through its ventral border. Just under the internal segment the fibers turn toward the midline; their aggregate was prominent in Figure 99. Then, on reaching the medial margin of the internal capsule, the fibers turn sharply dorsalward, and arriving in that way atop the supralenticular limb of the internal capsule, they join the comb-system fibers, which got there by perforating the capsule.* The resulting communal fiber bundle is called the subthalamic fasciculus, or sometimes the fasciculus lenticularis. It is in fact the collective output channel for the internal pallidal segment. The fasciculus promptly turns caudalward. At first it lies just dorsal to the medial margin of the internal capsule. Then, in Figure 100, it gets lifted away from the capsule (which has become the cerebral peduncle) by the advent of the subthalamic nucleus. In that way it becomes a fiber sheet investing the dorsum of the nucleus. In this part of its trajectory the fasciculus forms field H-2 of Forel — Auguste Forel, a Swiss neurologist and psychiatrist. Forel intended the "H" to stand for *Haube,* the term then employed in the German nomenclature to signify the tegmentum. (*Haube* means hood or bonnet.) The H fields are therefore the *Haubenfelder,* the tegmental fields. Forel was perhaps the first to realize that the subthalamus amounts to a continuation of the midbrain tegmentum into the forebrain. In Figure 100 the fields of Forel are invaded on their lateral side by a tongue of gray matter. The gray tongue is known as the zona incerta. Its inputs now seem to come from the cerebellum and from the motor cortex, and not, as was understandably thought, from the ansa lenticularis. Its outputs have long remained obscure. It appears to project chiefly to the midbrain reticular formation. The fiber stratum dorsal to the zona incerta is field H-1 of Forel, also called the thalamic fasciculus. The fiber stratum ventral to the zona incerta is field H-2 of Forel. A medial, nodal area left unsplit by the zona incerta is field H.

The fibers that arise in the internal segment of the globus pallidus assemble, then, in field H-2. Some will continue their caudalward course and enter the midbrain tegmentum. They form no circumscribed bundle. They will terminate in the pedunculopontine nucleus, a tegmental cell group near the caudal border of the mesencephalon. Most, however, describe a hairpin turn through field H into field H-1, and coursing rostralward in field H-1, commingled there with a multitude of fibers from the brachium conjunctivum and the medial lemniscus, they arrive from below at the thalamus. Their main destinations are the ventral anterior nucleus and the ventral lateral nucleus, which compose the V.A.-V.L. complex. Not until 1939 was the bizarre trajectory of the ansa lenticularis demonstrated definitively. In 1912, the

---

*The discovery of the ansa lenticularis was really a set of discoveries spanning 23 years. It began with the ventral division; that is to say, the first known contingent of fibers leaving the globus pallidus was the one that curves around the internal capsule. Indeed, the term ansa lenticularis, coined in 1872 by Theodor Meynert, who discovered the ventral division, was inspired by the loop the division makes. Next, in 1895, the Swiss histologist Constantin von Monakow recognized the perforant, dorsal division. At the same time he described the fiber contingent projecting to the subthalamic nucleus from the external pallidal segment. He named it the middle division. In hindsight it seems a miraculous discovery. None of the experimental methods of axon tracing available today were known in Monakow's time.

German neurologist Cécile Vogt had recognized the hairpin curve, but neither she nor later she and her husband, the neuropathologist Oskar Vogt, could determine whether the fibers ran from the globus pallidus to the thalamus or in the opposite direction. One imagines that investigators in the time of Forel must have looked at the *Haubenfelder* in bewilderment, seeing only masses of white matter cloven by gray and never imagining that a single fiber system might enter one of Forel's fields, traverse another, enter the third, and finally enter the thalamus.

Centrum Medianum

The seventh cut in Figure 95 exposes the frontal section shown photographically in Figure 101. It exhibits the caudal pole of the lentiform nucleus. On the right side of the section the putamen alone remains; on the left a sliver of the external pallidal segment is visible as well. The tail of the caudate nucleus appears twice, once in the lateral wall of the lateral ventricle (in Figure 101, the cella media) and again in the roof of the temporal horn of the ventricle. More notably, Figure 101, like Figure 100 (and for that matter Figure 89), displays the continuity of the cerebral peduncle with the internal capsule. Cut in cross section, the capsule appears to bifurcate. The arc of the capsule under the putamen toward the white core of the temporal lobe is the sublenticular limb of the capsule. It includes the auditory radiation, directed from the medial geniculate body of the thalamus toward the primary auditory cortex on the superior temporal gyrus. It also includes the loop of Meyer-Archambault, or more simply Meyer's loop, a ventral part of the visual radiation, directed, like the rest of the radiation, from the lateral geniculate body to the primary visual cortex. The loop makes a forward swing through the white matter of the temporal lobe and then describes a curve that sweeps it back toward occipital cortex. The arc of the internal capsule over the putamen toward the white core of the frontal lobe and the parietal lobe is the supralenticular limb of the capsule. It includes the thalamocortical radiations directed toward central regions of neocortex: that is, the motor cortex, on the precentral gyrus, and the primary somatic sensory cortex, on the postcentral gyrus. It also includes the pyramidal tract, descending from the motor cortex. Dorsal to the cerebral peduncle the rostral pole of the substantia nigra appears, dislodging the subthalamic nucleus from its position abutting the dorsum of the peduncle. The diencephalon is giving way to the midbrain. Next in dorsalward sequence are the fields of Forel: first field H-2, the subthalamic fasciculus, and then, above it, field H-1, the thalamic fasciculus. The zona incerta is no longer present between them. The small disk of gray matter in the medial part of the H fields is the rostral pole of the red nucleus.

Then comes the thalamus. As before, the internal medullary lamina divides it into an inner, mediodorsal district and an outer, ventrolateral district. The mediodorsal district is dominated by the mediodorsal nucleus; the ventrolateral district is dominated by the ventral nucleus. Here again the upper part of the ventral nucleus is the ventral lateral nucleus; the darker-staining lower part is the ventrobasal nucleus. The darkness of the latter results from the dense, heavily myelinated neuropil placed in it by the medial lemniscus. A slender, sickle-shaped subdivision in the ventral part of the ventrobasal nucleus is notable, however, for its striking poverty in myelin. It has several names: the semilunar nucleus, the arcuate nucleus, and (most tellingly) the thalamic gustatory nucleus. It does indeed process taste sensation. Its sensory afferents are the gustatory lemniscus, which arrives from the rostral third of the nucleus of the solitary tract after synaptic interruption in the parabrachial nuclei. Lateral to it, the rest of the ventrobasal nucleus represents, in ventral-to-dorsal order, somatic sensation from the face, the arm, and the leg. In Figure 101 the internal medullary lamina is greatly widened by the presence of the largest intralaminar nucleus, the centrum medianum. The centrum medianum was given its name by the French physician Jean Luys, who also described the subthalamic nucleus. While performing brain autopsies he had found that a transverse cut exactly halfway between the frontal and the occipital pole always exposed a large, circumscribed cell group plainly delineated in the thalamus even in unfixed, unstained brain tissue. His term for the nucleus — *centre médian* — referred to its halfway placement and so is an exception to the rule that median denotes a position at the midline. Its inputs and outputs are curious. A massive input to the centrum medianum issues from the internal segment of the globus pallidus as part of the ansa lenticularis. It arrives, therefore, as a constituent of field H-1 of Forel. A second input issues from the motor cortex. There is, in other words, a convergence of the pyramidal and the extrapyramidal motor system on this common thalamic target. As for output, the centrum medianum projects to the striatum, mainly to the putamen, thus closing a circuit from the putamen to the globus pallidus to the thalamus and finally back to the putamen. Remarkably, the centrum medianum appears to have no projection to cerebral cortex.

Hippocampus

The eighth cut in Figure 95 exposes the frontal section shown photographically in Figure 102. The lentiform nucleus is no longer a part of the section. In its place the section includes a large triangle of white matter: the retrolenticular limb of the internal capsule. Its dorsal part, continuous with the supralenticular limb of the capsule, carries primarily the thalamocortical traffic between the pulvinar and the posterior parietal cortex; its ventral part, continuous with the sublenticular limb of the capsule, consists primarily of the optic radiation. Some final islands of the putamen's gray matter are visible inside the retrolenticular limb, especially on the left side of the section. A more notable inclusion is visible on the right. There the ventral part of the retrolenticular limb shows the rostral pole of the lateral geniculate body. (Recall that the caudal thalamus, with the lateral geniculate body at its tip, curves ventrally, then rostrally, around the retrolenticular limb of the internal capsule.) In the corresponding position on the left side of the section one still sees only the optic tract. At its lateral corners the retrolenticular limb becomes continuous with the corona radiata. Meanwhile, at the opposite, medial corner, the limb expands downward and toward the midline to become the cerebral peduncle, at the ventral surface of the midbrain. The peduncle underlies the substantia nigra, which quite plainly has a ventral district, the pars reticulata, and a dorsal district, the pars compacta. At the medial side of the nigra the pars compacta continues into the ventral tegmental area. It in turn is overlain by the red nucleus, seen here almost at its fullest. The patch of myelinated fibers immediately lateral to the red nucleus comprises the medial lemniscus, on its way to the ventrobasal nucleus of the thalamus, and the brachium conjunctivum, on its way to the V.A.-V.L. complex. In short, the patch is the caudal continuation of field H-1 of Forel.

In Figure 102 the bulk of the cross section of the thalamus — in fact all of it except the lateral geniculate body — is in its characteristic position atop the internal capsule. The mediodorsal nucleus is nearing its caudal pole. Ventral and lateral to it the centrum medianum is plain, especially on the left, where the internal medullary lamina forms a capsule around it. Much of the rest of the thalamic cross section consists of the ventral nucleus: in particular, the ventral lateral nucleus and below that the ventrobasal nucleus. The latter is heavily myelinated, except for the gustatory nucleus. Again the myelination reflects mostly the neuropil attending the arrival of the medial lemniscus. Dorsolaterally in the thalamus a further nucleus appears; it was in evidence even in Figure 101. It is the lateral posterior nucleus. It projects to parietal association cortex. In the next, more caudal section in our series it will expand to form the pulvinar, which is perhaps the largest thalamic nucleus in the human brain.

One thing more about the thalamus. On the medial face of the mediodorsal nucleus in Figure 100 and Figure 101 a compact, well-myelinated fiber bundle is visible precisely at the line along which the choroid roof of the third ventricle attaches itself to the thalamus. It is the stria medullaris. The stria has a dual origin. A large part of it arises in the stylus septi, the thickened part of the septum along the rostral margin of the columna fornicis, dorsal to the anterior commissure. The rest arises nearer the base of the forebrain, in the lateral hypothalamus and the nucleus of the diagonal band as well as in the olfactory tubercle and the ventral pallidum. The bundle courses caudalward; it appears to contain no fibers carrying signals in the opposite direction. In Figure 102 it terminates in the habenular nuclei (or simply the habenula), a set of cell groups forming a small but conspicuous protrusion on the medial face of the mediodorsal nucleus, again at the roof of the third ventricle. The habenular nuclei are regarded by many as composing a separate division of the diencephalon, the so-called epithalamus. (*Epi-* signifies "upon.") In any case the name habenula is somewhat slipshod. It means "the reins" — the reins of a horse. The nuclei happen to lie at a point where the pineal gland is attached to the dorsum of the thalamus by a pair of stalks that resemble a set of reins. Yet the nuclei send no axons into the reins; that is, they do not innervate the pineal gland.* Instead the habenula releases a compact fiber bundle, the fasciculus retroflexus of Meynert, which descends toward the base of the midbrain, circumventing the red nucleus. The fasciculus is dramatically visible in Figure 102, especially on the left side of the section. Its main destination is the raphe of the mesencephalon; we have come on the principal input affecting the serotonergic cell groups of the midbrain, and hence the serotonergic innervation of the entire cerebral hemisphere. What does it signify? All one can say is that the conduction route from the forebrain to the mesencephalic raphe nuclei by way of the habenular nuclei (and the mesencephalic cell group known as the interpeduncular nucleus) contrasts with a less traveled ventral route, which employs the medial forebrain bundle and engages the hypothalamus as an intermediary processing station. The two routes undoubtedly use different combinations of neurotransmitters. For example, the fasciculus retroflexus includes a cholinergic fiber contingent that appears to be lacking in the descending axonal population of the medial forebrain bundle.

Figure 102 shows the mode of inrolling by which the margin of the cortical sheet becomes the hippocampal formation. Both sides of the section show it. First, at the medial side of the top of the temporal lobe, the cortical sheet folds toward the temporal horn of the lateral ventricle, whose medial wall it forms. Then it folds over itself. To this point, therefore, it describes a figure S. Next, at the end of the upper fold, it turns under itself and extends into the hilus (the mouth) of a small final gyrus, U shaped on cross section, the dentate gyrus, or fascia dentata. The bulk of the structure — the figure S and its underturning into the hilus of the fascia — is Ammon's horn, or the cornu Ammonis. That is the Latin term denoting the horn of plenty. Little wonder, all in all, that Broca decided he had found the edge of the cerebral cortex, at

---

*The pineal gland, named for its resemblance to a pinecone, apparently gets no fibers whatsoever from the brain. Instead it receives postganglionic sympathetic innervation. The path is now well established, at least in animals such as the rat. It begins in the retina, which projects, by way of the so-called accessory optic tract, to a hypothalamic cell group called the suprachiasmatic nucleus in recognition of its position dorsal to the optic chiasm. The suprachiasmatic nucleus evidently employs its visual afferentation to generate a circadian, or day-night, rhythm for the brain. In addition it emits a descending projection, which influences preganglionic sympathetic motor neurons of the lateral horn. They in turn influence postganglionic sympathetic motor neurons of the superior cervical ganglion, which emits the fibers that reach the pineal. The fibers release the postganglionic sympathetic transmitter, norepinephrine: less of it during daylight than at night. In response the pineal converts the amino acid tryptophan first into serotonin and then, in two chemical steps catalyzed by enzymes not present in the serotonergic neurons of the midbrain raphe, into the hormone melatonin, produced exclusively by the pineal. The function of melatonin remains elusive. Investigators, however, are impressed by its pattern of release from the pineal: more at night than in daylight; more in winter than in summer, when days are long; a notably large amount in the years preceding puberty. Accordingly, investigators including Richard Wurtman and his colleagues at the Massachusetts Institute of Technology are seeking links between melatonin, the timing of puberty, and certain forms of psychological depression commonest in winter.

least in the temporal lobe, and little wonder that he initially chose to call his discovery the great lobe of the hem. Here, in the temporal lobe, the edge is clearly arrayed in a way suggesting the strategy of a seamstress who finishes off the hem of a garment by folding its material several times and even placing over its end an extra piece of fabric before stitching it all together. One aspect of the anatomy is confusing at first. The hippocampal white matter is at the surface of the brain and therefore gives the impression of not being subjacent to the cortical gray — of no longer being, in other words, the cable basement of the cerebral cortex. But this is simply because the upper fold of Ammon's horn makes the subjacent white matter occupy its seemingly inappropriate position. To put the matter baldly, the eversion of the hippocampus turns the white matter belly up. The largest aggregation of hippocampal white matter appears in Figure 102 as a mooring for the choroid membrane of the temporal horn near the dentate gyrus. It is called the fimbria fornicis, meaning the fringe of the fornix, and it is in fact the marshaling ground for the fibers of that bundle. In a well-fixed brain it can be retracted to reveal the medial edge of the dentate gyrus, with the row of "dentition" embossed thereupon. The fibers composing the fimbria originate throughout Ammon's horn and assemble in a thin sheet of white matter that covers the horn's ventricular surface. It is known as the alveus, meaning (in Latin) the belly. Perhaps the anatomy really did remind early observers of the curving whitish belly of a fish and of many mammals.

It should be said that both Ammon's horn and the dentate gyrus have only a single cell layer. Thus they are quite unlike neocortex, which covers most of the cerebral hemisphere. In a word, they are archicortex. Their curious architecture results from a tendency on the part of the cortical sheet to undergo a stepwise simplification of its laminar pattern as it nears its temporal margin. The sequence shows itself best in a Nissl preparation; we display one in Figure 104. Note first, at the bottom right of the figure, the medial climb of cortex toward the vertex of the parahippocampal gyrus. In the lower part of the climb the gray matter has a pattern in which the cortical lamination is unusually distinct. In it five cell layers are marked off from one another by bands poor in cell bodies. The pattern characterizes the entorhinal area, the gateway for neocortical input to the hippocampus. At the vertex of the parahippocampal gyrus, the cell layers begin to fuse. The result is called the presubiculum. It is an essentially two-cell-layered cortex. Soon, at a fairly sharp border, the presubiculum gives way to the subiculum, or subiculum hippocampi, the first stretch of cortex with only a single cell layer (if only toward the left of its extent in Figure 104). The subiculum forms much of the lowest turn of Ammon's horn; hence its name, which signifies the hippocampal foundation or underpinning. The subiculum contributes fibers to the fornix; on that ground it is a part of the hippocampus. Next, at approximately the end of the lower limb of the *S* of Ammon's horn, there comes a point where the sole remaining cell layer becomes thinner and the cells in the layer become far more densely packed. There the subiculum gives way to the CA (cornu Ammonis) fields of Lorente de Nó — Rafael Lorente de Nó, a pupil of

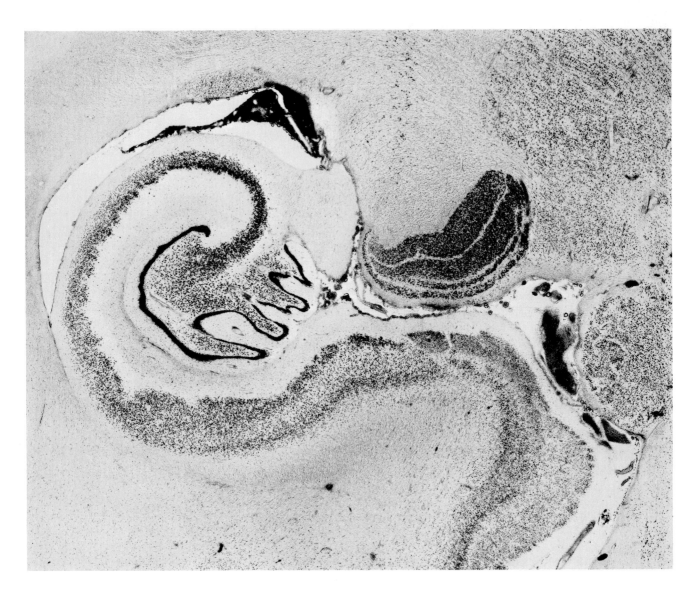

Figure 104: **Hippocampus,** along with the sequence of cortical regions leading into the hippocampus, occupies most of this Nissl-stained frontal section, which shows tissue from the temporal lobe of a human brain. The sequence begins at the bottom right, where temporal cortex climbs the medial face of the temporal lobe. Its initial part is the entorhinal area, the final link in projections from the neocortex to the hippocampus. The area bulges briefly, producing a field called the parasubiculum. Then, at the end of the bulge, where the cortex curves toward the horizontal, the thickness of the cortical sheet abruptly diminishes and some of the cell layers coalesce, producing the presubiculum. About two-thirds of the way across the horizontal stretch of the temporal cortex (under the lateral geniculate body, which shows four of its six laminae), the presubiculum gives way to the subiculum, the first of a series of single-cell-layered fields composing the hippocampus itself. The single cell layer becomes consolidated toward the left of the field of view. At the extreme left the layer narrows and curves toward the vertical. The resulting field is called CA1. Toward the top of the curve, clusters of large neurons mark field CA2. By the top of the curve the large neurons are densely packed, marking CA3. The latter curves into the mouth of the dentate gyrus, where it forms field CA4. For its part the dentate gyrus has a single cell layer so densely packed with neuronal cell bodies that the layer shows up as a thick black line. At the top of the hippocampus, in the ventral wall of the temporal horn of the lateral ventricle, the fimbria, or fringe, of the fornix stains lightly. Above it, in the dorsal wall of the temporal horn, the oval region stippled with neuronal cell bodies is the tail of the caudate nucleus. The round mass of cells at the extreme right (to the right of the cross section of a dark-staining vein) is the medial geniculate body.

Santiago Ramón y Cajal. First comes CA1, then CA2 (whose limits are indistinct), then CA3, and finally CA4, where the dentate gyrus folds over the end of the CA progression, thus forming the true edge of the cortical sheet. Regarding projections: Cascades of corticocortical fibers converge on the entorhinal area. The entorhinal area projects to the CA fields. Its main projection, however, is to the dentate gyrus. In turn the dentate gyrus projects to CA3, by means of extremely thin axons known as mossy fibers. (They are not to be confused with another class of mossy fibers, which enter the cerebellum.) In CA3 a part of the fornix begins. In particular, the axons originating in CA3 join the alveus, and so become part of the fornix. Before that, they give off collaterals (the so-called Schaffer collaterals), which distribute to CA1 and the subiculum. In turn CA1 and the subiculum contribute to the fornix. It is now known that the fibers joining the fornix from the CA fields have only two targets: the septum and the contralateral CA fields. (The traffic to the latter composes the hippocampal commissure.) The remaining fornix fibers, which end in the nucleus accumbens, the anterior nucleus of the thalamus, and the mammillary body, arise in the subiculum.

Caudal Thalamus

The ninth cut in Figure 95 exposes the frontal section shown photographically in Figure 103. In it the thalamus has changed. For much of its length the internal medullary lamina gave it two great subdivisions. Now, at this caudal level, the lamina is gone. Instead one sees three thalamic nuclei. The pulvinar is the most dorsal of the three. Then, underneath it, the medial geniculate body and the lateral geniculate body disrupt the continuity between the cerebral peduncle and the retrolenticular limb of the internal capsule. The medial geniculate body is a fairly uniform mass. Still, its cell architecture is not homogeneous. In contrast, the lateral geniculate body is strikingly laminated: its neurons are arrayed in six concentric, *U*-shaped bands whose mouths all open downward. The bands are known as layers 1 through 6; the numbering advances from the innermost (and ventralmost) of the *U*'s. The fibers of the optic tract entering the lateral geniculate body distribute themselves so that crossed fibers, representing the nasal half of the contralateral retina, terminate in layers 1, 4, and 6, while uncrossed fibers, representing the temporal half of the ipsilateral retina, terminate in layers 2, 3, and 5. The layers are in register; hence a line passing dorsoventrally like the spoke of a wheel through all six layers crosses cells all representing the same part of the visual field. To put it another way, the output of the retinas is mapped in the lateral geniculate bodies so that two conditions are simultaneously satisfied: the data from each eye are segregated, yet the topology of the binocular visual field is preserved. Two chapters from now we shall describe a different strategy by which the primary visual cortex attains the identical end. At the lateral side of the lateral geniculate body the visual radiation emerges, on its way to the visual cortex. On the right side of the section the emergence is clear: the fibers invade the retrolenticular limb of the internal capsule. One contingent of the radiation first courses forward in the sublenticular limb of the capsule, so that its continuation in the corona radiata shows up as early as Figure 101 and even Figure 100.

The transformation of the thalamus to its appearance in Figure 103 reflects the evolution of the structure. In nonprimate mammals it is ovoid. In primates, however, and most of all in the human brain, its caudal pole augments in volume and extends itself over the back of the cerebral peduncle in a hook-shaped curve that moves laterally and ventralward to flank the rostral half of the mesencephalon along a trajectory that parallels the curve of, say, the caudate nucleus. The hook rapidly attenuates in girth; the attenuation is composed of the medial geniculate body and the lateral geniculate body and is sometimes called the metathalamus (Greek for "that which follows the thalamus"). At the vertex, not the tip, of the downward curve is the pulvinar. Its volume is particularly responsible for the augmentation of the caudal pole of the human thalamus. The term pulvinar derives from the Latin *pulvinus,* or pillow; but then, the thalamus in a primate does look much like a pillow slung over the back of a chair. (The chair is the cerebral peduncle.) The pulvinar is a corner of the pillow—a corner sagging downward. It makes the entire analogy vivid.

The sight of the brainstem in Figure 103 is rather disconcerting. The reason is simple. A transverse cut through the forebrain entails an oblique cut through the rest. Take the cerebral peduncle as a start for some excursions. At the ventromedial end of the peduncle the pontine gray matter begins. The grotto above it is not a ventricle. It is the foramen cecum. In essence it is a deep intunneling of the surface of the brain, and hence the subarachnoid space. Above the cerebral peduncle the substantia nigra is prominent, and also the red nucleus. A triangular, heavily myelinated region extending from the nucleus in a lateral direction includes mostly the medial lemniscus and the part of the brachium conjunctivum that bypasses the red nucleus and is destined for the thalamus. Finally, toward the dorsal side of the brainstem, the third ventricle narrows into the cerebral aqueduct. Here, and throughout the midbrain, the central gray substance surrounds it. In turn the central gray substance is sharply delineated from the surrounding midbrain tegmentum by its dearth of myelin. (The oculomotor nuclei, in the ventral part of the central gray substance, are even more lacking in myelin.)

Lateral to the central gray substance, ventral and medial to the pulvinar, and rostral to the superior colliculus (though Figure 103 cannot reveal the last of these anatomical relations) one sees the pretectal area. Like the superior colliculus, it is heavily played on by fibers from the visual cortex and fibers from the retina. But in one of the area's cell groups, neurons have been identified that do not respond to stimuli from any particular part of the visual field. They respond to every part. In brief, they have no "receptive field," unless it be the entire visual field. Apparently they monitor the overall intensity of the light impinging on the retina. They are light meters, so to speak, and that is exactly what is required of an area of the brain that serves the adjustment of the pupil of the eye. Each side of the pretectal area receives retinal input only from the contralateral eye. Yet each side of the pretectal area projects to the Edinger-Westphal nuclei on both sides of the brain. The crossing projection employs the posterior commissure, a sizable fiber bundle quite visible in Figure 103 in the part of the central gray substance that forms the roof of the cerebral aqueduct. The posterior commissure also contains true commissural fibers, which connect the contralateral pretectal areas. Shine light in either eye, and both pupils will constrict. Robert Whytt, a Scottish physician, described the tandem constriction, now called the consensual pupillary reflex, two centuries ago.

The tenth cut in Figure 95 exposes a final frontal section, one we do not show photographically. At last the pattern is simple again: all that remains of the cerebral hemispheres is the occipital lobes, and under them is the brainstem. The section therefore is dominated by cortex: that of the cerebrum and that of the cerebellum. The first is arrayed in the broad folds known as gyri, the second in the narrow folds known as folia. In Figure 95 there is nothing but space between the two. In the skull, however, they are separated by a dural sheet, the tentorium cerebelli. The cerebral hemispheres do show some final details. For example, the white core of each occipital lobe offers a final view of the lateral ventricle, specifically the occipital horn of the ventricle. Its medial wall is pressed inward by the fundus of a deep fissure that invades from the medial side. It is the calcarine fissure. The bulge the invasion produces is called the calcar avis, meaning the spur of the bird, because of its resemblance to the posterior toe of a bird: the toe with which the animal grasps the branch on which it is poised. The walls of the calcarine fissure are primary visual cortex. So are the continuation of the ventral wall, on the lingual gyrus, and that of the dorsal wall, on the cuneus. The spans of the continuations amount to little more than half the depth of the calcarine fissure; hence one can judge that more than half the visual cortex is hidden inside the fissure. The brainstem also shows some details. The pair of protuberances flanking the midline on the brainstem's ventral surface are the medullary pyramids, each raised by a pyramidal tract; the cut has gone caudal to the pons. The cranial nerve at the ventral surface is the statoacoustic. The heavily myelinated fiber bundle framing the anterior recess of the fourth ventricle is the brachium conjunctivum, just leaving the cerebellum. The part of the cerebellum forming the roof of the anterior recess is the vermis. The rest of the cerebellum is formed by the cerebellar hemispheres.

Chapter Fifteen

Cerebellar Cortex

A simple conception of the brain is that it consists of blobs and sheets. The blobs are cell groups: the ones in the brainstem, the ones in the thalamus, the ones in the hypothalamus, the ones in the amygdala, and the ones in the corpus striatum. They taunt you with their disorder. Their neurons send off dendrites in seemingly random directions. Moreover, the shape of each neuronal cell body seems characteristic only of itself. It is particularly disconcerting to contemplate such a tangle, say in a Golgi preparation, and reflect that the blob may be involved, as some blobs undoubtedly are, in a function as precise and crucial as the control of body temperature or the concentration of oxygen in the blood. The sheets are a more pleasant sight. They include, in the hindbrain, the inferior olivary nucleus; in the cerebellum, the dentate nucleus; in the midbrain, the superior colliculus; and in the thalamus, the lateral geniculate body. Above all else, they seem to be well ordered. Here, too, the tissue is fundamentally neurons embedded in neuropil. Often, however, one sees a pattern in the tissue. Different-looking cells — large versus small, for example — may tend to be at different depths in the sheet, and at different packing densities. Levels poor in cell bodies may accentuate the laminated appearance. In the brain of a mammal the most impressive sheets are the cortices: that of the cerebellum and that of the cerebrum. They satisfy the four criteria laid out in Part I. First, they are at the surface of the brain. Second, they are layered. Third, the outermost layer, at the very surface of the brain, is a fiber layer largely devoid of cell bodies. Fourth, a substantial proportion of the processes emitted by the cells strike off in particular directions, so that the tissue (in the appropriate preparations) may resemble a palisade. The cerebellar cortex is especially impressive. Nothing there is disordered. Dendrites and axons are aligned in specific patterns. Moreover, the cells are of indisputable types: the shape and the connectivities of each of the multitude of neurons make it a granule cell, a Purkinje cell, a stellate cell, a basket cell, or a Golgi cell. Nowhere else in the central nervous system does one find such stereometry: such three-dimensional regularity. To anatomists and physiologists the cerebellar cortex has thus become a darling. After all, the manifest order of the cerebellar cortex seems to promise that a detailed understanding of the function of the organ cannot be far behind. It is sobering, then, to confess that it remains unclear just what the relation between structure and function in the cerebellum is. In essence a blob is daunting in its seeming disarray; the cerebellar cortex is daunting in its lack of disarray. The intent in the following paragraphs is to explore the difficulties.

Main and Auxiliary Paths

The axons entering the cerebellum from the spinal cord, the vestibular nuclei, the pons, and elsewhere tend to give off collaterals to the deep cerebellar nuclei. In the main, however, they distribute their branches to the deepest layer of the cerebellar cortex, the granular layer, which is characterized by granule cells: extremely small neurons with a packing density matched almost nowhere else in the brain. In the granular layer the branches (called mossy fibers because they end in large, somewhat lobulated terminals) make synapses with the short, clawlike dendrites the granule cells deploy (Figure 105). In turn, the granule cells emit thin, unmyelinated axons that rise into the most superficial layer of the cerebellar cortex, the molecular layer. In obedience to the generic definition of cortex it is a stratum occupied largely by neuronal processes to the exclusion of neuronal cell bodies. In the molecular layer each arriving axon bifurcates into a left and right collateral. That is, it assumes the shape of a *T*. Each collateral runs parallel to the long axis of the folium (the cerebellar convolution) in which the parent fiber arrived. Thus it runs parallel to its myriad fellows. Such collaterals are called parallel fibers. In the cat, and presumably in primates, they are several millimeters long. Now, the granule cells are so numerous that the sum of the parallel fibers packs the molecular layer (Figure 106). There is room nonetheless for the dendrites of the Purkinje cells: large neurons (first described by the 19th-century Czech physiologist Johannes Purkinje) whose flask-shaped cell bodies are found at intervals of about 100 micrometers in a file at the interface between the granular layer below them and the molecular layer above. The file constitutes a third layer of the cerebellar cortex. Each Purkinje cell has one or, more commonly, two or three dendritic trunks. The trunks rise into the molecular layer. There they produce an extraordinary tree, all in a single plane perpendicular to the long axis of the folium, and thus to the parallel fibers (Figure 107). The tree is notable for a wealth of short, thick dendritic spines; the spines are preferential sites for synapses. Here they are sites at which each

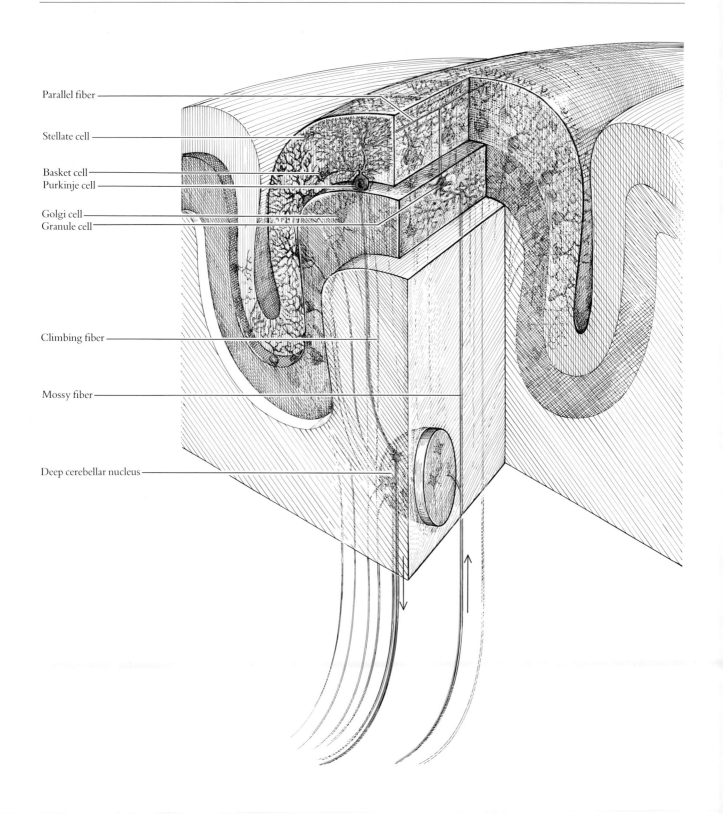

Parallel fiber

Stellate cell

Basket cell
Purkinje cell

Golgi cell
Granule cell

Climbing fiber

Mossy fiber

Deep cerebellar nucleus

Purkinje cell receives excitatory signals from the multitude of parallel fibers that pass through its dendritic plane. The Purkinje cell's efferent channel — its axon — leaves the cerebellar cortex and makes synapses in the deep cerebellar nuclei. The deep cerebellar nuclei project to the red nucleus, the V.A.-V.L. complex, and other places beyond the cerebellum. That is the main cerebellar circuitry.

There are, however, detours. In particular, the information channeled into the basic pathway from mossy fiber to granule cell to Purkinje cell to deep cerebellar nucleus encounters auxiliary circuits. Consider a stellate cell. Its cell body is stationed high in the molecular layer. Plainly, then, it is one among few, because it and its fellows do little to contradict the impression that the molecular layer is devoid of cell bodies. Its dendritic tree is flattened into a plane athwart the traffic of parallel fibers. Thus the stellate cell, like the Purkinje cell, gets its input from parallel fibers. Its axon is distinctive: it passes above Purkinje cells and makes synapses with their dendritic trees. Its influence is inhibitory.

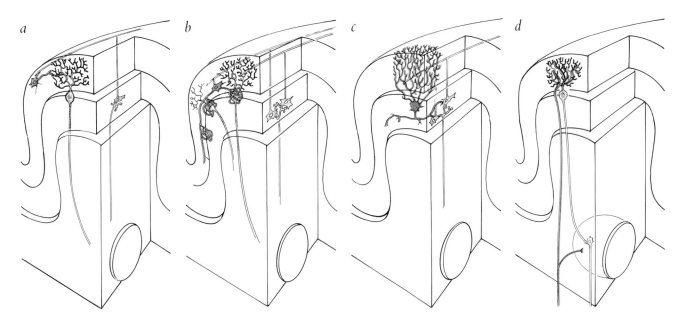

Figure 105: **Cerebellar circuitry** is notable both for its unchanging composition (the circuit is the same throughout the cerebellar cortex) and for its stereometry (the neuronal elements composing the circuit are arranged in an impressive three-dimensional order). At the left the basic circuit (*color*) occupies a somewhat schematic representation of a folium, or cerebellar convolution. The cerebellar afferents called mossy fibers enter the inner, or granular, layer of the cerebellar cortex. There they synapse with the dendrites of granule cells. In turn the granule cells emit the axons called parallel fibers, which fill the outer, molecular layer. Purkinje cells gather input from parallel fibers. They project to the deep cerebellar nuclei. Two classes of cerebellar neurons — the stellate cells (*a*) and the basket cells (*b*) — gather input from parallel fibers and inhibit Purkinje cells. In contrast, the Golgi cells (*c*) gather input from parallel fibers but inhibit granule cells. Finally, the cerebellar afferents called climbing fibers (*d*) disinhibit Purkinje cells. Two parts of the cerebellar circuit (parallel fibers and the Purkinje cell) are shown photographically in the next two illustrations.

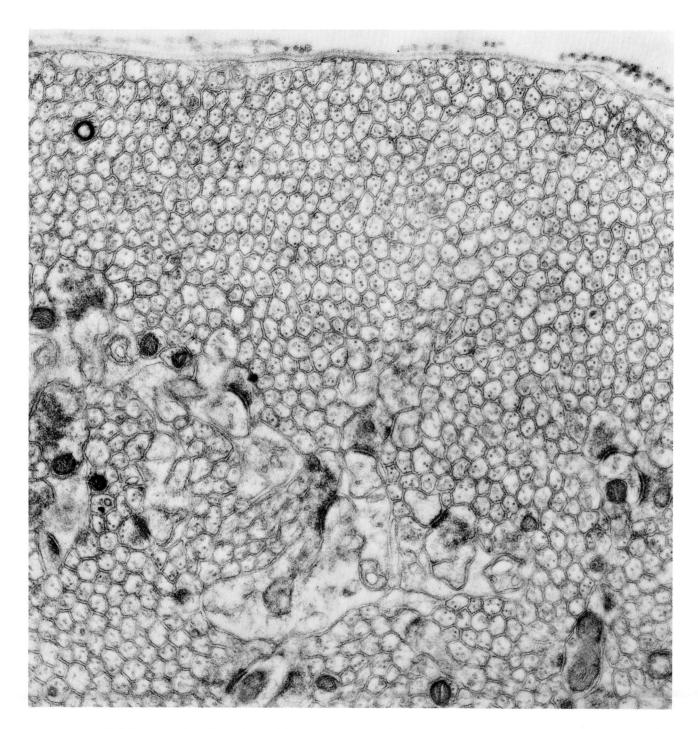

Figure 106: **Parallel fibers** pack the molecular layer of the cerebellar cortex. The field encompasses the cross section of a cerebellar folium on a plane between the territories of two consecutive Purkinje-cell dendritic trees. It is occupied almost exclusively by parallel fibers; even glial cells are lacking. Toward the bottom of the field a few neuronal processes appear. They are the dendritic spines of cerebellar neurons that gather input from parallel fibers. The electron micrograph, made by Sanford L. Palay of the Harvard Medical School, shows tissue from the cerebellum of a rat at an enlargement of approximately 30,000 diameters.

A second class of auxiliary circuits in the cerebellar cortex is established by basket cells. Again the dendritic tree is in a plane across the width of a folium. It, too, gathers input from parallel fibers. The cell body, however, lies deep in the molecular layer. The axon, too, is unique. Over a length of about a millimeter it courses across the width of a folium, emitting collaterals that descend to weave axonal baskets around the cell bodies of as many as 12 Purkinje cells. Hence the name basket cell. Side branches emerge from the trunk of the axon and also from the collaterals. They weave baskets around still other Purkinje cells. In this way a single basket cell participates in weaving axonal baskets around the cell bodies of a hundred or even two hundred Purkinje cells. Conversely, the basket around any one Purkinje cell is woven by several basket cells. The arrayal of the baskets means, of course, that the synapses of basket cells on Purkinje cells occupy the cell bodies of the latter. In fact, some of the synapses are axoaxonal: they occupy a Purkinje cell's initial axon segment. Their placement suggests a potent inhibition — indeed, the ability to veto the Purkinje cell's output at the very site where it is produced. One infers that the basket cell is a dominant inhibitor of the Purkinje cell's activity, far more so than a stellate cell, with its inhibitory synapses placed high in the Purkinje cell's dendritic tree.

A third class of auxiliary circuits in the cerebellar cortex is established by Golgi cells. In this case the cell body is high in the granular layer, just under the file of Purkinje cells. It spreads its dendrites throughout a spherical volume whose radius is perhaps half a millimeter; then most of the dendrites veer upward and invade the molecular layer. The Golgi cell is thus the only type of cell in the cerebellar cortex that seeks input in the molecular layer but fails to flatten its dendrites into a plane. Still, the dendrites get their input from parallel fibers. The crucial difference between the Golgi cell and the other auxiliary neurons of the cerebellar cortex (the stellate cell and the basket cell) is that the Golgi cell does not inhibit Purkinje cells. It inhibits granule cells. Specifically, the rich and widespread ramifications of the axon of a typical Golgi cell grip the claws of granule-cell dendrites, just as the claws of granule-cell dendrites grip the endings of mossy fibers. It can be said, then, that impulses traveling along parallel fibers are conveyed to the dendrites of four types of cells: Purkinje cells, which are the only projection cells in the circuit, since only their axons leave the cerebellar cortex; basket cells, whose axons exert a powerful inhibition on the cell bodies and initial axon segments of Purkinje cells; stellate cells, whose axons exert a more graded inhibition high in the dendritic trees of Purkinje cells; and Golgi cells, whose axons exert an inhibition at the places where impulses arrive in the cerebellar cortex.

One final piece of circuitry remains to be superimposed on what we have now described. It is the climbing fiber, a special line to the cerebellar cortex in that climbing fibers are the only cerebellar afferents that transmit their influence to Purkinje cells without the intervention of granule cells. On entering the cerebellum each climbing fiber, like a mossy fiber, gives off collaterals to the deep cerebellar nuclei. Then, however, it passes straight through the granular layer of the cerebellar cortex, and straight through the Purkinje-cell layer as well. In the molecular layer it establishes a quite remarkable terminal: its ramifications cling to the main dendritic trunks of a single Purkinje cell like a vine clinging to a trellis. The entire extent of the clinging is packed with synaptic vesicles. Indeed, the clinging might well be taken to establish a single gigantic synapse. Physiological findings concur. Each climbing fiber tends to be quiescent for some time, and then to give the Purkinje cell an excitation so intense it erases all preexisting inhibition imposed on that cell by the axons of basket cells and stellate cells. One wishes, of course, to know the parentage of this potent disinhibition. How does it serve the animal? What neural events bring it on? The answers are shrouded by the fact that climbing fibers appear to originate largely, perhaps exclusively, in the inferior olivary nucleus. True, the inferior olive gets somatic sensory input from the spinal cord by way of two paths, the spinothalamic tract and a projection from the dorsal column nuclei. (Whether the latter is a set of fibers independent of the medial lemniscus or simply collaterals emitted by certain fibers in the lemniscus is not known.) Yet each of these connections reaches no more than a limited part of the olive. Apparently the most massive fiber system afferent to the olive is the central tegmental tract, descending from brainstem levels rostral to the olive and originating in large part high in the midbrain reticular formation. It is entirely obscure just what the nature of the information it conveys to the olive might be.

A Curious Mismatch

Our survey of the cerebellar circuitry is done. Some details have been omitted. For example, axon collaterals loop from one Purkinje cell to another, and axon collaterals from the deep cerebellar nuclei loop back to the cerebellar cortex. But the basics are there. Surely the three-dimensional pattern is plain. Parallel fibers are axial in each folium, the dendrites of Purkinje cells are transverse, and so on. Perhaps most investigators would agree that these arrangements enable the cerebellum to help in governing the temporal order in bodily movement. In particular, the cerebellum seems to be a time-chopping device. After all, the parallel fibers each make synapses in great number as they pass at a right angle through a succession of Purkinje-cell dendritic

Figure 107: **Purkinje cell,** the projection cell of the cerebellar cortex, is shown in Golgi-stained tissue from the cerebellum of a rat. The view is obliquely downward. The dendritic tree of the cell fills much of the field of view; it consists of a few dendritic trunks, whose ramifications are all confined to a plane. The parts in sharp focus show that the tree is studded with dendritic spines. The Golgi treatment has left unstained the multitude of parallel fibers passing through its meshes. The flask-shaped cell body characteristic of a Purkinje cell is at the right. From its right-hand edge comes a faint, dark-staining wisp: the axon of the cell, which is not in sharp focus. The micrograph was made, at an enlargement of 1,000 diameters, by Sanford Palay.

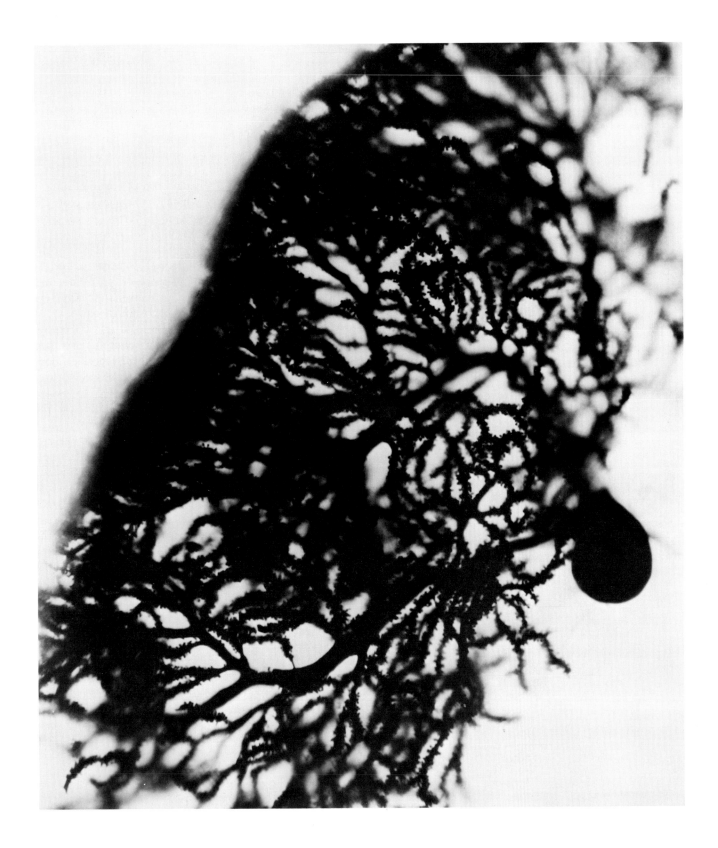

trees. Hence when an impulse from a granule cell travels into the molecular layer by way of a parallel fiber, certain alignments of Purkinje cells receive the synaptic message in strict sequential order. The concomitant spread of inhibition by stellate cells, basket cells, and Golgi cells must also proceed sequentially, though in a more complex fashion, arriving, as time goes on, at an ever widening field of Purkinje cells.

What, then, is so vexing about the cerebellar cortex? For one thing, a curious mismatch between the pattern by which the cerebellar cortex is afferented and the pattern by which disorders of movement result from various lesions. In brief, the mossy fibers conveying somatic sensory data from the spinal cord distribute themselves chiefly to the rostral half of the vermis; a second field of distribution is just lateral to the caudal part of the vermis. Either way, the somatic sensory afferents reach only a paramedian zone of the cerebellar cortex. Yet a lesion situated medially in the cerebellum affects only, or almost only, the trunk: it brings on trunk ataxia. A lesion situated laterally, where no somatic sensory fibers seem to end, affects the limbs. Conversely, the lateral expanse of the cerebellar hemisphere receives most of its mossy-fiber input from the pons, which in turn receives input from the entire expanse of the neocortex. Why should a disorder of movement peculiar to the limbs result from a lateral lesion?

A resolution is available: it is suggested by three findings. First is the clinical finding that when great regions of cerebellar cortex are destroyed by a lesion, a clear-cut disorder of bodily movement sometimes fails to emerge. Yet a much smaller lesion directly affecting the deep cerebellar nuclei brings on pronounced ataxic disorders. Second is the anatomical finding that the deep cerebellar nuclei receive afferents direct from the incoming fiber systems, mossy and climbing alike. Third is the finding, again anatomical, that the axons of Purkinje cells converge on the deep cerebellar nuclei. Their influence is inhibitory. All things considered, it seems conceivable that the pattern of connections in the deep cerebellar nuclei may prove to account for the pattern of movement disorder. That is to say, a somatotopic map in the depths of the cerebellum may prove to be more significant than the map known to exist at the surface. With that hypothesis, however, the intricate circuitry of the cerebellar cortex must be taken to provide no more than a fine tuning of what goes on deep in the organ. Why, then, should the cerebellar cortex have augmented so markedly in the course of evolution? Why should a large and varied set of structures in the central nervous system — including all of the neocortex — send data there? And why should the circuitry be the same throughout the cerebellar cortex, when the inputs to the cortex are so extraordinarily varied? Just what does the circuitry do? The lack of answers, despite the wealth of knowledge about the cerebellar circuitry, is both challenging and appalling.

Chapter Sixteen

Neocortex

The manifest regularity found in the cerebellar cortex makes it a striking contrast to the other, more prominent cortex, namely the cerebral cortex. In the former the basic circuit is known. Indeed, one dares think that nothing major remains to be learned about the pattern of neuronal interconnection. Yet function is elusive: no one can say just what the circuit does. In the latter — the cerebral cortex, and in particular neocortex — the situation is much the opposite. The circuit is poorly understood. No general pattern of neuronal interconnection has yet emerged; it may be that none exists. In fact, no one is certain how many types of neuron are there. The most conservative scheme distinguishes only three: the pyramidal cell, the stellate cell, and the fusiform cell. (Stellate cells, however, are often termed spiny or smooth.) Other schemes distinguish as many as 60. Yet discoveries are being reported; in not only the primary sensory fields but even association cortex, functional organizations are now being probed.

Neocortical Layers; Neocortical Axons

Figure 108 shows neocortical tissue in a Golgi preparation. The enlargement is modest; hence the figure serves to suggest the pervasiveness of neocortical neurons whose cell bodies are shaped like elongated triangles. They are the pyramidal cells of the cortex. The axon emerging at the base of each such pyramid characteristically descends into the cortical cable basement: the white matter under the cortex, which consists of axons that enter the cortex

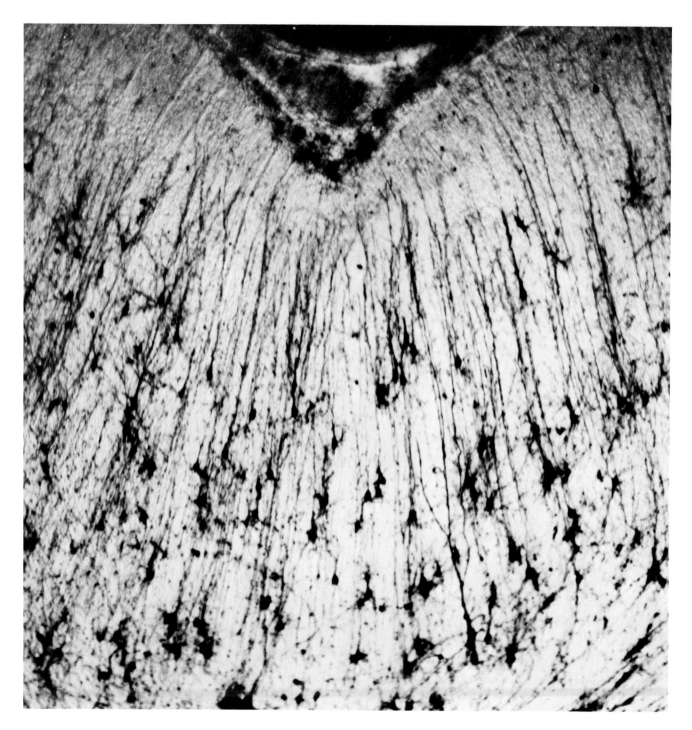

Figure 108: **Golgi-stained neocortex** demonstrates the pervasiveness of neocortical neurons shaped like an elongated pyramid. From each such cell an apical dendrite rises toward, and often into, the tissue's outermost, plexiform layer. The micrograph at the left spans the height of a field of parietal association cortex from the brain of a cat. At the top center the cortical surface dips; a few millimeters from the plane of the section the halves of the field become two neighboring gyri. The dark encrustations at the surface are artifacts unavoidable in a Golgi preparation. The lack of sharp focus is also unavoidable. In order to capture the palisadic appearance conferred on the

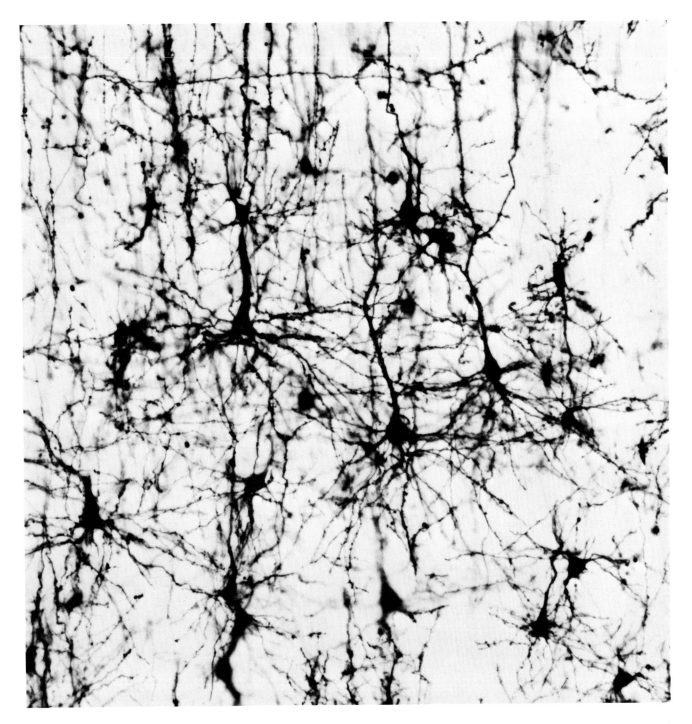

cortex by apical dendrites the section had to be about 100 micrometers thick, well beyond the depth of field of the microscope's optics; otherwise the full extent of any one apical dendrite would tend to stray out of the section. The micrograph at the right displays (at greater magnification) some Golgi-stained neurons from middle depths—layers 3, 4, and 5—of the cat's parietal cortex. Pyramidal cells are joined by stellate cells, which make up a second great class of neocortical neurons. The cell bodies of stellate cells are often distinctly nonpyramidal; the processes of the cells strike off in all directions. Thus a stellate cell has no apical dendrite.

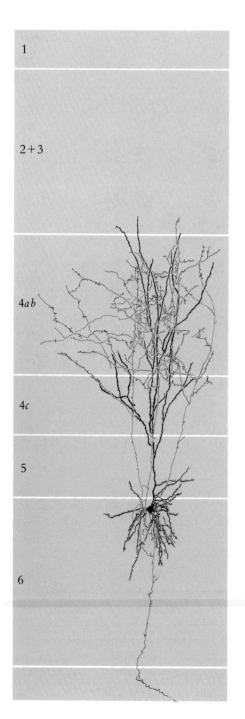

1

2+3

4ab

4c

5

6

(from the thalamus, for instance) and others that leave the cortex. The apex of each of the pyramids emits an apical dendrite. Often one can follow it into the plexiform layer, where it ramifies into what are called terminal arches. Neurons with apical dendrites are found throughout the cortex: that is, in every neocortical cell-containing layer, and in all neocortical fields. Still, many cortical dendrites do not join in the climb toward the plexiform layer. For one thing, the typical pyramidal cell (Figure 109) emits several dendrites at its base, and these processes, called basilar dendrites, are more or less parallel (not perpendicular) to the surface of the brain. In general they are shorter than apical dendrites. Furthermore, the neocortex has multitudes of neurons whose processes all remain quite local in distribution. Such neurons are the stellate cells of the cortex (Figure 110).

Figure 111 is a kind of counterpoint to Figure 108. It shows two fields of neocortex in a Nissl preparation, again with little enlargement. Now the cell layers are plain. To begin with, the tissue under the cortex is the cortical cable basement. Next, just above that white matter, is a densely stippled layer. It is the deepest layer—layer 6—of the neocortex. Each stipple reveals a cell. Some are glial cells. The glia tend to be masked, however, by the more impressive presence of neurons. In particular, layer 6 is notable for its content of large pyramidal cells, and also fusiform cells: spindle-shaped neurons found in no other layer. Immediately above it, layer 5 contains large (in some parts of the neocortex, very large) pyramidal cells. Then comes a layer characterized by a crowding of very small stellate cells, which are here called granule cells. This is layer 4; it is conspicuous throughout much of the neocortical expanse. Superficial to layer 4 is a broad zone of cells that are more loosely packed. This is layer 3; it is composed in large measure of small and medium-size pyramidal cells. Above it is the last cell layer, the second, containing small pyramidal cells as well as granule cells. Then, finally and outermost, comes the plexiform layer, in which sporadic neurons appear.

The number of layers in the cerebral cortex varies. A terminology introduced by Cécile and Oskar Vogt reflects the broadest distinction. In it the neocortex, with five cell layers under the plexiform layer, is denoted isocortex, from the Greek *isos,* meaning "the same." (In all mammals the neocortex is the largest of the cortical expanses.) In contrast, the two-cell-layered olfac-

Figure 109: **Pyramidal cell** in the primary visual cortex of a rhesus monkey exemplifies the individuality and complexity of neocortical neurons; this one deploys its processes from a cell body high in layer 6. Dendrites studded with spines emerge from the base of the cell body, and at the opposite end of the cell an apical dendrite ascends, emitting collaterals that all remain more or less vertical. In this cell the apical dendrite does not attain the plexiform layer; indeed, it gathers its input almost exclusively in layer 4. The axon descends; it is thinner than the dendrites. It, too, emits collaterals: recurrent collaterals that turn upward to layer 4. The main branch of the axon leaves the cortex. Since the cell is in layer 6, the axon descends to the thalamus, in particular the lateral geniculate body, from which the visual cortex gets its sensory input. The cell represents a corticothalamic feedback loop. The camera-lucida drawing was made by Charles Gilbert of the Rockefeller University.

tory cortex, also called paleocortex, and the one-cell-layered hippocampal cortex, also called archicortex, are denoted allocortex, from *allos,* meaning "other." The neocortical total of six is often contested: some investigators subdivide layers that others judge to be unitary. In any case, six layers can readily be distinguished in many parts of the neocortex, and this enables one to say that neocortex is the most highly evolved form of cortex, at least in terms of a count of layers. Besides, six-layered cortex is unique to the mammals, and so is the newest form of cortex to have arisen in evolution.

The six-layered neocortical pattern is not, however, unchanging. Nissl-stained sections of neocortex from different parts of the cerebral hemisphere establish that the neocortical layers vary from place to place in thickness, prominence, and composition. Layer 4 is perhaps the most inconstant. It is especially well developed in the primary sensory fields: the somatic, the auditory, and most notably the visual. Indeed, granule cells crowd so densely in layer 4 of a primary sensory field that Nissl preparations show the layer as a prominent dark band. (Examine Figure 24 and the right side of Figure 111.) Often one can see it without the aid of magnification. Accordingly, the primary sensory fields are termed koniocortex, or literally dusty cortex, from *konios,* the Greek word meaning dust. The term designates the extreme of a category called granular cortex. In contrast, layer 4 is poorly developed in the anterior half of the cingulate gyrus and most of the posterior half of the frontal lobe. They are thus termed dysgranular cortex. Finally, layer 4 is barely recognizable in the rearmost part of the frontal convexity; that is, in the motor cortex, which is hence termed agranular cortex. (Examine the left side of Figure 111.) In light of its varying pattern, the neocortex is construed to be a quiltwork consisting of areas or fields, each more or less uniform in cytoarchitecture and more or less distinct from its neighbors. Among the more distinct are the primary sensory fields, with their koniocortical pattern. The most distinct of all is the primary visual cortex, at the posterior pole of the brain. There, in man and most of the primates, layer 4 is in fact a pair of cell layers with a cell-poor stratum between (Figure 112). At the perimeter of the primary visual cortex the pair abruptly coalesce, as if to announce that one has entered a surrounding cortical belt in which a different form of information processing is embodied. Other parts of the cortical quilt are much more difficult to delimit. In the frontal association cortex, at the anterior pole of the brain, one investigator finds several fields where another sees only a single, homogeneous expanse of granular cortex. The commonly accepted patterns for neocortical parcellation are the map of Brodmann and the map of von Economo and Koskinas. They show considerable similarity. Nevertheless, the former uses numbers to designate more than 40 fields (Figure 113); the latter uses letters to designate roughly 80. That alone suggests there are differences of opinion.

One aspect of neocortical organization is common to all of the fields. Neocortical cross sections stained to demonstrate myelin show that the axons passing at a right angle through the cortical layers tend to aggregate at intervals into slender, tapering bundles that extend into the cortical gray

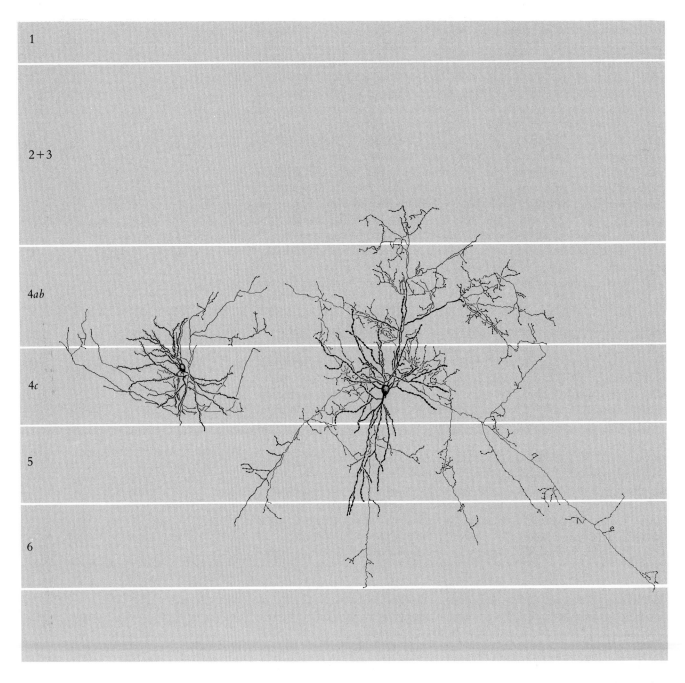

Figure 110: **Two stellate cells** in the primary visual cortex of a rhesus monkey were also drawn by Charles Gilbert. Both are in sublayer 4c, the deepest of the three strata composing layer 4 in a primate's visual cortex. Sublayer 4c is remarkable in that it includes no pyramidal cells. That is, all of its neurons are stellate. The cell on the left is a spiny stellate cell: its dendrites are studded with spines. It is typical of neurons in sublayer 4c. Its axon, thinner than its dendrites, ramifies somewhat more widely than the dendrites. The cell on the right is a smooth stellate cell: its spines are sparse. In some smooth stellate cells spines are totally absent.

matter like spikes from the underlying white (Figure 114). They are the radial fascicles of the cerebral cortex. Gradually tapering in girth, they can be followed to layer 3, in which they lose their identity. Most of the fibers in the fascicles turn out to be the axons of pyramidal cells in layer 3 and layer 5, and of pyramidal cells and fusiform cells in layer 6. The axons descend from the cells; thus the fascicles are the visible expression of a tendency among neocortical exit fibers to group themselves in compact bundles. The presence of the fascicles means that the deeper neocortical layers assume a radial organization. That is, the fascicles are more or less cell-free cortical radii, with cell-rich cortical radii intercalated between them.

The fibers in the fascicles obey the following pattern. The ones that descend from layer 5 and layer 6 are true projection fibers. The ones from layer 6 terminate in the thalamus; the ones from layer 5 terminate in the other subcortical stations to which the neocortex projects. In contrast, the fibers descending from layer 3 return to the neocortex. Some stay on one side of the brain: they are called ipsilateral corticocortical fibers or ipsilateral cortical association fibers. They make up a wealth of connections linking neocortical fields. The shortest among them connect neighboring gyri by curving through the floor of the intervening sulcus. They are aptly called U fibers. Others are longer, and in the subcortical white matter in the brain of a primate they tend to be grouped into massive bundles (Figure 115). A straightforward dissection can reveal their presence. Take a well-fixed human brain and pull apart the temporal and parietofrontal parts of the cerebral hemisphere, whose opercula, or lips, compose the Sylvian fissure. The white matter under the cortex will cleave in a quite predictable way, and the white matter exposed at the cleavage will have striations suggesting the orientation of the fibers. (In general, a cleavage deep enough to expose the corona radiata will show striations radial with respect to the insula. The association bundles are less deeply placed; thus a shallow cleavage will show striations more or less longitudinal in the forebrain.) Cortical association fibers projecting to neocortex on the opposite side of the brain also begin their course as constituents of the radial fascicles. They are called contralateral corticocortical fibers, contralateral cortical association fibers, cortical commissural fibers, or callosal fibers. The last term signifies that most such fibers pass from one hemisphere to the other through the corpus callosum, a massive commissure. (The remainder occupy the anterior commissure, a far smaller bundle.) The callosal fibers interconnect homotopic fields in the left and right cerebral hemisphere. Several regions, however, make no such cross-connection. In the monkey, for example, the part of the primary somatic sensory cortex that represents the hand (or rather the forepaw) is exempt from callosal participation. One is reminded of the biblical injunction that the left hand not know what the right hand doeth. But physiological experiments suggest that callosal fibers linking homotopic fields not far from the somatic sensory cortex on each side of the brain carry signals representing somatic sensation from the hand.

Neocortical cross sections stained to demonstrate myelin show not only

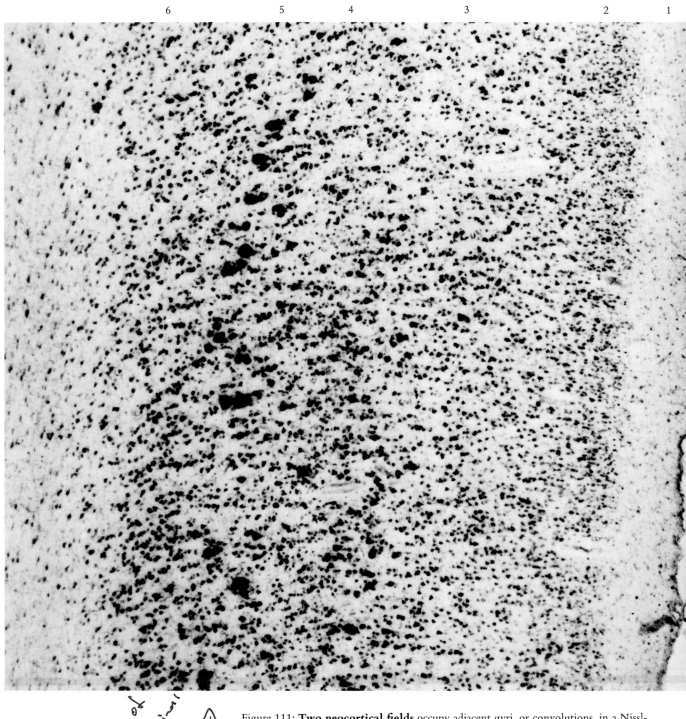

6   5   4   3   2   1

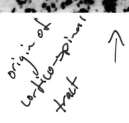

origin of cortico-spinal tract

Figure 111: **Two neocortical fields** occupy adjacent gyri, or convolutions, in a Nissl-stained human brain. Specifically, they form the walls of the central sulcus, the chasm at the center of this low-power micrograph. The fields are both six-layered. Moreover, the outermost layer — layer 1, the plexiform layer — is free of neuronal cell bodies. Beyond that, the fields are distinctly different. At the left, on the precentral gyrus, is motor cortex.

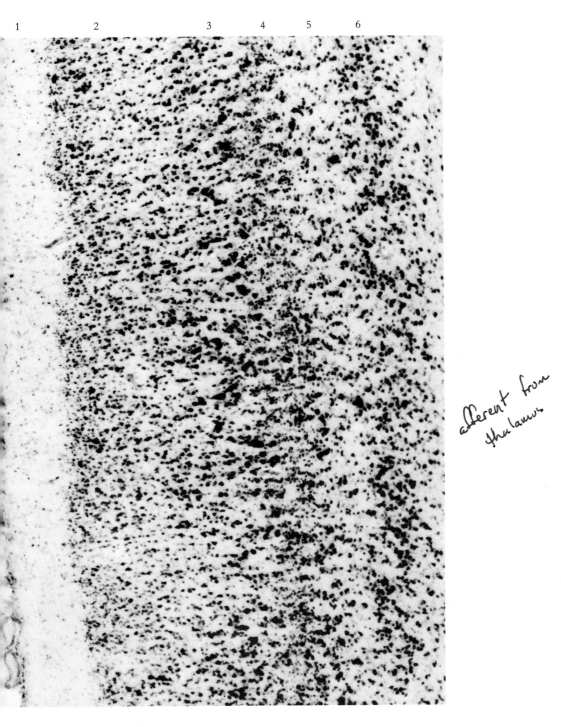

1   2   3   4   5   6

afferent from thalamus

The largest neurons there (that is, the largest stipples in the micrograph) are pyramidal cells in layer 5. They are the giant pyramids of Betz, unique to motor cortex. At the right, on the postcentral gyrus, is somatic sensory cortex. It is thinner than motor cortex. In somatic sensory cortex the largest neurons are in layer 3; layer 5 looks rather empty. In contrast, layer 4 is notable for a packing of small stellate cells.

radial fascicles but also tangential nets of fibers: nets consisting of axons whose course is parallel to the surface of the brain. Each net is thus at a constant depth in the cortical sheet. One such net forms the upper part of layer 3; it is called the stripe of Kaes-Bechterew: Theodor Kaes (a German neurologist) and Vladimir Bechterew. A second net forms a wider band that fills the thickness of layer 4; it is the outer stripe of Baillarger, named for the French neurologist Jules Gabriel François Baillarger, who was the first to

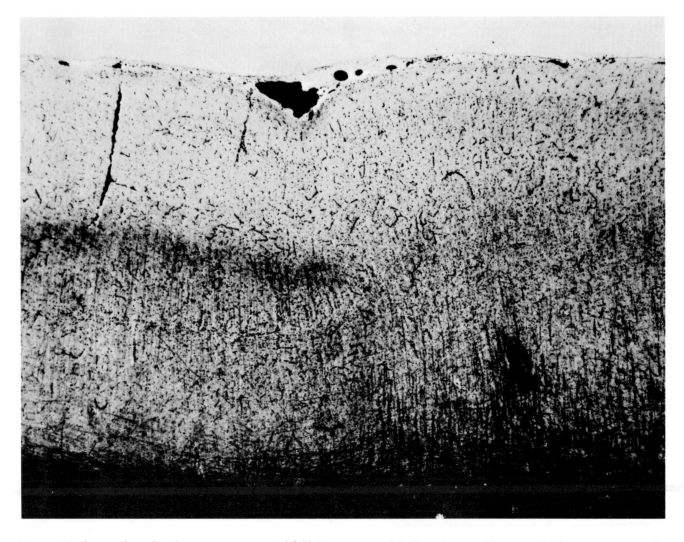

Figure 112: **Sharpest boundary** between two neocortical fields is the one between area 17, the primary visual cortex, and area 18, a surrounding band receiving fibers from the primary visual cortex. Here the boundary is shown in a human brain — specifically in sec- tions of the lingual gyrus of the occipital lobe. Two staining techniques were employed. The section at the left is Weigert stained: it was stained, that is, for myelin. The dark band at the middle of the thickness of the cortex in the left half of the field is the axon plexus

propose (in 1840) that cortical gray matter is six layered. In the primary visual cortex the stripe is prominent: it cleaves layer 4 into the pair of sublayers mentioned above. Hence in the primary visual cortex it is given a special name: it is called the line of Gennari, after Francesco Gennari, the Italian medical student who examined sections of a frozen human brain and so discovered the line, in the occipital gray matter, in 1776. A third and final net, the inner stripe of Baillarger, lies deep in layer 5. All three nets consist

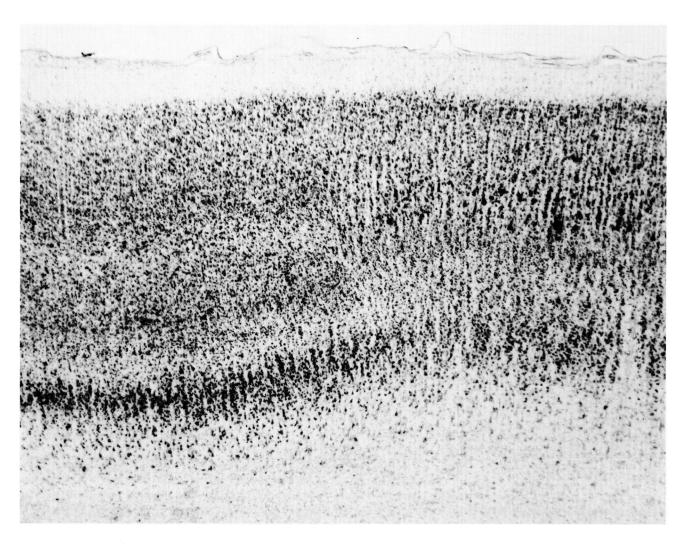

called the line of Gennari; it marks the primary visual cortex. Its upper boundary is the border between sublayers 4*a* and 4*b*; its lower boundary is somewhere in sublayer 4*c*. The section at the right is Nissl stained: it was stained, that is, for neuronal cell bodies. At the depth of the line of Gennari in the primary visual cortex (again the left half of the field) one sees a somewhat cell-poor zone: sublayer 4*b*. Above and below it, the rest of layer 4 is densely stippled with granule cells.

primarily of intrinsic cortical fibers. Almost certainly they include collaterals emitted by the axons descending from pyramidal cells. It is known that many of the axons emitted by large pyramidal cells in layer 5 and layer 6 give off branches that travel horizontally a short distance and then ascend through the cortex. The collaterals traverse layer 6 and layer 5 to attain layer 3 and layer 2, and sometimes even the plexiform layer. Then, too, the undercutting of the primary visual cortex, with the resulting Wallerian degeneration of fibers ascending from the lateral geniculate body, fails to notably diminish the line of Gennari. That means the line cannot consist substantially of the terminal ramifications of incoming sensory fibers.

Columnar Organization

The fiber architecture of the neocortex strongly suggests, therefore, the superposition of two patterns of organization, one radial, the other tangential, in the fashion of a skein. This makes it curious that investigators often center their attention on the former, the cortical woof, so the speak, without reference to the latter, the cortical warp. Surely the workings of neocortex are a reflection of both. On the other hand, the development of the microelectrode as a device for probing the physiological activity of individual neurons has made possible some dramatic discoveries about the radial pattern. In particular it has led to the discovery that neurons with remarkably similar response characteristics (a term from neurophysiology) are aligned throughout the primary sensory fields in columnar volumes of neocortex extending vertically through all six cortical layers. The first such finding was reported in 1957 by Vernon B. Mountcastle of Johns Hopkins University, who studied the primary somatic sensory area in the cat and in the monkey and found that cells in columnar volumes are responsive to stimuli applied to particular places on the surface of the body. The cells in a given column tend uniformly to be rapid or slow to adapt (that is, to stop responding) to a stimulus. Evidently the cells are preferentially sensitive not only to a particular site of somatic stimulation but also to a particular somatic sensory submodality. In the case of rapid adaptation, Mountcastle proposed that the sensory input to the column derives from touch sensation. Touch sensation is notoriously transient. One rapidly becomes unaware, for example, of the feel of the clothes one is wearing.

In the primary auditory cortex, columnar assemblies soon turned out each to be "tuned" to a particular frequency of sound. But it was in the primary visual cortex that a columnar organization and its significance became most strikingly apparent, mostly owing to studies conducted on the primary visual cortex of the cat by David H. Hubel and Torsten N. Wiesel at the Harvard Medical School. In the primary visual cortex of the cat the majority— perhaps the totality — of the cells in a given column responded preferentially to a bar of light that the investigators projected to a particular place on a dark wall confronting the animal. Many of the cells responded best when the bar was oriented a particular way or moved in a particular direction. Neighboring columns showed a similar preference for the location of the bar but different preferences for its orientation. A certain small locus of the primary visual cortex thus turns out to encompass a set of columns representing orientations at a given point in visual space. The locus evidently derives its information from one eye. Adjacent to it one finds a second locus containing a second collection of columns. They represent orientations at the same point in visual space, but they derive their information from the opposite eye. The two sets of columns compose a macrocolumn. It is approximately 800 micrometers in diameter, and it gives binocular representation to a point in visual space. Still, the data from each of the eyes are rigorously segregated. In fact, the macrocolumns are arranged so that input from each eye reaches alternating serpentine bands of the primary visual cortex. The overall pattern resembles the stripes on a zebra (Figure 116). To be sure, the layout of the primary visual cortex is topologically accurate: a line traced in any direction across the surface of the primary visual cortex will intercept the cortical representations of a connected sequence of parts of visual space. The point is that certain sinuous pathways over the cortical surface will lead one's microelectrode to successively encounter, in a series of penetrations, only columns representing afflux with parentage in the left (or right) retina, whereas a direction chosen

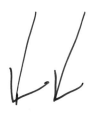

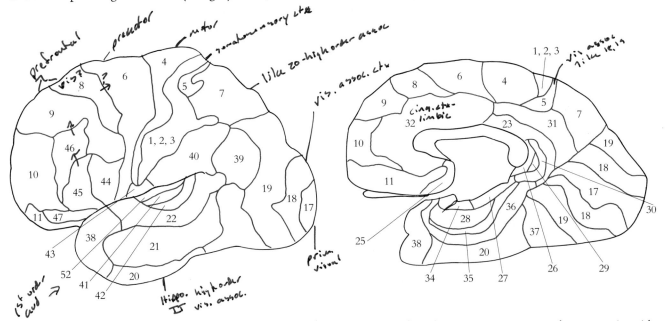

Figure 113: **Neocortical quiltwork** of areas or fields was mapped in 1909 by the German neurologist Korbinian Brodmann; his scheme is the one now favored for neocortical parcellation. In it the primary visual cortex is area 17; the primary auditory cortex (largely hidden on the upper face of the temporal lobe in the Sylvian fissure) is area 41; the primary somatic sensory cortex is areas 1, 2, and 3; the motor cortex is area 4. The speech areas are harder to place. Broca's area, not far from the motor cortex, is more or less coextensive with area 44; Wernicke's area, not far from the primary auditory cortex, is the convergence of three of Brodmann's areas: 22, 39, and 40. The cortical level for eye-movement control is even more elusive. The electrical stimulation of three areas—8, 19, and 22—can cause the eyes to turn in unison toward the contralateral side of the visual world.

at a right angle to any part of this pathway will reveal alternating bands of cortical columns, representing first one eye, then the other, and then again the first. The arrangement illustrates the capacity of cortical tissue to simultaneously map several variables. In 1982, Hubel, working with Margaret Livingstone at the Harvard Medical School, found still another map. Blob-shaped districts spaced at even intervals in layer 3 of the primary visual cortex contain cells preferentially sensitive to particular contrasting colors in partic-

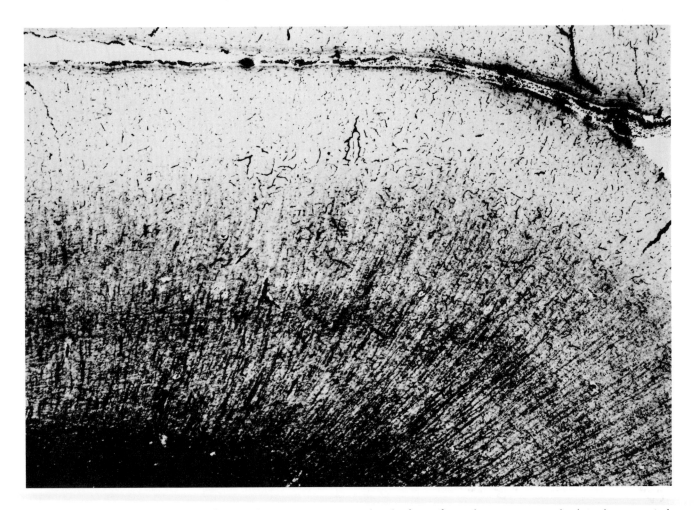

Figure 114: **Neocortical warp and woof** (that is, the superposition of radial and tangential organizations of neocortical axons) are found throughout the neocortex; here they are seen in a human brain, in Weigert-stained motor cortex. The radial organization takes the form of radial fascicles, which are especially clear toward the right. They are spikelike aggregations of neocortical efferent fibers descending through the cortical layers. The tangential organization takes the form of axonal nets at constant depth in the neocortical sheet. In motor cortex the most prominent example is the inner stripe of Baillarger, a dark-staining band found deep in layer 5. Above it, in layer 3, at the tips of the radial fascicles, the stripe of Kaes-Bechterew is much harder to see. A third net, the outer stripe of Baillarger, quite prominent in visual cortex, where it is called the line of Gennari, can barely be noted in motor cortex.

ular parts of visual space. It seems unarguable that the cortical representation of the topology of the retinas is determined by the rigorously topologic dispersal of fibers from each retina to the lateral geniculate body and the equally rigorous dispersal of fibers from the lateral geniculate body to the cortex. On the other hand, the sensitivity of cortical neurons to the pattern of brightness and motion of a visual stimulus, or to contrasts in color, is likely to be determined by a succession of local neuronal circuits in the retina, in the lateral geniculate body, and in the visual cortex itself.

How widespread are neocortical columns? They are ubiquitous, perhaps. For one thing, the orderly aggregation of neocortical efferent fibers into radial fascicles is found throughout the neocortex. Moreover, the projection of one neocortical field to another is remarkably well ordered. In a study done at the Massachusetts Institute of Technology Patricia Goldman-Rakic injected tritiated leucine into the neocortex on the convexity of the cerebral hemisphere a short distance behind the frontal pole of the brain of a monkey. Autoradiography then established that some of the corticocortical fibers originating on the convexity near the frontal pole made their synapses on the medial face of the cerebral hemisphere, in the retrosplenial area of the cingulate gyrus, just behind the corpus callosum. The synapses lay in a series of columnar volumes 200 to 500 micrometers in diameter that were segregated from one another by volumes of roughly similar width in which no such synapses were found (Figure 117). Neither the origin nor the target in this projection is a primary sensory field. Indeed, each is quite well insulated from the impact of sensory data newly arrived in the neocortex. For example, the origin—the cortex near the frontal pole—is a minimum of three synaptic steps (that is, three sequential projections) from the somatic sensory cortex; thus the target—the retrosplenial cortex—is a further step away. Moreover, each gets massive input from a thalamic cell group that has no lemniscal afferentation. The frontal cortex receives fibers from the mediodorsal nucleus; the retrosplenial cortex receives fibers from the anterior nucleus. One cannot so much as guess at the transformations imposed on neural signals when they encounter such way stations. And yet the prospect remains: if neocortical projections map neatly from column to column in even the most distant parts of the association cortex, a columnar organization may turn out to be basic to neocortex.

Association Fields

But what could be the significance of a columnar organization at a place remote from fresh sensory data? What form of information processing—and what kind of topologic map—could it serve at an advanced stage of the cascading neocortical circuitry? How can the topology of the binocular visual field remain the ordering principle throughout the full sequence of corticocortical projections that carries information of retinal origin into association cortex? How can frequency remain the ordering principle for auditory traf-

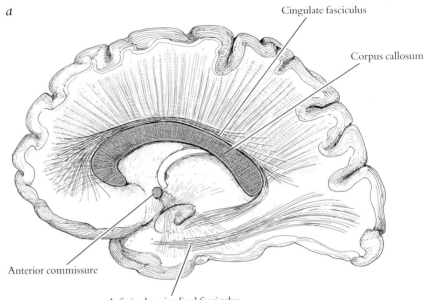

a

Cingulate fasciculus

Corpus callosum

Anterior commissure

Inferior longitudinal fasciculus

b

U fibers

Superior occipitofrontal fasciculus

Superior longitudinal fasciculus

Arcuate fasciculus

Uncinate fasciculus

Figure 115: **Association fibers** link neocortical fields. Some are simply *U* fibers, connecting neighboring gyri. Others, often far longer, produce systematic patterns of striation in the white matter under the neocortical sheet. In the aggregate the longer fibers are termed association bundles or fascicles. The drawings suggest the pattern exposed by a parasagittal, or lengthwise, cut made rather medially in the cerebral hemisphere (*a*) and the pattern exposed by a cut made somewhat more laterally (*b*). The drawings also include the two neocortical commissures, the anterior commissure and the corpus callosum (*color*).

fic? How can the topology of the body surface remain the ordering principle for somatic sensory traffic? What, then, is the ordering principle in a cortical field where traffic with antecedents in all three primary sensory fields comes into gross-anatomical overlap? By one recent count, eight maps of visual space are known in the cerebral cortex of the rhesus monkey. Thirteen are known in the cat, six in the rat, and four in the mouse. The more one looks, the more one seems to find. A physiological experiment revealing "visual areas" requires, however, that experimental animals be anesthetized when the microelectrode is in place. Under such a condition visual information continues to arrive in the neocortical sheet, but other brain function is surely abnormal. The argument can be continued in several ways. To begin with, researchers studying the neocortex always find cells that fit no easy physiological category: cells that have no simple sensitivity to light or to sound or to a touch on the skin. Moreover, fields of neocortex beyond the primary sensory fields have no single dominant input. They tend instead to have many inputs competing. This has a physiological correlate. In a primary sensory field, gross changes in the pattern of neuronal activity come in response to gross changes in sensory input, and beyond that come only with gross changes in the state of the animal, such as a transition from wakefulness to deep sleep. The cells in a primary sensory cortex are strongly driven by sensory input. In contrast, the patterns of neuronal activity beyond the primary sensory fields are continually changing, even when nothing seems to have changed in the animal's surroundings. What induces the modulation can only be described as the animal's motivational set. All things considered, many "sensory maps" in the neocortical sheet may lie in areas far more abstract in function than is suggested by any map of sensory input.

Some experiments done by Mountcastle and his colleagues at Johns Hopkins are almost a parable on these themes. The work concerns in part the superior parietal lobule, or area 5 of Brodmann, an association field just behind the somatic sensory cortex. It gets input direct from the latter. The work began with the training of monkeys. Each animal was taught to depress a telegraph key whenever a small light went on. The light would then dim slightly. The monkey was to keep the key depressed for a particular length of time. If the task was done correctly, the light would go out, and the monkey would get a reward: a small amount of orange juice. After an interval another trial would begin. Monkeys that learned to perform correctly were given further tasks. The monkeys would be trained to release the key and press a panel, or pull a lever, or choose between two levers. For a set of experiments described by Mountcastle and his colleagues in 1975, four monkeys mastered a full range of tasks after training sessions lasting well over a month. Single-cell recordings then were made for almost a thousand cells in area 5. Roughly two-thirds of the cells responded when the experimenter changed the position of one of the animal's limbs. Another tenth were driven by mechanical stimulation of the skin. They were much like cells of the somatic sensory cortex, yet in several ways they differed. For one thing, they tended to become undriveable when the animal was drowsy: arriving sensory data had no clamp on these cells comparable to the clamp such data exert on the primary sensory fields. Also, the cells responsive to mechanical stimulation had large receptive fields: in one case, the entire palm and much of the forearm and upper arm. These were hardly the neurons to make fine-grained sensory distinctions about the world. Then there were cells that could not be driven by sensory stimulation. They simply were not sensory cells. They accounted for roughly a tenth of the total. Some discharged when the animal reached out, but only if the animal reached "for an object he desires, such as food when he is hungry." The pattern of discharge was independent of the

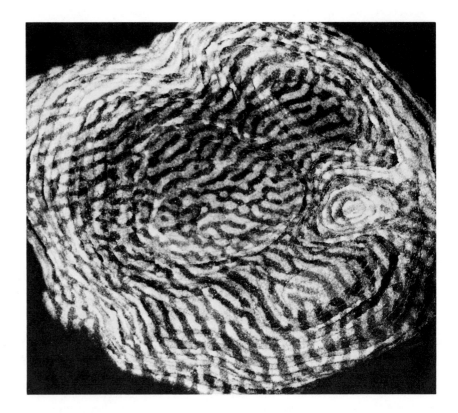

Figure 116: **Ocular dominance stripes** in layer 4 of the primary visual cortex demonstrate the ability of visual cortex to map the visual world while maintaining the segregation of the data from each eye. In the experiment that yielded this montage of dark-field autoradiographs a macaque monkey received in one of its eyes an injection of an amino acid (proline) labeled with tritium, or radioactive hydrogen. During the next two weeks the radioactivity was transported to the lateral geniculate body and then to layer 4 of the primary visual cortex, where the distribution of arriving axons confined it to a series of bands (*white stripes*). The intervening bands get their visual input from the opposite eye. The montage encompasses about a fourth of the total extent of area 17 on one side of the brain (the side ipsilateral to the labeled eye). The width of each stripe is about 350 micrometers. The experiment was done by Simon LeVay at the Harvard Medical School.

particular trajectory of the arm. Other cells discharged when the hand manipulated the object. One begins to suspect that the parietal association cortex concerns itself with *space*—the space that surrounds the animal and whose limit is defined by the reach of the animal's arm. Such space is an abstraction from sensory data; doubtless it is computed by the brain from vision, from touch, and from the arrayal of the body from instant to instant. Still, a problem persists. The curious neurons of area 5 fail to respond when objects are "uninteresting." So the brain must be deciding that certain objects are of greater interest than others. How, and where, are such decisions made?

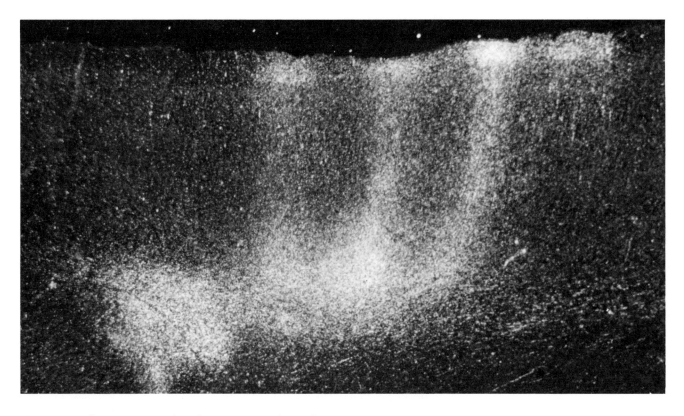

Figure 117: **Columns in retrosplenial cortex** suggest that a columnar organization may be basic to all neocortex, not just the primary sensory fields. Patricia Goldman-Rakic, who was then at the Massachusetts Institute of Technology, injected a tritiated amino acid (leucine) into association cortex near the frontal pole of the brain of a monkey. Autoradiography of the retrosplenial area (association cortex on the medial face of the cerebral hemisphere behind the splenium of the corpus callosum) then revealed that axons arriving from frontal cortex terminate in columnar volumes no more than 500 micrometers in diameter. Here three columns can be seen; the radioactive labeling is notably dense and circumscribed in the plexiform layer of the cortex. Further work by Goldman-Rakic has established that the intervening regions are the places where callosal fibers from the homotopic field on the opposite side of the brain make their synapses.

Chapter Seventeen

Prospects

Santiago Ramón y Cajal was born on the first of May, 1852, in the Spanish village of Petilla. His training in anatomy began in his fifteenth year; his teacher was his father, Don Justo Ramón Casasús, a noted surgeon (a step below physician) in the district of Aragon. The first lessons were osteological: father and son climbed the walls of a cemetery to pick out bones "half buried in the grass." The young Cajal "felt a special delight in taking apart and putting together again, piece by piece, the organic clock, and hoped some day to understand something of its intricate mechanism." (The quotes are from his autobiography.) Upon the completion of his secondary education, he undertook, at the Aragonese Medical School in Zaragoza, to become a doctor. He became in fact an army surgeon. By 1877 he had returned to Zaragoza; he had contracted malaria in a Cuban jungle. Through the kindness of a friend he was named to the post of temporary assistant in anatomy; two years later he became a temporary auxiliary professor. By then he had purchased (on installment, with his army savings) a microscope and a microtome. The microtome was poor; he reverted to using a barber's razor. His first investigations concerned the microscopic structure of cartilage, the cornea, the lens of the eye, and muscle fibers. The latter induced him to study nerve endings in muscle. Eventually, he turned to the nervous system itself. For that, the staining methods in wide use in the 1880's were inadequate. As Cajal later wrote: "The great enigma in the organization of the brain was the way in which the nervous ramifications ended and in which neurons were mutually connected. It was a case of finding out how the roots and branches of these trees in the gray matter terminate, in that forest so dense that there are no spaces in it, so that the trunks, branches, and leaves touch everywhere." Yet the ramifications were lost in the "dismal fog." The only recourse was to soften a block of tissue and then attempt with needles on the stage of a microscope to draw one nerve cell out from the forest. The occasional, triumphant result was the sight of a neuron. Even then, one learned only that neurons emit processes; that axons, for example, are not independent cellular entities.

A new staining technique — "the instrument of revelation" — already existed; it was the Golgi technique, discovered some years earlier by Camillo Golgi at Pavia in Italy. Cajal learned of it in 1887. In 1888 — "my greatest year, my year of fortune" — he employed it to establish the doctrine that neurons do not fuse but nonetheless transmit the nerve impulse by contact with one another. In 1892 he assumed the Chair of Normal Histology and Pathological Anatomy at Madrid. It was a time, he later remembered, of "devouring activity," as he "hunted cells with delicate and elegant forms, the mysterious butterflies of the soul, the beatings of whose wings may some day — who knows? — clarify the secret of mental life." By that time his investigations centered on cerebral cortex. In particular, he extended his studies to the human cerebral cortex, seeking to find a qualitative difference between the brains of people and animals; suspecting otherwise, it seemed to him, was "a little unworthy of the dignity of the human species." He began with the primary visual cortex; later came studies of other cortical fields. "The functional superiority of the human brain," he finally decided, "is intimately linked up with the prodigious abundance and unaccustomed wealth of forms of the so-called neurons with short axons." It is linked, that is, to the intricate interconnections of local-circuit neurons. That was the essence of the problem of cerebral cortex. "I desired to determine as far as possible its fundamental plan. But, alas! my optimism deceived me. For the supreme cunning of the structure of the gray matter [in cerebral cortex] is so intricate that it defies and will continue to defy for many centuries the obstinate curiosity of investigators."

Forms of Cunning

Was Cajal correct? Will centuries be required? Or will the brain be just as cunning then? At the end of this account of neuroanatomy it seems appropriate to suggest a few of the issues. We have three in mind. They are: specificity versus nonspecificity, the direction of information flow, and systems in the brain.

Specificity versus nonspecificity. The term nonspecific signifies a brain structure whose inputs are inhomogeneous, or multimodal. In practice, therefore, it signifies a structure whose cells are converged on by numerous projections. Examples are many. In the reticular formation the neurons are nonspecific, at least in their afferentation. (They may be quite choosy about where they send their axon.) Conversely, the term specific signifies a brain structure whose inputs are unimodal. Examples are few. The ones most often cited are the specific sensory relay nuclei of the thalamus. Yet even they are not truly specific. They, too, are likely to have auxiliary inputs with a modulatory function. For one thing, the monoaminergic projections arising in the brainstem are invaders of even the cell groups one most wants to think of as unimodal. Both specificity and nonspecificity would seem to have a role in the organization of the brain. Specificity, for instance, would allow the preservation of a sensory map; nonspecificity would allow the brain to distill from its sensory input a baseline state of activity. In this regard, the ventromedial nucleus (the most medial part of the ventral lateral nucleus of the thalamus) is remarkable. The ventromedial nucleus receives input from the substantia nigra, and it dispatches two projections to neocortex. One of them follows the pattern of a specific thalamocortical projection both by distributing its terminals in a well-defined part of the neocortical sheet (in particular, a part of the frontal association cortex) and by terminating preferentially in certain neocortical cell layers (in particular, layer 3, layer 4, and layer 6). The second projection is blatantly nonspecific. It is extensive: it ignores the boundaries between neocortical fields. Indeed, in the rat it distributes its fibers in gradually diminishing number from the frontal pole far enough to the rear so that some of them enter even the primary visual cortex. Then, too, the projection confines its terminals to layer 1, the plexiform layer. In fact, it confines its terminals to the upper half of layer 1, just under the pia mater. Thus the terminals influence the very farthest reaches of the apical dendrites of pyramidal cells in all neocortical layers. Two projections to neocortex, specific and nonspecific but produced by a single cell group. It suggests how hollow one's pronouncements can sound when they come up against the particulars of the brain.

The direction of information flow. The investigator tracing pathways in the brain is most certain of the significance of a discovery when the tracing begins at a sensory surface and works its way inward from there. In such an undertaking, the investigator can offer the brain a sensory stimulus—a touch of the skin, an auditory tone, a spot of light on the retina—and feel assured that it resembles what sensory neurons are primed to respond to. In a motor path the situation is less accommodating. The tracing is countercurrent: it goes against the direction of impulse traffic. Hence a peripheral excitation has no physiological significance. Suppose the investigator just chooses a neuron and applies electric current. In effect, the investigator raises an electrical storm: crude electrical activity having essentially no resemblance to the complex convergence of neural influences acting at, say, a local motor apparatus. In any case, it suits the understanding of the brain to trace signals from an array of sensory receptors to a processing station in the spinal cord or the brainstem, to trace from there a lemniscal ascent to the thalamus, and from the thalamus a final link to the cerebral cortex. It then seems sensible to say that the organism has felt something, or heard something, or seen something, and that the organism is poising itself to make appropriate responses to its environment.

Plainly the conduction paths that allow for such responses are essential for survival. Yet an organism may have equal need for information flowing in the opposite direction. A fairly straightforward example is the projection by which a primary sensory field in the neocortex reciprocates its thalamic afferentation. The somatic sensory cortex extends the reciprocation by directing some of its descending fibers to the dorsal-column nuclei, the source of the medial lemniscus. Still, the fibers are on the sensory side of the organization: they could enable the neocortex to screen its sensory input. A more recondite example is the projection by which the amygdala plays on the temporal association fields from which it gets neocortical input. Here one can argue that the amygdala participates in the neocortical appreciation of the world. Perhaps the neocortical appreciation of the world is being assayed for its potential impact on the organism. An intriguing example involves the superior colliculus. That structure emits two projections. One, directed downward, is tectobulbar and tectospinal. Clearly it is motoric: it suggests the superior colliculus is involved in directing the gaze. The other projection, directed upward, attains the district of the pulvinar called the lateral posterior nucleus, which projects in turn to large expanses of association cortex, thus creating the "second visual pathway" shown in Figure 38. Why has nature installed this second path? An answer is implicit in one of the brilliantly simple observations the German physicist and physiologist Hermann von Helmholtz offered more than a century ago. Helmholtz noted that when the eyes move, or the head, the image of the world must sweep across the retina. Yet the visual world stands still. (In fact, a person engaged in the act of turning infallibly remarks the rabbit moving through an otherwise motionless landscape.) In contrast, the poke of an eye with a finger makes the visual world seem to jump. Evidently the oculomotor stations of the brain are capable of warning the visual sensory stations that the eyes are about to be moved. It is as if certain motor stations can instruct sensory stations to turn their map of the world so as not to get befuddled.

Systems in the brain. The nomenclature devised by neuroanatomists sometimes seems to suggest that the brain can be divided into modules or systems, like well-designed electronics. Take the telencephalon — the endbrain, or cerebral hemisphere. Broadly speaking, it consists of three anatomical realms: the neocortex, the limbic system, and the extrapyramidal motor system. But is it three distinct kingdoms? Not really. The neocortex and the limbic system merge in numerous places. The amygdala is limbic, but it communicates with temporal neocortex. The frontal association fields are neocortical, but they communicate with the hypothalamus. The limbic system and the extrapyramidal motor system merge in numerous places. The nucleus accumbens is a part of the striatum, but it projects to the hypothalamus. Dopamine cell group A-10 in the ventral tegmental area is a part of the substantia nigra; with the rest of the dopaminergic cell population of the nigra it innervates the striatum, but it lies in the path of the principal limbic highway, the medial forebrain bundle. The extrapyramidal motor system and the neocortex merge in at least one place: the extrapyramidal system is a great looping circuit by which a distillate of neocortical activity can be brought to bear on the motor cortex after passing sequentially through the striatum, the pallidum, and the thalamus.

The extrapyramidal motor system, with its center, the striatum, exemplifies the problematic nature of brain "systems." Surely no other part of the brain has a more varied set of inputs. After all, the striatum receives afferents from every field of the neocortex. It receives afferents from both of the principal limbic structures, the hippocampus and the amygdala. It receives afferents from the nonspecific nuclei of the thalamus. It receives dopaminergic afferents from the substantia nigra and serotonergic afferents from the mesencephalic raphe nuclei. Could all that be intended purely as input for a "motor system"? Could it serve only to fine-tune the contraction of skeletal muscle? It seems a poor design, especially since much of the striatal outflow appears to be channeled back to the domain of its origin: to the neocortex or to the limbic system. What, then, is the striatum? Consider that bodily movement and goal-directed thought both require motivation: an effort to get them started, an effort to keep them "on track." They share a need for feedback: an allowance for corrective adjustment. They are physiologically coupled: ideation often initiates unintentional changes in bodily posture and facial expression. Finally, they seem to have inverse relations to dopamine, which is, among other things, the nigrostriatal transmitter. The ideational disorder characteristic of schizophrenia often responds to drugs that block neural signal transmission from dopaminergic neurons. Yet such drugs, administered chronically, can bring on somatic motor disorders resembling parkinsonism. It is as if schizophrenia and parkinsonism were derangements at opposite chemical poles, schizophrenia resulting from an excess of dopamine and parkinsonism from a dearth.

Is the striatum a place where brain mechanisms of movement, thought, and motivation intersect? It is difficult to say. Movement itself resists our understanding. One imagines that thought or motivation must be harder things to probe. Yet after a century of intensive brain research one cannot even say where in the brain the impulse to a deliberate bodily movement arises, or by what sequence of steps it becomes expressed in the necessary patterns of motor-neuronal activation and inhibition.

Complexity at Each Level

What in fact does it mean to "understand the brain?" In 1977, David Marr and Tomaso Poggio, at the Massachusetts Institute of Technology, formulated three levels of understanding. The first is the level of computation. In addressing this level one asks: What tasks must the brain accomplish? That is, why must the brain map information from one form into another? The second is the level of algorithm. One asks: What sequence of operations puts information into a useful form? The third is the level of hardware. One asks: How might the apparatus available in the brain — that is, the neurons and their synaptic interconnections—execute an algorithm and thus perform a computation? No level accounts for everything. (As Marr writes, one cannot understand flight by studying the structure of a feather.) Yet each level constrains the others. In particular, an algorithm is constrained by the nature of the computation it is intended to perform. Also, it is constrained by the hardware with which it is implemented. It is constrained, therefore, by what neurons can do.

Some examples may help; they come from the study of vision. Item: The reconstruction of the three-dimensional visual world from the two-dimensional images that the world casts on the retinas is a computation. The sequence of operations that extracts useful clues from the two-dimensional images (including shadings, textures, and binocular disparities) is an algorithm. The neuronal networks that execute the algorithm are hardware. Presumably the networks begin in the retina with neurons sensitive to patterns of illumination along particular lines of sight, and continue first in the lateral geniculate body and then in the primary visual cortex, with neurons that extract "edges" of brightness from visual data. Item: The recognition of a face is a computation. The representation of the face in a form that frees it from the changeable circumstances of illumination and viewing angle, so that the face can be compared with remembered faces, requires an algorithm. Again, neuronal networks are the hardware.

Neuroanatomy, along with neurophysiology and neurochemistry, is of course the study of hardware: the third of the levels at which the brain must be understood. But since the levels are coupled, the anatomy resonates. It is certainly the level at which computations and algorithms must find their embodiment in the brain, and the level at which understanding must be tested. Consider, then, a block of primary visual cortex subjacent to one square millimeter of the surface of the brain. How many neurons are in that block of cortex? The answer is readily available. T. P. S. Powell and his colleagues at Oxford University have shown that the number of neurons in a cylindrical volume of neocortex 30 micrometers in diameter extending vertically through all six cortical layers is virtually constant, at about 110, in motor cortex, in somatic sensory cortex, and in frontal, parietal, and temporal association fields, in spite of the variations these places show in architecture, and presumably in function. (Human motor cortex is roughly five millimeters thick. Visual cortex is less than half that.) Equally surprising, the number is the same in the brain of mouse, rat, cat, monkey, and man. There is, however, a single exception. It is the primary visual cortex of a primate, where the number more than doubles, despite the relative thinness of the neocortical sheet in the primary visual area. The doubling is surely a consequence of the extraordinary crowding of stellate cells into layer 4 of the primary visual cortex. There are from 260 to 270 neurons in a block of the visual cortex with surface dimensions of 25 by 30 micrometers. A simple calculation gives the figure for a block with surface dimensions of a millimeter square. It is roughly 300,000.

Examine layer 4 of the block. The cortical afferents arising in the lateral geniculate body terminate densely there, with collaterals terminating in layer 1 and layer 6. Layer 4 is therefore crucial. In a primate's visual cortex it consists of three sublayers, designated *a, b,* and *c* by Brodmann. Examine sublayer 4*c*. It is notable in two ways. First, it contains no pyramidal cells, but only stellate cells. Second, it receives the thalamocortical axons emitted by *X* cells in the lateral geniculate body. The *X* cells are slow-adapting: the activity they generate in response to a visual stimulus tends to be long-lived. (In contrast, the *Y* cells of the lateral geniculate body are rapid to adapt: they respond fleetingly to their stimuli.) All in all, sublayer 4*c* is a rather circumscribed compartment of the primary visual cortex. Sublayer 4*c* is roughly 140 micrometers thick. The primary visual cortex is more than 10 times thicker. But let sublayer 4*c* have 15 percent of all the neurons in the primary visual cortex; we are trying to be conservative. It has, then, 40,000 cells for each square millimeter of its extent.

What about their input? Most investigators would agree that the number of neurons in the lateral geniculate body is not much greater than the number of optic-nerve fibers arriving there from the eyes. The latter figure is a million. Let all the cells in the lateral geniculate body project to the visual cortex; again, we are trying to be conservative. And let the surface area of the primary visual cortex be 1,500 square millimeters. Curiously, that number is the most uncertain one in this sequence of calculations. You will search without success for a diagram in the literature of neuroanatomy showing the neocortex flattened, much as the round earth is flattened by a geometer's ploy, to yield a map on which one can judge the size of the primary visual cortex and compare it with those of other fields, much as one would judge the size of Texas and compare it with that of France. Still, if a million fibers make their connections under 1,500 square millimeters of the neocortical surface, then each square millimeter, with its 300,000 cells, gets a mere 700 fibers. Even if they terminate entirely in sublayer 4*c* — which is not true, but imagine it is — they drive 40,000 cells.

How do the fibers make their connections? Each fiber resembles a string of rosary beads. The beads are terminal boutons. If each fiber has 1,000 boutons, then each square millimeter of sublayer 4*c* has 700,000, or roughly 15, on average, for each of its stellate cells. Now, just as the boutons are sites where the fiber gives off chemical signals, so are dendritic spines the sites where a neuron receives them. How many spines adorn a stellate cell? Say, 500; the number derives from a count made by Edward White at the Boston University School of Medicine. How many spines are met by each bouton? Say, four. The 15 boutons allotted to each cell and bringing it visual sensory data must then claim the attention, so to speak, of 60 dendritic spines, from the total of 500. That is only 12 percent. The cell has other inputs; indeed, the other inputs dominate, if only numerically. In every case the estimates seem to confound one's intuitions. One seems always to underestimate the complexity of the brain.

A final calculation now remains to be done. Consider once again the estimated 300,000 neurons beneath each square millimeter of surface in the primary visual cortex. How many of these neurons project their axons, which is to say, their output, beyond the primary sensory field? Two-thirds? Then some 200,000 fibers leave each square millimeter, when only 700 enter, freighted with visual data. The ratio of output to input is well over 200 to one. A daring guess might well have been five to one — a failure of intuition. The ratio is a reminder that the complexity of the brain is no less than fantastic. Another number is equally suggestive. Remember that sensory information spreads outward from the primary sensory fields. Some neocortical fields get fairly "pure" sensory data; others do not. Some progressions are linear; others are not. Still, the successive transformations performed on the sensory data summon up memories, words, behavior, emotion, expectations about the future. The transformations render the brain more successful at finding its way in the world. In the course of the transformations the time delays from field to field in the neocortex mount up into tenths of a second. But that is a number close to forever on the scale of neural activity; the time consumed by any single synaptic interruption in the path of a given signal can delay the processing of the signal by no more than a hundredth of that. What might the brain accomplish, on a time scale of tenths of a second? The asking of such a question evokes appreciation of the work that lies ahead.

Acknowledgments

Many people had a hand in the making of this book. Francis Crick's help came early: at the Salk Institute he read a preliminary draft of Part II and offered detailed comments; then, in 1979, his questioning of the investigators gathered in Woods Hole, Massachusetts, for a conference on cerebral cortex yielded the numerical estimates underlying the sequence of calculations regarding primary visual cortex that now concludes Part III. Among later readers of drafts of the book Floyd E. Bloom, now at the Scripps Clinic in La Jolla, California, and Sanford L. Palay of the Harvard Medical School were especially diligent and helpful. In addition they coached us on particular aspects of the neurosciences. In doing so they joined others who lent us their insight and expertise: A. J. Hudspeth of the School of Medicine of the University of California at San Francisco, Rodolfo R. Llinás of the New York University School of Medicine, Bryce L. Munger of the Hershey Medical Center of Pennsylvania State University, Pasko Rakic of the Yale University School of Medicine, James L. Roberts of the College of Physicians and Surgeons of Columbia University, Gordon M. Shepherd of the Yale University School of Medicine, and Richard J. Wurtman of the Massachusetts Institute of Technology. Illustrations came from several of those investigators, and from many others: David Barry of Bolt, Beranek & Newman, Inc., Milton W. Brightman of the National Institutes of Health, John E. Dowling of Harvard University, Charles R. Gerfen of the National Institutes of Mental Health, Charles Gilbert of the Rockefeller University, Patricia Goldman-Rakic of the Yale University School of Medicine, P. P. C. Graziadei of the Florida State University at Tallahassee, Miles Herkenham of the National

Institutes of Mental Health, David H. Hubel of the Harvard Medical School, Robert S. Kimura of the Massachusetts Eye and Ear Infirmary, Simon LeVay, who is now at the Salk Institute, M. M. Mesulam of the Harvard Medical School, Haring J. W. Nauta, who is now at the University of Texas Medical Branch in Galveston, Peter Paskevich of the Mailman Research Laboratories of McLean Hospital in Belmont, Massachusetts, Max Pavans de Ceccatty of the Université Claude Bernard in Lyon, Cedric S. Raine of the Albert Einstein College of Medicine of Yeshiva University, Arnold B. Scheibel of the School of Medicine of the University of California at Los Angeles, Peter S. Spencer of the Albert Einstein College of Medicine, Robert E. Waterman of the University of New Mexico School of Medicine, and Josiah N. Wilcox of the College of Physicians and Surgeons of Columbia University. Drawings came from three artists. The anatomical illustrations throughout the book were done by Carol Donner; the schematic drawings of brain circuitry in Part II were done by Gabor Kiss; a number of drawings (including the representations of neurotransmitter molecules in Figures 13, 14, and 15) were done by Edward Bell. Dozens of photographs are given no attribution. They come from M.I.T. There Diane Major made the histological preparations; Henry Hall did the photography. The Weigert-stained brainstem cross sections in Chapters 11 and 12 were the hardest of their tasks. Exceptionally well fixed human brain tissue was provided by Friedrich von Klützow of the Veterans Administration Hospital in Wichita. Two illustrations (the Nissl-stained motor neurons of Figure 7 and the astrocytes of Figure 18) posed special histological challenges; for them human brain tissue was provided by Neil W. Kowall of the Massachusetts General Hospital. At M.I.T. Ann M. Graybiel sheltered the photographic side of the effort. Also at M.I.T. Rigmor C. Clark smoothed our road in innumerable ways. The frontal sections appearing in color in Chapter 14 were selected from a unique collection of human brain sections presented to the Harvard Medical School by the late Paul I. Yakovlev. The Golgi preparations appearing in Figures 4, 6, and 108 were selected from a series of Golgi- and Nissl-stained sections of the brain of a cat, given to us by Enrique Ramón-Moliner of the University of Sherbrooke. At W. H. Freeman and Co., Michael Suh designed the book and heroically took on himself the layout of all of its pages. Perry Bassas steered the pages through the intricacies of production. A platoon of typists coped with successive drafts of the text. Gertrude Swope typed the final draft, and also the one after that.

Bibliography

Some Books for Further Reading:

Angevine, J. B., Jr., and Cotman, C. W. 1981. *Principles of Neuroanatomy.* Oxford University Press.

Brodal, A. 1981. *Neurological Anatomy in Relation to Clinical Medicine,* third edition. Oxford University Press.

Carpenter, M. B. 1976. *Human Neuroanatomy,* seventh edition. Williams & Wilkins Co.

Cooke, I., and Lipkin, M., Jr., editors. 1972. *Cellular Neurophysiology: A Source Book.* Holt, Rinehart and Winston, Inc.

Cooper, J. R., Bloom, F. E., and Roth, R. H. 1982. *The Biochemical Basis of Neuropharmacology,* fourth edition. Oxford University Press.

DeArmond, S. J., Fusco, M. M., and Dewey, M. M. 1976. *A Photographic Atlas: Structure of the Human Brain,* second edition. Oxford University Press.

Heimer, L. 1983. *The Human Brain and Spinal Cord.* Springer-Verlag, Inc.

Herrick, C. J. 1924. *Neurological Foundations of Animal Behavior.* Henry Holt and Co.

Kandel, E. R. 1976. *Cellular Basis of Behavior: An Introduction to Behavioral Neurobiology.* W. H. Freeman and Co.

Kandel, E. R., and Schwartz, J. H., editors. 1985. *Principles of Neural Science,* second edition. Elsevier Science Publishing Co.

Katz, B. 1966. *Nerve, Muscle and Synapse.* McGraw-Hill Book Co.

Kuffler, S. W., and Nicholls, J. G. 1985. *From Neuron to Brain: A Cellular Approach to the Function of the Nervous System,* second edition. Sinauer Associates.

Mountcastle, V. B., editor. 1980. *Medical Physiology,* 14th edition. C. V. Mosby Co. Two volumes.

Netter, F. H. 1983. *Nervous System. Part I. Anatomy and Physiology.* The CIBA Collection of Medical Illustrations, Volume I. CIBA Pharmaceutical Co., West Caldwell, N.J. 07006.

Nieuwenhuys, R., Voogt, J., and van Huijzen, C. 1978. *The Human Nervous System. A Synopsis and Atlas.* Springer-Verlag, Inc.

Peters, A., Palay, S. L., and Webster, H. de F. 1976. *The Fine Structure of the Nervous System.* W. B. Saunders Co.

Shepherd, G. M. 1979. *The Synaptic Organization of the Brain,* second edition. Oxford University Press.

Shepherd, G. M. 1983. *Neurobiology.* Oxford University Press.

Siegel, G. J., and Albers, R. W. 1981. *Basic Neurochemistry,* third edition. Little, Brown and Co.

Stedman's Medical Dictionary, 23rd edition (1976) or 24th edition (1981). Williams & Wilkins Co.

Warwick, R., and Williams, P. L. 1973. *Neurology.* In *Gray's Anatomy,* 35th British edition. W. B. Saunders Co. Also published separately by Saunders, in 1975, as *Functional Neuroanatomy of Man.*

Weiner, H. L. 1978. *Neurology for the House Officer,* second edition. Williams & Wilkins Co.

Worden, F. G., Swazey, J. P., and Adelman, G., editors. 1975. *The Neurosciences: Paths of Discovery.* M.I.T. Press.

Selected References:

Invertebrate Nervous Systems

Bullock, T. H., and Horridge, G. A. 1965. *Structure and Function in the Nervous System of Invertebrates.* Two volumes. W. H. Freeman and Co.

Pantin, C. F. A. 1952. "The Elementary Nervous System." *Proceedings of the Royal Society of London, Series B,* 140:147–168.

Parker, G. H. 1919. *The Elementary Nervous System,* J. B. Lippincott Co.

Pavans de Ceccatty, M. 1974. "The Origin of the Integrative Systems: A Change in View Derived from Research on Coelenterates and Sponges." *Perspectives in Biology and Medicine,* Spring, 1974, 379–390.

Pavans de Ceccatty, M. 1974. "Coordination in Sponges: The Foundations of Integration." *American Zoologist* 14:895–903.

Young, J. Z. 1964. *A Model of the Brain.* Oxford University Press.

Embryology

Cowan, W. M. 1979. "The Development of the Brain." *Scientific American* 241(3):112–133.

Hamilton, N. J., and Mossman, H. W. 1972. *Human Embryology,* fourth edition. Williams & Wilkins Co.

Hughes, A. F. W. 1968. *Aspects of Neural Ontogeny.* Academic Press.

Jacobson, M. 1978. *Developmental Neurobiology,* second edition. Plenum Publishing Corp.

Rakic, P. 1978. "Neuronal Migration and Contact Guidance in the Primate Telencephalon." *Postgraduate Medical Journal* 54:25–40.

Rakic, P. 1979. "Genesis of Visual Connections in the Rhesus Monkey." In *Developmental Neurobiology of Vision,* Freeman, R. D., editor. Plenum Publishing Corp.

Rakic, P., and Riley, K. P. 1983. "Overproduction and Elimination of Retinal Axons in the Fetal Rhesus Monkey." *Science* 219:1441–1444.

Schmechel, D. E., and Rakic, P. 1979. "A Golgi Study of Radial Glial Cells in Developing Monkey Telencephalon: Morphogenesis and Transformation into Astrocytes." *Anatomy and Embryology* 156:115–152.

Sidman, R. L., and Rakic, P. 1982. "Development of the Human Central Nervous System." In *Histology and Histopathology of the Nervous System,* Haymaker, W., and Adams, R. D., editors. Charles C. Thomas, Pub.

Physiology

Brightman, M. W., and Reese, T. S. 1969. "Junctions between Intimately Apposed Cell Membranes in the Vertebrate Brain." *Journal of Cell Biology* 40:648–677.

Eccles, J. C. 1964. *The Physiology of Synapses.* Academic Press.

Hodgkin, A. L., and Huxley, A. F. 1952. "A Quantitative Description of Membrane Current and Its Application to Conduction and Excitation in Nerve." *Journal of Physiology* 117:500–544.

Llinás, R. R. 1984. "Comparative Electrobiology of Mammalian Central Neurons." In *Brain Slices,* Dingledine, R., editor. Plenum Publishing Corp.

Shepherd, G. M. 1972. "The Neuron Doctrine: A Revision of Functional Concepts." *Yale Journal of Biology and Medicine* 45:584–599.

Shepherd, G. M. 1978. "Microcircuits in the Nervous System." *Scientific American* 238(2):92–103.

Shepherd, G. M. 1981. "The Nerve Impulse and the Nature of Nervous Function." In *Neurons Without Impulses,* Society for Experimental Biology Seminar Series, Volume 6, Roberts, A., and Bush, B. M. H., editors. Cambridge University Press.

Sherrington, C. S. 1906. *The Integrative Action of the Nervous System.* Yale University Press.

Stevens, C. F. 1979. "The Neuron." *Scientific American* 241(3):55–65.

Chemistry; Anatomical Techniques

Bloom, F. E. 1981. "Neuropeptides." *Scientific American* 245(4):148–169.

Dahlström, A., and Fuxe, K. 1964. "Evidence for the Existence of Monoamine-Containing Neurons in the Central Nervous System." *Acta Physiologica Scandinavica, Supplement* 232:1–55.

Dale, H. 1935. "Pharmacology and Nerve Endings." *Proceedings of the Royal Society of Medicine* 28:319–332.

Gee, C. E., and Roberts, J. L. 1983. "In Situ Hybridization Histochemistry: A Technique for the Study of Gene Expression in Single Cells." *DNA* 2:157–163.

Gerfen, C. R., and Sawchenko, P. E. 1984. "An Anterograde Neuroanatomical Tracing Method That Shows the Detailed Morphology of Neurons, Their Axons and Terminals: Immunohistochemical Localization of an Axonally Transported Plant Lectin, *Phaseolus vulgaris* Leucoagglutinin (PHA-L)." *Brain Research* 290:219–238.

Herkenham, M., and Pert, C. B. 1982. "Light Microscopic Localization of Brain Opiate Receptors: A General Autoradiographic Method Which Preserves Tissue Quality." *Journal of Neuroscience* 2:1129–1149.

Hökfelt, T., Johansson, O., and Goldstein, M. 1984. "Chemical Anatomy of the Brain." *Science* 225:1326–1334.

Iversen, L. L. 1979. "The Chemistry of the Brain." *Scientific American* 241(3):134–149.

Kreutzberg, G. W. 1984. "100 Years of Nissl Staining." *Trends in Neurosciences* 7:236–237.

Lindvall, O., and Björklund, A. 1983. "Dopamine and Noradrenaline-Containing Neuron Systems: A Review of Their Anatomy in the Rat Brain." In *Chemical Neuroanatomy,* Emson, P. C., editor. Raven Press.

Mesulam, M. M., Mufson, E. J., Levey, A. I., and Wainer, B. H. 1984. "Atlas of Cholinergic Neurons in the Forebrain and Upper Brainstem of the Macaque Based on Monoclonal Choline Acetyltransferase Immunohistochemistry and Acetylcholinesterase Histochemistry." *Neuroscience* 12:669–686.

Roberts, J. L., Chen, C.-L. C., Dionne, F. T., and Gee, C. E. 1982. "Peptide Hormone Gene Expression in Heterogeneous Tissues." *Trends in Neurosciences* 5:314–317.

Roberts, J. L., Seeburg, P. H., Shine, J., Herbert, E., Baxter, J. D., and Goodman, H. M. 1979. "Corticotropin and Beta-endorphin: Construction and Analysis of Recombinant DNA Complementary to mRNA for the Common Precursor." *Proceedings of the National Academy of Sciences* 76:2153–2157.

Rothman, R. B., Herkenham, M., Pert, C. B., Liang, T., and Cascieri, M. A. 1984. "Visualization of Rat Brain Receptors for the Neuropeptide Substance P." *Brain Research,* 309:47–54.

Schwartz, J. H. 1980. "The Transport of Substances in Nerve Cells." *Scientific American* 242(4):152–171.

Snyder, S. H. 1980. "Brain Peptides as Neurotransmitters." *Science* 209:976–983.

Steinbusch, H. W. M. 1981. "Distribution of Serotonin Immunoreactivity in the Central Nervous System of the Rat—Cell Bodies and Terminals." *Neuroscience* 6:557–618.

Sutcliffe, J. G., Milner, R. J., Gottesfeld, J. M., and Reynolds, W. 1984. "Control of Neuronal Gene Expression." *Science* 225:1308–1315.

Neural Tissue; Neural Organization

Morell, P. 1984. *Myelin,* second edition. Plenum Press.

Morell, P., and Norton, W. T. 1980. "Myelin." *Scientific American* 242(5):88–118.

Nauta, W. J. H., and Karten, H. J. 1970. "A General Profile of the Vertebrate Brain, with Sidelights on the Ancestry of Cerebral Cortex." In *The Neurosciences: Second Study Program,* Schmitt, F. O., editor. Rockefeller University Press.

Rakic, P., editor. 1975. *Local Circuit Neurons. Neurosciences Research Program Bulletin* 13:291–446.

Ramón y Cajal, S. 1909, 1911. *Histologie du Système Nerveux de l'Homme et des*

Vertébrés. Paris: Maloine. Two volumes. Reprinted in 1952 by the Instituto Ramón y Cajal in Madrid.

Sensory Mechanisms

Boycott, B. B., and Dowling, J. E. 1969. "Organization of the Primate Retina: Light Microscopy." *Philosophical Transactions B* 255:109–184.

Dowling, J. E. 1979. "Information Processing by Local Circuits: The Vertebrate Retina as a Model System." In *The Neurosciences, Fourth Study Program,* Schmitt, F. O., and Worden, F. G., editors. M.I.T. Press.

Goldstein, M. H. 1980. "The Auditory Periphery." In *Medical Physiology,* 14th edition, Mountcastle, V. B., editor. C. V. Mosby Co.

Graziadei, P. P. C. 1971. "The Olfactory Mucosa in Vertebrates." In *Handbook of Sensory Physiology, Volume IV, Chemical Senses, Section 1, Olfaction,* Beidler, K., editor. Springer-Verlag, Inc.

Hudspeth, A. J., and Corey, D. P. 1977. "Sensitivity, Polarity, and Conductance Change in the Response of Vertebrate Hair Cells to Controlled Mechanical Stimuli." *Proceedings of the National Academy of Sciences* 74:2407–2411.

Maturana, H. R., Lettvin, J. Y., McCulloch, W. S., and Pitts, W. H. 1960. "Anatomy and Physiology of Vision in the Frog (*Rana pipiens*)." *Journal of General Physiology* 43:129–175.

Mountcastle, V. B. 1980. "Central Neural Mechanisms in Hearing." In *Medical Physiology,* 14th edition, Mountcastle, V. B., editor. C. V. Mosby Co.

Mountcastle, V. B. 1980. "Neural Mechanisms in Somesthesia." In *Medical Physiology,* 14th edition, Mountcastle, V. B., editor. C. V. Mosby Co.

Munger, B. L. 1977. "Neural-Epithelial Interactions in Sensory Receptors." *The Journal of Investigative Dermatology* 69:27–40.

Munger, B. L. 1983. "The Sensory Innervation of Primate Facial Skin. I. Hairy Skin." *Brain Research Reviews* 5:45–80. "II. Vermillion Border and Mucosa of Lip." *Brain Research Reviews* 5:81–107.

Norgren, R. 1976. "Taste Pathways to Hypothalamus and Amygdala." *Journal of Comparative Neurology* 166:17–30.

Norgren, R., and Leonard, C. M. 1973. "Ascending Central Gustatory Pathways." *Journal of Comparative Neurology* 150:217–237.

Polyak, S. 1941. *The Retina.* University of Chicago Press.

Rasmussen, G. L., and Windle, W. F., editors. 1960. *Neural Mechanisms of the Auditory and Vestibular Systems.* Charles C. Thomas, Pub.

Spencer, P. S., and Schaumberg, H. H. 1973. "An Ultrastructural Study of the Inner Core of the Pacinian Corpuscle." *Journal of Neurocytology* 2:217–235.

The Somatic Motor System

Evarts, E. V. 1979. "Brain Mechanisms of Movement." *Scientific American* 241(3):164–179.

Evered, D., and O'Connor, M. 1984. *Functions of the Basal Ganglia.* CIBA Foundation Symposium 107. London: Pitman Publishing, Ltd.

Graybiel, A. M. 1978. "Organization of Oculomotor Pathways in the Cat and Rhesus Monkey." In *Control of Gaze by Brainstem Neurons. Developments in Neuroscience, Volume 1,* Baker, R., and Berthoz, A., editors. Elsevier North Holland Biomedical Press.

Haber, S. N., Groenewegen, H. J., Grove, E. A., and Nauta, W. J. H. 1985. "Efferent Connections of the Ventral Pallidum: Evidence of a Dual Striato-pallidofugal Pathway." *Journal of Comparative Neurology* 235:322–335.

Henneman, E. 1980. "Motor Functions of the Cerebral Cortex." In *Medical Physiology,* 14th edition, Mountcastle, V. B., editor. C. V. Mosby Co.

Henneman, E. 1980. "Motor Functions of the Brainstem and Basal Ganglia." In *Medical Physiology,* 14th edition, Mountcastle, V. B., editor. C. V. Mosby Co.

Kuypers, H. G. J. M. 1981. "Anatomy of the Descending Pathways." In *Handbook of Physiology, Section 1, The Nervous System, Volume 2, The Motor System, Part 2.* American Physiological Society.

Lundberg, A. 1975. "Control of Spinal Mechanisms from the Brain." In *The Nervous System, Volume 1: The Basic Neurosciences,* Tower, D. B., editor. Raven Press.

Székely, G. 1963. "Functional Specificity of Spinal Cord Segments in the Control of Limb Movements." *Journal of Embryology and Experimental Morphology* 11:431–444.

Székely, G. 1968. "Development of Limb Movements: Embryological, Physiological and Model Studies." In *Growth of the Nervous System,* Wolstenholme, G. E. W., and O'Connor, M., editors. London: Churchill Livingstone, Inc.

The Visceral Domain; The Limbic System

Anderson, P. 1975. "Organization of Hippocampal Neurons and Their Interconnections." In *The Hippocampus, Volume I: Structure and Development,* Isaacson, R. L., and Pribram, K. H., editors. Plenum Publishing Corp.

Bard, P. 1928. "A Diencephalic Mechanism for the Expression of Rage, with Special Reference to the Sympathetic Nervous System." *American Journal of Physiology* 84:490–515.

Ben-Ari, Y., editor. 1981. *The Amygdaloid Complex.* Elsevier North Holland Biomedical Press.

Cannon, W. B. 1929. *Bodily Changes in Pain, Hunger, Fear, and Rage.* D. Appleton & Co.

Gloor, P. 1972. "Temporal Lobe Epilepsy: Its Possible Contribution to the Understanding of the Functional Significance of the Amygdala and of Its Interaction with Neocortical-Temporal Mechanisms." In *The Neurobiology of the Amygdala,* Eleftheriou, B. E., editor. Plenum Publishing Corp.

Isaacson, R. L. 1982. *The Limbic System,* second edition. Plenum Publishing Corp.

Milner, B. 1966. "Amnesia Following Operation on the Temporal Lobes." In *Amnesia,* Whitty, C. W. M., and Zangwill, G. L., editors. Butterworth & Co.

Milner, B. 1972. "Disorders of Learning and Memory after Temporal Lobe Lesions in Man." *Clinical Neurosurgery* 19:421–446.

Nauta, W. J. H., and Domesick, V. B. 1981. "Ramifications of the Limbic System." In *Psychiatry and the Biology of the Human Brain,* Matthysse, S., editor. Elsevier North Holland Biomedical Press.

Nauta, W. J. H., and Haymaker, W. 1969. "Hypothalamic Nuclei and Fiber Connections." In *The Hypothalamus,* Haymaker, W., Anderson, E., and Nauta, W. J. H., editors. Charles C. Thomas, Pub.

Olds, J. 1975. "Mapping the Mind onto the Brain." In *The Neurosciences: Paths of Discovery,* Worden, F. G., Swazey, J. P., and Adelman, G., editors. M.I.T. Press.

Papez, J. W. 1937. "A Proposed Mechanism of Emotion." *American Medical Association Archives of Neurology and Psychiatry* 38:725–743.

Ricardo, J. A., and Koh, E. T. 1978. "Anatomical Evidence of Direct Projections from the Nucleus of the Solitary Tract to the Hypothalamus, Amygdala, and Other Forebrain Structures in the Rat." *Brain Research* 153:1–26.

Saper, C. B., Loewy, A. D., Swanson, L. W., and Cowan, W. M. 1976. "Direct Hypothalamo-Autonomic Connections." *Brain Research* 177:305–312.

Scharrer, E., and Scharrer, B. 1940. "Secretory Cells within the Hypothalamus." *Research Publications, Association for Research in Nervous and Mental Disease* 20:170–194.

Swanson, L. W. 1975. "The Hippocampus." *Trends in Neurosciences* 2:9–12.

Willoughby, J. O., and Martin, J. B. 1978. "The Role of the Limbic System in Neuroendocrine Regulation." In *Limbic Mechanisms: The Continuing Evolution of the Limbic System Concept,* Livingstone, K. E., and Hornykiewicz, O., editors. Plenum Publishing Corp.

Spinal Cord

Brown, A. G. 1981. *Organization in the Spinal Cord: The Anatomy and Physiology of Identified Neurons,* Springer-Verlag, Inc.

Fields, H. L., and Basbaum, A. J. 1978. "Brainstem Control of Spinal Pain-Transmission Neurons." *Annual Review of Physiology* 40:217–248.

Henneman, E. 1980. "Organization of the Spinal Cord and Its Reflexes." In *Medical Physiology,* 14th edition, Mountcastle, V. B., editor. C. V. Mosby Co.

Mountcastle, V. B. 1980. "Central Nervous Mechanisms in Sensation." In *Medical Physiology,* 14th edition, Mountcastle, V. B., editor. C. V. Mosby Co.

Perl, E. R. 1968. "Myelinated Afferent Fibers Innervating the Primate Skin and Their Response to Noxious Stimuli." *Journal of Physiology* 197:593–615.

Rexed, B. 1952. "The Cytoarchitectonic Organization of the Spinal Cord in the Cat." *Journal of Comparative Neurology* 96:415–495.

Rexed, B. 1954. "A Cytoarchitectonic Atlas of the Spinal Cord in the Cat." *Journal of Comparative Neurology* 100:297–379.

Wall, P. D. 1980. "The Substantia Gelatinosa, a Gate Control Mechanism Set Across a Sensory Pathway." *Trends in Neurosciences* 3:221–224.

Willis, W. D., and Coggeshall, R. E. 1978. *Sensory Mechanisms of the Spinal Cord.* Plenum Publishing Corp.

Brainstem

Brodal, A. 1957. *The Reticular Formation of the Brainstem: Anatomical Aspects and Functional Correlations.* Edinburg: Oliver and Boyd, Ltd.

Brodal, A. 1965. *The Cranial Nerves: Anatomy and Anatomic-Clinical Correlations,* second edition. Oxford: Blackwell Scientific Publications, Ltd.

Moruzzi, G., and Magoun, H. W. 1949. "Brainstem Reticular Formation and Activation of the EEG." *Clinical Neurophysiology* 1:455–473.

Nauta, W. J. H., and Kuypers, H. G. J. M. 1958. "Some Ascending Pathways in Brainstem Reticular Formation." In *Reticular Formation of the Brain,* Jasper, H. H., et al., editors. Little, Brown and Co.

Scheibel, M. E., and Scheibel, A. B. 1958. "Structural Substrates for Integrative Patterns in the Brainstem Reticular Core." In *Reticular Formation of the Brain,* Jasper, H. H., et al., editors. Little, Brown and Co.

Cerebellum

Gilman, S., Bloedel, J. R., and Lechtenberg, R. 1981. *Disorders of the Cerebellum.* F. A. Davis Co.

Llinás, R. R. 1975. "The Cortex of the Cerebellum." *Scientific American* 232(1):56–71.

Llinás, R. R. 1981. "Electrophysiology of the Cerebellar Networks." In *Handbook of Physiology, Section 1, The Nervous System, Volume 2, The Motor System, Part 2.* American Physiological Society.

Palay, S. L., and Chan-Palay, V. 1973. *Cerebellar Cortex: Cytology and Organization.* Springer-Verlag, Inc.

Palay, S. L., and Chan-Palay, V., editors. 1982. *The Cerebellum: New Vistas.* (*Experimental Brain Research,* Supplement No. 6.) Springer-Verlag, Inc.

Neocortex

Bizzi, E., and Schiller, P. H. 1970. "Single-Unit Activity in the Frontal Eye Fields of Unanaesthetized Monkeys during Eye and Head Movements." *Experimental Brain Research* 10:151–158.

Geschwind, N. 1967. "The Apraxias." In *Phenomenology of Will and Action,* Straus, E. W., and Griffith, R. M., editors. Duquesne University Press.

Geschwind, N. 1969. "Problems in the Anatomical Understanding of the Aphasias." In *Contributions to Clinical Neuropsychology,* Benton, A. L., editor. Aldine Publishing Co.

Geschwind, N. 1974. "The Organization of Language and the Brain." In Geschwind, N., *Selected Papers on Language and the Brain.* D. Reidel Publishing Co.

Graybiel, A. M. 1972. "Some Ascending Connections of the Pulvinar and Nucleus Lateralis Posterior of the Thalamus in the Cat." *Brain Research,* 44:99–125.

Hécaen, H., and Albert, M. L. 1978. *Human Neuropsychology.* John Wiley & Sons, Inc.

Hubel, D. H., and Wiesel, T. N. 1968. "Receptive Fields and Functional Architecture of Monkey Striate Cortex." *Journal of Physiology* 195:215–244.

Hubel, D. H., and Wiesel, T. N. 1977. "Ferrier Lecture: Functional Architecture of Macaque Monkey Visual Cortex." *Proceedings of the Royal Society of London, Series B,* 198:1–59.

Hubel, D. H., and Wiesel, T. N. 1979. "Brain Mechanisms of Vision." *Scientific American* 241(3):150–162.

Hubel, D. H., Wiesel, T. N., and Stryker, M. P. 1978. "Anatomical Demonstration of Orientation Columns in Macaque Monkey." *Journal of Comparative Neurology* 177:361–379.

Jones, E. G., and Powell, T. P. S. 1969. "Connexions of the Somatic Sensory Cortex of the Rhesus Monkey. I. Ipsilateral Cortical Connexions." *Brain* 92:477–502.

Jones, E. G., and Powell, T. P. S. 1970. "An Anatomical Study of Converging Sensory Pathways within the Cerebral Cortex of the Monkey." *Brain* 93:793–820.

Klüver, H. 1937. " 'Psychic Blindness' and Other Symptoms following Bilateral Temporal Lobectomy in Rhesus Monkeys." *American Journal of Physiology* 119:352–353.

Klüver, H. 1941. "Visual Functions after Removal of the Occipital Lobes." *Journal of Psychology* 11:23–45.

LeVay, S., Connolly, M., Houde, J., and Van Essen, D. C. 1985. "The Complete Pattern of Ocular Dominance Stripes in the Striate Cortex and Visual Field of the Macaque Monkey." *Journal of Neuroscience* 5:486–501.

Lorente de Nó, R. 1943. "Cerebral Cortex: Architecture, Intracortical Connections, Motor Projections." In Fulton, J. F., *Physiology of the Nervous System*, second edition. Oxford University Press.

Luria, A. R. 1966. *Higher Cortical Functions in Man.* Plenum Publishing Corp.

Luria, A. R. 1972. *Man with a Shattered World: A History of a Brain Wound.* Basic Books, Inc.

Mountcastle, V. B. 1957. "Modality and Topographic Properties of Single Neurons of Cat's Somatic Sensory Cortex." *Journal of Neurophysiology* 20:408–434.

Mountcastle, V. B., Lynch, J. C., Georgopoulos, A., Sakata, H., and Acuna, A. 1975. "Posterior Parietal Association Cortex of the Monkey: Command Functions for Operations within Extrapersonal Space." *Journal of Neurophysiology* 38:871–908.

Nauta, W. J. H. 1971. "The Problem of the Frontal Lobe: A Reinterpretation." *Journal of Psychiatric Research* 8:167–187.

Pandya, D. N., and Kuypers, H. G. J. M. 1969. "Corticocortical Connections in the Rhesus Monkey." *Brain Research* 13:13–36.

Szentágothai, J. 1973. "Synaptology of the Visual Cortex." In *Central Processing of Visual Information, Handbook of Sensory Physiology, Volume VII/3B.* Jung, R., editor. Springer-Verlag, Inc.

Teuber, H. L. 1966. "Alterations of Perception after Brain Injury." In *Brain and Conscious Experience,* Eccles, J. C., editor. Springer-Verlag, Inc.

Wiesel, T. N., Hubel, D. H., and Lam, D. M. K. 1974. "Autoradiographic Demonstration of Ocular-Dominance Columns in the Monkey Striate Cortex by Means of Transneuronal Transport." *Brain Research* 79:273–279.

Zurif, E. B., and Blumstein, S. E. 1978. "Language and the Brain." In *Linguistic Theory and Psychological Reality*. Halle, M., Bresnan, J., and Miller, G. A., editors. M.I.T. Press.

Prospects

Crick, F. H. C. 1979. "Thinking about the Brain." *Scientific American* 241(3):219–232.

Marr, D. 1982. *Vision*. W. H. Freeman and Co.

Marr, D., and Poggio, T. 1977. "From Understanding Computation to Understanding Neural Circuitry." *Neurosciences Research Program Bulletin* 15:470–488.

Marr, D., and Poggio, T. 1979. "A Computational Theory of Human Stereo Vision." *Proceedings of the Royal Society of London, Series B,* 204:301–328.

McCulloch, W. S. 1965. *Embodiments of Mind.* M.I.T. Press.

Poggio, T. 1984. "Vision by Man and Machine." *Scientific American* 250(4):106–116.

Ramón y Cajal, S. 1906. "The Structure and Connexions of Neurons." In *Nobel Lectures: Physiology or Medicine, 1901–1921.* Elsevier Science Publishing Co. (1967).

Ramón y Cajal, S. 1937. *Recollections of My Life.* Craigie, E. H., translator. Memoirs of the American Philosophical Society. Two volumes. Republished in 1966 by M.I.T. Press.

Index